WHERE
MEDICINE
FAILS

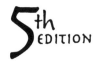

5th EDITION

WHERE MEDICINE FAILS

CAROLYN L. WIENER & ANSELM L. STRAUSS
EDITORS

With a new introduction by Carolyn L. Wiener

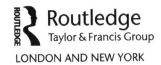

Routledge
Taylor & Francis Group

LONDON AND NEW YORK

First published 1970 by Transaction Publishers

Published 2017 by Routledge
2 Park Square, Milton Park, Abingdon, Oxon OX14 4RN
711 Third Avenue, New York, NY 10017, USA

Routledge is an imprint of the Taylor & Francis Group, an informa business

New material this edition copyright © 1997 by Taylor & Francis.
Previous editions copyright © 1970, 1973, 1979, 1984 by Taylor & Francis.

Library of Congress Catalog Number: 96-13279

Library of Congress Cataloging-in-Publication Data

Where medicine fails / edited by Carolyn L. Wiener and Anselm L. Strauss ;
   with a new introduction by Carolyn L. Wiener. — 5th ed.
     p. cm.
   Includes bibliographical references.
   ISBN 1-56000-869-5 (pbk. : alk. paper)
   1. Medical care—United States. 2. Medical policy—United States.
3. Medical ethics—United States. I. Wiener, Carolyn L., 1930–   .
II. Strauss, Anselm L.
RA395.A3W48   1996
362.1'0973—dc20   96-13279
                                                              CIP

ISBN 13: 978-1-56000-869-9 (pbk)

Contents

Introduction to the Fifth Edition

Carolyn L. Wiener

In the preface to the 1984 edition of *Where Medicine Fails,* Anselm Strauss expressed the hope that the national failures in health care, so poignantly covered in the first four editions, would have received more forthright and equitable attention when time for the fifth edition came around. Since then, attention, of a sort, has been paid but with scant results. And equitable distribution of health care remains elusive. The 1993 Clinton "health plan" died aborning, followed by a press postmortem that was almost as lengthy as the bill itself. A *New York Times* obituary captures the essence of the legislative collapse: "Though unfinished, the history of health care legislation is a striking measure of the complexity of legislating major change in an era of intense partisanship, with a public that distrusts Washington as never before, a campaign technology applied to whipping around voters' opinions, and news reports that emphasize conflict, not explanation."[1] Health care reform was a bonanza for pollsters, pundits, number crunchers, lobbyists, and advertising agencies, but did not improve the lot of the people it was supposed to help.

The so-called debate over health care that surrounded the proposed legislation only served to heighten the public fear of change. Change, however, was already occurring, to some extent in anticipation of legislation but largely preceding political discussion of health reform. Historians have cited several previous turning points in health care: Successful breakthroughs in bacteriology, the introduction of aseptic surgical techniques, the professionalization of medicine, advances in anesthesia, and discoveries in immunology. A revolution of equal import can now be seen to have occurred in the 1980s with the introduction of Medicare's Prospective Payment System, which accelerated reappraisal by the insurance industry of traditional fee-for-service reimbursement for all beneficiaries, not just the elderly. Despite the public fear of "managed care," as proposed in the Clinton legislation, capitated payment (a flat per person fee) in the form of Health Maintenance Organizations and Preferred Provider Organizations is a rapidly growing phenomenon. This shift is a reflection of the cost-conscious 1990s, wherein hospitals and physicians are being asked to carefully monitor and control costs in order to survive, and is spurred to a great extent by employer groups anxious to control the rising toll of employee health benefits. As characterized by journalist Malcolm Gladwell, "We are now in a period during which medicine has been chastised repeatedly for its extravagance, and heroics are reserved not for spending money but for saving it."[2]

In this climate, where do the issues raised in the previous four editions of *Where Medicine Fails* stand? Sad to say, Strauss' "Medical Ghettos," save for an updating of the statistics on poverty, is as relevant as when it was written. The acute phases of chronic illnesses—cancer, diabetes, hypertension, arthritis, and pulmonary, heart, and renal diseases—are still what brings people to health care facilities. The list of chronic illnesses now includes AIDS, as described by the authors of "AIDS and Health Care Deficiencies" in this volume and health care delivery is still driven by the intertwining of chronic illness, specialization, and the technological imperative, as the same authors in "What Price Chronic Illness?" attest. Facing up to the reasons behind the health care price tag would mean replacing our concern over health care's portion of the gross national product (the argument used most frequently) with the decision that health is a social good, not a commodity.

Instead, emphasis in the health care arena is being placed on amassing a huge volume of statistical data—administrative and epidemiological, current and retrospective—in the name of quality of care. Databases that were set up for financial purposes are now expected to shed light on clinical practice. The basic assumption is that health care is a matter of economics. Health care facilities are told by governmental and private payers to think of themselves as part of an industry. Improved efficiency will lead to better care. Competition will weed out the losers. The growing field of health informatics (i.e., health care information technology) will enable payers, patients, and providers, and most importantly, employer groups as purchasers of health plans, to assess the relationship between price and quality for a specific physician, procedure, laboratory, treatment outcome, or hospital. Vigorous development and marketing efforts on the part of software companies attest to the problems of adapting an industrial model to patient care. As these companies attempt to adjust for "risk" and "severity of illness" (i.e., the human variables that challenge categorizing), the best method of measurement remains a matter of debate. Congress has established the Agency for Health Care Planning and Research, which for the last five years has spent $200 million on "outcomes research." So far, the goal of pinpointing which medical interventions produce the best outcomes remains uncertain, to say the least. Furthermore, adhering to an industrial model has brought about a questionable integration of financial and clinical concerns. As psychiatrist Thomas Szasz has said, "Final diagnoses on the discharge summaries of hospitalized patients are often no longer made by physicians, but by bureaucrats skilled in the ways of Medicare, Medicaid, and private health insurance reimbursement—based partly on which medical terms for his ailment and treatment ensure the most generous reimbursement for the services rendered."[3]

Meanwhile, there are still vast inequities in American health care delivery. All of the imbalances previously catalogued in this volume—disparate access to health care services, inappropriate distribution of resources, emphasis on acute rather than chronic care—still exist. We still have 40 million uninsured citizens, a statistic that fluctuates in response to unemployment. The most recent figures at this writing reveal that many families of seriously ill patients experience severe care-giving and financial burdens and families of younger, poorer, and more functionally dependent patients are most likely to report loss of most or all of the family's savings.[4] This figure could be exacerbated if, in the cost crunch, employers decide to drop health coverage for dependents. Clearly, today's health care still raises difficult ethical, financial, and social issues.

Out of a total of twenty-seven essays in this revised edition, seventeen are new, having appeared in *Society* since 1983. The book has been divided into three sections somewhat arbitrarily since there is considerable overlap among the issues touched upon. While the aforementioned imbalances are a unifying theme, there is greater emphasis in this edition on the dominance of the marketplace. In Part I, the authors of "AIDS and Health Care Deficiencies" examine the moral and economic issues highlighted by this disease. Guillemin's "Planning To Die" and Markson's "Moral Dilemmas" deal with the perplexities surrounding technologized dying. In "Turf Battles on Medicine Avenue," Field scrutinizes the professional implications of medical advertising in an era when "power in the hospital, which in the past rested squarely with the doctors, is slowly passing to the managers and administrators." Thorne addresses the commercialization of fetal-tissue transplants for a range of chronic diseases, asserting that the present organ-transplant activity is a cottage industry compared to the industry that is likely to emerge around fetal-tissue transplant. Four articles published previously, those by Strauss, Wiener et al., Smith et al., and Bard, reappear in Part I. The first, while not specifically dealing with economic and moral issues, is a classic introduction to the chronic illness theme that runs throughout the book. Although this article and the one that follows it assert that infectious and parasitic diseases are under control—a position seemingly belied by the appearance of AIDS and of new deadly organisms and mutating viruses that are antibiotic resistant—the major elements of both of these articles remain relevant. "The Health of the Haight-Ashbury" is not only important historically but illuminates the ongoing issue of class differences in health care and attitudes toward treatment of Americans marginal to mainstream medicine. Bard's article on cancer patients kept alive by modern technology questions the trade-off between cancer survival and "psychological invalidism," which, if anything, is even more salient today as treatment technology proliferates.

Part II is devoted to the fissures in the American hospital. By carefully searching the past as prologue, these articles ground our health care problems in the specific aspects of American entrepreneurship and individualism. The first six articles in this section are new and continue the threads already touched upon in Part I: changes in physician standards of clinical treatment, the impact of external financial incentives, insufficient access for the poor, and health care as a right or as a commodity. These issues, however, are viewed through the prism of a critique of American hospitals. The article by Cohen and Estner, on the reasons for the rate of cesarian births in the United States continues to be significant in the 1990s, as this figure remains high. The last article in this section, by Hochbaum and Galkin, examines the skewed incentives that contribute to using nursing homes as America's "final resting place."

The need for restructuring runs throughout the preceding sections, but the essays in Part III are more explicit regarding health policy and reform. Strauss' "Medical Ghettos" serves as an introduction as do the subsequent articles which are new in this edition. In the first paper in this section, "A Century of Health Reform," Ginzberg examines the embedment of our health care system in American cultural, political, economic, ideological, and social institutions. In so doing, he alludes to the link between housing and health care, an issue addressed with fervor in the brief statement from Altman et al. that originally appeared in a *Society* issue devoted to the Institute of Medicine's report, *Homelessness, Health and Human Needs*. Wallace and Estes focus on "Health Policy for the Elderly." Their discussion demonstrates the durability of the conflict regarding the proper distribution of federal, state, and local roles, an issue that has been revitalized in the conservative political swing of the 1990s. Poplin provides an overview of the intricacies of "managed care," concluding that whoever pays the piper ultimately calls the tune. Friedman, in "The All-Frills Yuppie Health Care Boutique," looks at some of the absurdities that have resulted from our zest to make health care conform to consumerism and offers recommendations for reform. Kirp examines toxic hazards in the work place. The last three essays in this section, debating the possible causative relevance of environment to cancer, appeared in the previous edition. Alas, the debate continues as does the prevalence of the disease.

It has become increasingly apparent, especially in the failure once again to achieve a national health plan, that the health care that citizens of any country receive is reflective of national characteristics. The United States, federal *and* democratic in form of government, covering a vast continent, enormously heterogeneous in population, capitalist but with elements of welfare, and still to a great extent class-driven, has drifted into a health care system that is a many-sided market. Profit-motivated corporations, both within the health care arena and outside of it as major purchasers of insurance, are dominating this drift. Espousing a philosophy of Federalism, called "devolution" in the 1990s, is a way to shift responsibility from the federal level to the states to the counties, with less and less money available at each level and less and less inclination to worry about the poor, who have no effective lobbying groups to protect them. Amid the current rhetoric regarding American values, little attention is paid to inherent paradoxes. We buy the mythology regarding American mobility but ignore the fact that mobility can be downward as well as upward. We value individualism but in our antipathy toward the poor interpret individualism as the right to ask, "I made it, why can't they?" We value equity but as Stevens correctly observes in this volume, "In retrospect, the egalitarian expectations for Medicaid appear as an aberration in a long history of class discrimination in hospital care in the United States." We extol frugality, especially for others to practice and especially if it does not affect the services to which we have a right. What is going to happen when Americans can no longer see their physician of choice because their health plans have responded to employers' demands for a rollback in premiums by reducing the number of physicians on their lists? What is going to happen when the light dawns from the vantage point of a hospital bed that "re-designing" means reducing nursing staff and assigning new responsibilities to lesser-paid and lesser-trained unlicensed staff? These changes are occurring very rapidly but Americans are just beginning to feel the impact.

Strauss concluded his introduction to the previous edition of *Where Medicine Fails* with the following: "There are increasingly fewer Americans with no chronic illnesses at all; there will be fewer still in the next decade." Friedman, in this edition, wonders what will happen to health care reform when even the most health-minded Yuppies (young upwardly mobile professionals) become, in columnist Art Hoppe's phrase, Grumpies (grown up mature people) needing health care. While it might be assumed that personal experience will lead to increased compassion for the health care needs of politically powerless and socially unpopular groups, increased demand could as well encourage a less communitarian attitude. We now have a society where the average CEO makes 149 times the average factory worker's pay and the average pay increase was 30 percent in 1994 for the 23 CEOs whose corporations eliminated the most American jobs—and, by contrast, a society in which the number of children growing up in poverty has increased by 50 percent since 1973.[5] Yet we continue to worry about the welfare burden and balk at the mention of increased taxes to support social programs. If the essays in this volume encourage a serious examination of the current structure of health services and of the complicated facets of proposed health care reform they will have served a useful purpose.

Notes

1. A. Clymer, R. Pear, and R. Toner, "For Health Care, Time Was A Killer," *New York Times* (29 August 1994): p. A1.
2. M. Gladwell, "How Safe are Your Breasts?" *The New Republic* 211, no. 17 (1994): 22–28, p. 28.
3. T. Szasz, "Mental Illness Is Still a Myth," *Society* 31 (1994): 34–39, p. 37.

4. K. Covinsky, L. Goldman, E. Francis Cook, R. Oye, N. Desbiens, D. Reding, W. Fulkerson, A. Connors, J. Lynn, and R. Phillips, "The Impact of Serious Illness on Patients' Families," *Journal of the American Medical Association* 272 (1994): 1839–44.
5. R. Barnet, *Global Dreams: Imperial Corporations and the New World Order* (New York: Touchstone Books, Simon & Schuster, 1995).

Part I

Economics vs. Moral Issues

Chronic Illness

Anselm L. Strauss

Smallpox, diphtheria, polio, measles—conquered through immunization. Tuberculosis, leprosy, plague, yellow fever, malaria—defeated or checked by sanitation, improved living conditions, and effective treatment.

In the old days, people who died from diseases contracted them quickly, reached crisis shortly thereafter, and either died or pulled through. Modern medical researchers have changed this dramatic pattern by taming many once-devastating ailments. Improved conditions of living, along with effective medical skills and technology, have altered the nature of illness in scientifically advanced societies. While patients suffering from communicable diseases once filled most hospitals, treatment centers now serve mainly those afflicted with chronic ailments.

Many who would have died soon after contracting a disease now live and endure their affliction. Today most illnesses are chronic diseases—slow-acting, long-term killers that can be treated but not cured. A 1964 survey by the Department of Health, Education, and Welfare indicates that about 40 percent of all Americans suffer from one or more chronic diseases; one out of every four so afflicted have lost some days at work because of disabling symptoms.

A large and growing body of medical literature presents detailed discussions of etiology, symptomatology, treatments, and regimens. This outpouring of information, however, generally ignores a basic aspect of chronic illness—how to deal with such ailments in terms that are *social*—not simply medical. How can patients and professionals cope with health-related problems of family disruption, marital stress, role destruction and adjustment, stigmatization, and even loss of body mobility?

Each chronic condition brings with it multiple problems of living. Among the most pressing are preventing and managing medical crises (that go even to death), managing regimens, controlling symptoms, orga-

11

nizing one's time efficiently, preventing or living with social isolation, adjusting to changes in the disease trajectory, and normalizing interaction and life, despite the disease. To handle those problems, people develop basic strategies which call for an organization of effort (including that of kinsmen, neighbors, and health professionals). To establish and maintain this organization requires certain resources (financial, medical, familial, and so forth), as well as interactional and social skills in order to make the necessary arrangements.

Medicine and the health professionals are very much included in this scheme but are neither at the scheme's focal point nor even constitute its primary elements. What is primary is simply the question of living: the difference between chronic sufferers and "normal people" merely being that the former must live with their diseases, their symptoms and often with their regimens. Medicine may contribute, but it is secondary to "carrying on."

Coping with Crises

Some chronic diseases carry a constant threat of grave medical crises. Diabetics may fall into insulin coma and die; epileptics can go into convulsions (which of themselves are not lethal) and be killed in a fall or a traffic accident. In order to prevent crises, minimize their effects, get the critically ill person into the hands of a physician or a hospital staff—and if need be actually save him—the person himself and possibly his kinsmen must be organized and prepared to handle all contingencies.

Relevant to the question of crises is how far they can go (to, or short of, death), how fast they appear, the clarity of advance warning signals to laymen or even to health professionals, the probability of recurrence, the predictability of their appearance, the complexity of the saving operations, and the speed and completeness of recovery from them.

The ability to read signs that portend a crisis is the first important step in managing chronic illness. Thus, diabetics or the parents of diabetic children learn how to recognize the signs of oncoming sugar shortage or insulin shock and what to do in case of actual crisis. Likewise, epileptics and sickle cell disease sufferers, if they are fortunate enough to have warning signs before their crises, learn to prepare themselves: if they are in public they get themselves to a place of safety and sit or lie down. Diabetics may carry instructions with them and may also carry those materials, like sugar or candy or insulin, which counteract the crisis; and epileptics may stuff handkerchiefs between their teeth just before convulsions.

When signs aren't properly read, are read too slowly or are interpreted as meaning something else, then people die or come close to dying. This may happen the first time a cardiac patient experiences severe chest pains and doesn't yet know their cause or treatment. (After the first sequence the patient may put his doctor's name close to the telephone for emergency use.) Even physicians may misread signs and so precipitate a crisis—even death. If an unconscious sickle cell anemia sufferer is brought bleeding to a hospital he may die if the natural immediate effort is made to stop his bleeding. Patients who carry instructions with them can sometimes avoid difficulties. Whenever an unconscious individual is brought into the emergency room of the nearest hospital, the physicians there understandably may treat him for the wrong disease. Inexperienced patients who are on kidney dialysis machinery may not realize that their machinery is working incorrectly and that their bodies are nearing crisis. The complexity of the human body can cause even experienced persons to misread important signs.

Any breakdown or disruption of the crisis-preventing or crisis-coping organization can be disastrous. Family strain can lead to the abandonment of or lessening control over regimens, and temporary absence of "protective agents" or of "control agents" (such as mothers of diabetic children who are prone to eat too much candy) can also be traumatic. A divorce or separation that leaves an assisting agent (a mother helping her cystic fibrosis child with absolutely necessary exercises) alone, unrelieved with her task, can gradually or quickly lead to a crisis. (One divorced couple arranged matters so that the father relieved the mother on weekends and some evenings.) Even an agent's illness can lead to the relaxation of regimens or the elimination of activities that might otherwise prevent crisis.

There is also a post-crisis period, in relation to the organization of effort. Some failure of organization right in the hospital can be seen when the staff begins to pull away from a cardiac patient, recently saved from a heart attack, but now judged "less critical" than other patients. Back home, of course, some patients require plenty of family organization to prevent additional attacks. What is not so evident is that the patient and his family may read signs of improvement where few exist, or that contingencies may arise which render faulty the organization for crisis prevention and crisis management. Relevant variables here are the length and rapidity of recovery—since both of these may vary for different disease conditions.

During an extended period of crisis the family may need to make special arrangements about their time (for visiting the hospital, for nursing the patient at home) and their living space (having the bed downstairs rather than upstairs, living near the hospital during the peak of the crisis). They may have to juggle the family's finances or spell each other in nursing the patient during his crisis. Even the patient himself—in trying to get better rather than giving up—may have to contribute to the necessary organization of effort to bring the family through the crisis period.

Unless the physician is absolutely helpless in the face of a given chronic disease, he will suggest or command some kind of regimen. Adhering to regimens, though, is a very complex matter, for regimens can sometimes set problems so difficult that they may present more hardships than the symptoms themselves.

Patients do not adhere to regimens automatically. Those who accept and maintain a regimen must have abiding trust in the physician, evidence that the requirements work without producing distressing or frightening side effects (or that the side effects are outweighed by symptom relief or fear of the disease itself), and the guarantee that important daily activities, either of the patient or of people around him, can continue relatively uninterrupted.

In addition to the time it takes and the discomfort it causes, an important property of a given regimen is whether it is visible to other people, and what visibility may mean to the patient. If the regimen means that a stigmatized disease can be suspected or discovered, the person is unlikely to carry it out in public. (Tuberculosis patients sometimes have this problem.) If the visible regimen is no more than slightly embarrassing or is fully explainable, then its visibility is much less likely to prevent its maintenance in public or private.

Another property is also important: if the regimen appears to work for the patient, then that may convince him that he should continue with it. But continuance is problematic, not only because the other properties noted above may counteract his best intentions or his good sense, but because once a regimen has brought symptom relief, the patient may forego the routine—no matter what the physician says. This is exactly what happens when tuberculosis patients see their symptoms disappear, and figure that now they can cut out—partially or totally—their uncomfortable regimen.

The very properties of the regimen, then, constitute contributing conditions for adhering, relaxing, or even rejecting the prescribed activities. Thus, if the patient simply denies that he has the disease (as with tuberculosis, where many patients experience no symptoms), he may not carry out his regimen. Instructions for a treatment routine may leave him confused or baffled: cardiac patients told to "rest" or "find their own limits" can be frustrated because they don't really know what "sufficient rest" means.

Patients and kinsmen inevitably enter into negotiations with each other, and sometimes with the physician, over relaxing or otherwise changing (substituting one drug for another, one activity for another) the regimen. They are negotiating not only over such matters as the elimination of discomfort and side effects, but also the possibility of making the management of ordinary life easier or even possible. Physicians, of course, recognize much of this bargaining, but they may not realize just how high the stakes can be for the patient and his family. If a doctor ignores those factors, his patients may go shopping for another physician or, at the least, he may quietly alter his regimen or substitute part of it with something recommended by an amateur—pharmacist, friend, or relative.

Symptom Management

The control of symptoms is obviously linked with adherence to effective regimens. Like adherence to regimen, symptom control is not merely a matter of medical management. Most of the time, the patient is far from medical facilities, so he and his family must rely upon their own judgment, wisdom, and ingenuity in controlling symptoms—quite aside from faithfully following the prescribed regimens. Some physicians—probably not many—recognize that need for judgment.

Whatever the sophisticated technical references may be, the person who has symptoms will be concerned primarily with whether he hurts, faints, trembles visibly, has had his mobility or his speech impaired, or is evidencing some kind of disfigurement. How much they interfere with his life and social relationships depends on whether they are permanent or temporary, predictable or unpredictable, publicly visible or invisible; also on their degree (as of pain), their meaning to bystanders (as of disfigurement), the nature of the regimen called for to control the symptom; and of course on the kinds of life-style and social relations which the sufferer has been accustomed to.

Even minor, occasional symptoms may lead to some changing of habits, and major symptoms may call for the redesigning or reshaping of important aspects of a patient's life-style. Thus, someone who begins to suffer from minor back pains is likely to learn to avoid certain kinds of chairs and even discover to his dismay that a favorite sitting position is precisely the one he must forego. Major adjustments could include moving to a one-story house, buying clothes that cloak disfigurement, getting the boss to assign jobs that require less strength, using crutches or other aides to mobility. In one case a mailman suffering from colitis lived "on a leash," having arranged never to be very far from that necessary toilet. Emphysema patients learn to have "puffing stations" where they can recoup from lack of breath while looking like they have stopped normally.

Ideas for redesigning activities may come from others, too. A community nurse taught an emphysema patient how to rest while doing household chores; a sister taught a patient afflicted with brittle bones (because of a destructive drug) how to get up from the toilet, minus a back brace, without breaking bones in her back. Another woman figured out how her cardiac-arthritic grandfather could continue his beloved walks on his farm, by placing wooden stumps at short distances so that he could rest as he reached each one. Unfortunately, kinsmen and health professionals can function in just the opposite fashion: for instance, a woman with multiple sclerosis had carefully arranged her one-room apartment so that every object she needed was literally within arm's reach; but the public health nurse who visited her regarded the place as in a terrible shambles and proceeded to tidy things up herself.

Perhaps inventiveness, just as much as finances or material resources, is what makes the difference between reaching and not reaching some relatively satisfying redesign of life. The cancer patient with lessened energy who can ingeniously juggle her friends' visits and telephone calls can maintain a relatively unimpaired social life. Arthritic farm women who can get neighbors to bring in groceries can live on their farms during the summer although they must move to town for the winter months. One multiple sclerosis patient who is a student not only has rearranged her apartment but persuaded various people to help her manage despite her increasingly restricted mobility. A veritable army of people have come to her aid: the university architect redesigned certain of the public toilets for her wheelchair and also put in some ramps; the handymen around the university help her up and down stairs, by appointment; they also have rebuilt her cupboards so that she can reach them from her wheelchair; and so on.

Lack of imagination about useful redesigning makes symptom control harder. This lack of imaginative forethought can be seen in many homes for the elderly where stiff-jointed or low-energy people must struggle to rise from sitting positions on low sofas and chairs, or must painstakingly pick their way along highly polished corridors—minus handrails.

The reshaping of activities pertains also to the crucial issue of "interaction." A variety of judicious or clever maneuvers can keep one's symptoms as unobtrusive as possible. Sometimes the tactics are very simple: a college teacher with bronchitis, whose peak load of coughing up sputum is in the morning, arranges his teaching schedule so that he can stay at home, or at least in his office, until after lunchtime. Another person who tends continually to have a runny allergic nose always carries tissue in her hand when in public. Another with a tendency to cough carries cough drops with him—especially important when he attends concerts. An epileptic may have to persuade acquaintances that his epileptic fits are not communicable! Emphysema sufferers learn to sit down or lean against buildings in such a fashion that they are not mistaken for drunks or loiterers.

Agents of various kinds can also be useful—wives who scout out the terrain at a public meeting to find the least obtrusive spot, and then pass on the information to their husbands in wheelchairs or on crutches. Spouses may have prearranged signals to warn each other when a chronic symptom (for example, runny nose) starts appearing. In a more dramatic instance a couple was attending a party when the husband noticed his wife's temporarily slurred speech—a sign of her tiredness and pain from cancer. Since they did not want to have their friends know of her illness, he acted quickly to divert the others' attention and soon afterward manufactured an excuse so that they could leave the party.

When visible symptoms cannot easily be disguised, misleading explanations may be offered—fainting, for instance, is explained away by someone "in the know" as a temporary weakness due to flu or to some other reasonable cause. When a symptom cannot be minimized, then a wife may attempt to prepare others for the distressing sight or sound of her husband's affliction. The sufferer himself may do this, as when a cancer patient who had lost much weight warned friends, over the phone, that when they visited they would find her not looking like herself at all. Each friend who visits is very likely, in turn, to warn other friends what to expect.

Various chronic diseases lead to such disruption that they call for some temporal re-ordering. One all-too-familiar problem is too much time. It may only be temporary, as with persons who are waiting out a post-crisis period, but, for the disabled elderly or victims of multiple sclerosis, it may be a permanent condition. Among the consequences are boredom, decreased social skills, family strains, negative impact on identity, and even physical deterioration.

Just as common is not enough time. Not only is time sopped up by regimens and by symptom control, but those who assist the patient may expend many hours on their particular tasks. Not to be totally engulfed, they in turn may need to get assistants (baby-sitters, housecleaners, cooks) or redistribute the family workload. Occasionally the regimens require so much time, or crises come so frequently (some sickle cell anemia sufferers have been hospitalized up to 100 times), that life simply gets organized around those events; there is not enough time for much of anything else. Even just handling one's symptoms or the consequences of having symptoms may require so much time that life is taken up mainly with handling them. Thus, a very serious dermatological condition forced one woman to spend hour after hour salving her skin; otherwise she would have suffered unbearably. Unfortunately, the people who suffer cannot leave their bodies. Kinsmen and other assisting agents, however, may abandon their charges out of desperation for what the temporal engulfment is doing to their own lives. Abandonment, here, may mean shifting the burdens to a nursing home or other custodial institution, such as a state mental institution.

The term "dying trajectory" means the course of dying as defined by various participants in it. Analogously, one can also think of the course of the chronic disease (downward in most instances). Like the dying trajectory, that course can be conceived as having two properties. First, it takes place over time: it has duration. Specific trajectories can vary greatly in duration. Some start earlier, some end later. Second, a trajectory has shape. It may plunge straight down; it may move slowly but steadily downward; it may vacillate slowly, moving slightly up and down before diving downward radically; it may move slowly down at first, then hit a long plateau, then plunge abruptly even to death. Neither the duration nor shape of a dying trajectory is a purely objective physiological property. Both are perceived properties; their dimensions depend on when the perceiver initially defines someone as diseased and on his expectations of how the disease course will proceed. (We can add further that dying trajectory consists merely of the last phases of some chronic disease trajectories.) Each type of disease (multiple sclerosis, diabetes, and so forth) or subtype (different kinds of arthritis) may have a range of variation in trajectory, but they certainly tend to be patterned in accordance with duration and shape.

It would be much too simplistic to assert that specific trajectories determine what happens to a sense of identity; but certainly they do contribute, and quite possibly in *patterned* ways. Identity responses to a severe heart attack may be varied, but awareness that death can be but a moment away—everyday—probably cannot but have a different impact on identity than trajectories expected to result in slow death, or in leaving one a "vegetable" or perfectly alive but a hopeless cripple.

We have alluded to the loss of social contact, even extending to great social isolation, that may be a consequences of chronic disease and its management. This loss is understandable given the accompanying symptoms, crises, regimens and often difficult phasing of trajectories.

It is not difficult to trace some of the impact on social contact of varying symptoms, in accordance with their chief properties. The disfigurement associated with leprosy leads many to stay in leper colonies; they prefer the social ease and normal relationships that are possible there. Disease which are (or which the sufferer thinks are) stigmatizing are kept as secret as possible. But talking about his illness with friends who may understand can be comforting. Some may find new friends (even spouses) among fellow sufferers, especially through clinic visits or special clubs formed around the illness or disability (such as those formed by kidney failure victims and people who have had ileostomies). Some virtually make careers of doing voluntary work for those clubs or associations. People can also leave circles of friends whom they feel might now be unresponsive, frightened, or critical and move to more sympathetic social terrain. An epileptic who has used a warning tactic and has moved to a supportive terrain says:

I'm lucky, I still have friends. Most people who have epilepsy are put to the side. But I'm lucky that way. I tell them that I have epilepsy and that they shouldn't get scared if I fall out. I go to things at the church—it's the church people that are my friends. I just tell them and then it is okay. They just laugh about it and don't get upset.

Some people may chose to allow their diseases to advance rather than put up with their regiments. One cardiac patient, for instance, simply refused to give up his weekly evening playing cards with "the boys"— replete with smoking, beer drinking, and late hours—despite his understanding that this could lead to further heart attacks. Another cardiac patient avoided coffee breaks at work because everyone smoked then. He stayed away from many social functions for the same reasons. He felt that people probably thought him "unsociable," but he was not able to think of any other way to stop himself from smoking. Perhaps the extreme escape from—not minimization or prevention of—social isolation was exhibited by one woman with kidney disease who chose to go off dialysis (she had no possibility of getting a transplant), opting for a speedy death because she saw an endless time ahead, dependence on others, inability to hold down a job, increasing social isolation and a purposeless life. Her physicians accepted her right to make this choice.

Those who cannot face physically altered friends may avoid or even abandon them. One individual who was losing weight because of cancer remarked bitterly that a colleague of his had ducked down the street, across campus, to avoid meeting him. Spouses who have known great intimacy together can draw apart because of an illness: a cardiac husband may fear having sex or may be afraid of dying but cannot tell his wife for fear of increasing *her* anxiety. The awkwardness that others feel about discussing death and fear of it isolates many chronically ill people from their friends—even from their spouses. During the last phases of a disease trajectory, an unbridgeable gap may open up between previously intimate spouses.

Even aside from the question of death fears, friends may draw apart because the patient is physically isolated from the mainstream of life. One stroke patient who temporarily lost the ability to speak described what happened between himself and his friends: "I felt unguarded and my colleagues—who pretty soon found their conversation drying up in the lack of anything from me—felt bored, or at any rate I thought they were. My wife, who was usually present, saved the conversation from dying—she was never at loss for a word." A cardiac patient hospitalized away from his hometown at first received numerous cards and telephone calls, but once his friends had reached across the distance they chose to leave him alone, doubtless for a variety of reasons. He and his wife began to feel slightly abandoned. Later, when he had returned to part-time work, he found that his fellow executives left him relatively alone at first, knowing that he was far from recuperated. Despite his conscious knowledge that his colleagues were trying to help, he still felt out of things.

Friends and relatives may withdraw from patients who are making excessive demands or who have undergone personality changes caused by a crisis or the progress of a disease. Abandonment may be the final result. Husbands desert, spouses separate, and adult children place their elderly parents in nursing homes. In some kinds of chronic diseases, especially stigmatic (leprosy) or terribly demanding (mental illness), friends and relatives and even physicians advise the spouse or kinsmen quite literally to abandon the sick person: "It's time to put her in the hospital." "Think of the children." "Think of yourself—it makes no sense." "It's better for her, and you are only keeping her at home because of your own guilt." These are just some of the abandonment rationales that are offered, or which the person offers himself. Of course, the sick person, aware of having become virtually an intolerable burden, may offer those rationales also—though not necessarily alleviating his own sense of estrangement.

The chief business of a chronically ill person is not just to stay alive or to keep his symptoms under control, but to live as normally as possible despite his symptoms and his disease. In the case of chronically ill children, parents work very hard at creating some semblance of a normal life for their offspring. "Closed awareness" or secrecy is the ruling principle of family life. No one tells the child he is dying. Parents of children with leukemia, for example, have a very difficult time. For much of the time, the child actually may look quite well and live a normal life—but his parents have to work very hard at *acting* normal unless they can keep the impending death well at the back of their minds. The parents with children with longer life expectancies need not work so hard to maintain a normal atmosphere in their homes, except insofar as the child may rebel against aspects of a restrictive regimen which he feels makes *his* life abnormal. Some of the difficulties which chronic sufferers experience in maintaining normal interaction are reflected in the common complaint that blind and physically handicapped people make—that people assume they cannot walk and work like ordinary mortals, but rush up to help them do what they are quite as capable of doing as anyone else. The nonsick, especially strangers, tend to overemphasize the sick person's visible symptoms, so that they come to dominate the interaction. The sick person fights back by using various tactics to disavow his deviant status: he hides the intrusive symptom—covers it with clothes, puts the trembling hand under the table—or if it can't be hidden, then minimizes its impact by taking attention away from it—like a dying woman who has lost a great deal of weight but who forces visitors to ignore her condition by talking cheerfully and normally about their mutual interests.

Artful Striving

In setting guidelines for "acting normal" there is much room for disagreement between the ill person and those near to him about just how ill he is. The sick person may choose more invalidism than his condition really warrants. After a crisis or a peak period of symptoms, the sick person may find himself rushed by others—including his helping agents—who either misjudge his return to better health or simply forget how sick he might still be since he does not show more obvious signs of his current condition. All patients who have partial-recovery trajectories necessarily run that hazard. ("Act sicker than you look or they will quickly forget you were so ill" was the advice given to one cardiac patient who was about to return to his executive job.)

The more frequent reverse phenomenon is when the sick person believes his condition is more normal than others believe. His friends and relatives tell him, "Take it easy, don't rush things." His physician warns him that he will harm himself, even kill himself, if he doesn't act in accordance with the facts of his case. But it sometimes happens that the person really has a very accurate notion of just how he feels. One man who had had a kidney transplant found himself having to prove to his fellow workers that he was not handicapped—doing extra work to demonstrate his normality. A slightly different case is the ill person who may know just how ill he is but wishes others to regard him as less ill and allow him to act accordingly. One dying man who was trying to live as normally as possible right down through his last days found himself rejecting those friends, however well intentioned, who regarded him as "dying now" rather than as "living fully to the end."

As the trajectory of the ill person's health continues downward, he may have to come to terms with a lessened degree of normality. We can see this very clearly with those who are slowly dying, when both they and their friends or kinsmen are quite willing to settle for "something less" at each phase of the downward trajectory, thankful at least for small things. It is precisely when the chronically ill cannot settle for lower levels of functioning that they opt out of this life. When their friends and relatives cannot settle for less, or have settled for as much as they can stand, then they too opt out of his life: by separation, divorce, or abandonment. Those who are chronically ill from diseases like multiple sclerosis or other severe forms of neurological illness (or mental illness, for that matter) are likely to have to face this kind of abandonment by others. The chronically ill themselves, as well as many of their spouses, kinsmen, and friends, are remarkably able to accommodate themselves to increasingly lower levels of normal interaction and style; they can do this either because of immense closeness to each other or because they are grateful even for what little life and relationship remains. They strive manfully—and artfully—to "keep things normal" at whatever level that has come to mean.

We must not forget, either, that symptoms and trajectories may stabilize for long periods of time, or in fact not change for the worst at all: then the persons so afflicted simply come to accept, on a long-term basis, whatever restrictions are placed on their lives. Like Franklin D. Roosevelt, they live perfectly normal (even super-normal!) lives in all respects except for whatever handicaps may derive from their symptoms or their medical regimens. To keep interaction normal, they need only develop the requisite skills to make others ignore or deemphasize their disabilities.

Helping those afflicted with chronic diseases means far more than simply displaying compassion or having medical competence. Only through knowledge of and sensitivity to the *social* aspects of symptom control, regimen management, crisis prevention, handling dying, and death itself, can one develop truly beneficial strategies and tactics for dealing with specific diseases and chronic illness in general.

What Price Chronic Illness?

Carolyn Wiener, Shizuko Fagerhaugh,
Anselm Strauss, and Barbara Suczek

In recent years, the myth of the scientist-Magus has taken certain twists
in the health-care arena. While some people still consider modern technology a Faustian bargain—new knowledge resulting in huge costs—
others are looking elsewhere for villains. Our reimbursement system, the
tendency of physicians to practice "defensive medicine," consumer demand, extravagant claims made by the media, the emphasis in medical
education on specialization, the unwillingness of people to take responsibility for their own health—all of these come in for their share of the
blame regarding the rising cost of medical care. A closer look at this
debate reveals that participants are circling around a major issue, but not
directly grappling with it. That major issue is the increasingly *chronic*
and unresolved character of illness. By focusing on chronic illness, we
hope to demonstrate how contained is the current debate over cost.

To understand the explosive growth in medical technology, we need
first to understand that its source lies not only in greatly increased knowledge, but in the changed nature of illness. Since the 1940s, industrially
developed nations every where have manifested the same patterns of illness: as infectious and parasitic diseases have come under control, the
prevalence of various chronic illnesses has increased. The latter include
such highly visible illnesses as the cancers, cardiovascular illnesses, renal diseases, respiratory diseases, diabetes, arthritis—some dramatized
by heart transplant surgery, the use of pacemakers and dialysis machines,
chemotherapy and X-ray therapy for cancer, the "scanner" and so on.

Lewis Thomas, in *The Lives of a Cell,* has popularized a term for
these procedures, drugs, and machines, calling them "halfway technologies," meaning medical intervention applied after the fact in an attempt
to compensate for the incapacitating effects of disease whose course one

is unable to do much about. They are technologies designed to make up for the disease or postpone death. The outstanding example of this is the transplanting of organs. Thomas argues that this level of technology is by its nature highly sophisticated and at the same time primitive, continuing only until there is a genuine understanding of the mechanism involved in disease. (In caring for heart disease, for example, the technology that is involved is enormous: it involves specialized ambulances, specialized diagnostic services, specialized patient-care units, all kinds of electronic gadgets, plus an array of new skilled health professionals to maintain the machines and care for the patients on the machines.) Enormous cost, the continuing expansion of health facilities, and a need for more and more highly trained personnel are characteristic of this type of technology. Until the basic questions about the mechanisms of disease in the various chronic illnesses are answered, Thomas argues—correctly we believe—we must put up with halfway technologies.

That these illnesses cannot be "cured" but must be "managed" makes them different in many respects from acute illnesses, the model around which health care was traditionally built. A brief look at the salient qualities of chronic illness makes the differences apparent. Chronic illnesses are uncertain: their phases are unpredictable as to intensity, duration, and degree of incapacity. Chronic illnesses are episodic: acute flare-ups are followed by remissions, in many ways restricting a "normal" life. Chronic illnesses require large palliative efforts: symptomatic relief (from pain, dizziness, nausea, etc.) is often as necessary as the overall progress of treatment. Chronic illnesses are often multiple: long-term breakdown of one organ or physical system leads to involvement of others. One fact becomes obvious: halfway technologies are not only prolonging life but are stretching out the illness trajectories. By trajectories we mean not just the physical course of illness but all the work that patients, staff, and kin do to deal with the illness, and all the social/ psychological consequences that encircle the illness course (its intrusiveness on relationships, temperament, and so forth).

This medical technology is found in doctors' offices, hospitals, clinics, and increasingly in the homes of the chronically ill. It has prolonged life but has also made patients dependent on technology throughout the long years of their chronic illnesses. They cycle through the hospital, then go to the clinic or doctor's office, return home, go back to the hospital during acute episodes, and again back to their homes. The problems of coordinating the care given in the hospital, clinic, and home become immense. Accordingly, the explosion of technology has had a profound effect on the organization of health care and on the work of the implicated health professionals.

A special feature of medical specialization and technological innovation is that the two are parallel and interactive. If one looks at medical specialization, it is clear that it leads to technological innovation, which then involves industrial development, production, and distribution. In turn, this process creates further sophisticated specialization and associated medical work, and the establishing of associated organizations for medical work. We see this, for example, in the growth of intensive care units (ICUs), or critical care units. When first developed they were general ICUs, in which a variety of very ill patients, including cardiac patients, were cared for. Then, with further refinement of cardiovascular monitors and respirators, aided by large research funds for cardiac disease, separate intensive care cardiac units evolved. Simultaneously, specialized diagnostic cardiac units were developed, becoming further differentiated according to patient age—adult or pediatric. Corresponding with these developments, heart surgeons invented a sophisticated cardiac surgical technology. In large medical centers one finds that each specialty has begun to have its own intensive care unit—neurological ICUs, respiratory ICUs, and so on.

Discussion of indirect costs due to chronic illness rarely goes beyond suggesting loss of work time and restriction of activity. There are, however, other costs, equally hard to measure (and many borne principally by patients and their families):

- Help in the home for patients who are incapacitated, as, for instance, stroke patients.
- Transportation to and from clinics, hospitals, and physicians' offices.
- Increased burden on middle-aged, middle-class working tax payers (for Medicare, Medicaid, and increased insurance premiums).
- Counseling to cope with disease-induced stress.
- Tutoring for children with chronic illness.
- Technical services (in the use and maintenance of home equipment, such as dialysis machines and respiratory equipment).
- Inflationary cost of products as employers respond to increased benefit packages offered employees.

The impact of specialization is also greater than the most extravagant criticism of it. An example on the research level is the burgeoning field called neuroscience, which blends specialists in biochemistry, anatomy, psychology, and pharmacology in an international effort to chart the brain, thereby to discover means to suppress pain and treat mental illness. Each aspect of this effort requires highly specialized knowledge and skill and is dependent on highly specialized equipment. While the neuroanatomist is exploring the limits of autoradiography—a technique of photographing slices of animal brain tissue after first treating it with radioactive substances—the biological psychiatrist is using computerized laboratory equipment to study the blood plasma of patients who are especially sensitive to pain. Similar combinations of expertise are to be found in the development of electronic prosthetic devices (an implantable electronic inner ear, electronic vision) brought about by the increased miniaturization of electronic circuitry and the combined work of engineers, chemists, and biologists. Or consider the artificial pancreas, a still nascent development dependent on all kinds of basic science: mathematical models constructed through experimentation in a metabolic research unit; enzymatic methods for measuring blood sugar; improvement of chemical films that allow immobilization of enzymes despite the risk of infection; computer analysis to measure insulin levels; production of refined bio-materials; creation of a machine which measures a patient's blood sugar over a twenty-four-hour period. This machine finally confirmed what the researchers had long suspected: that the diabetic taking insulin everyday is never fully under control; that no diabetic is being treated very well. Thus, the work of specialized research scientists becomes joined to the highly specialized world of medical instrumentation.

Obviously, the expanded medical knowledge and the technology which evolves through the combined efforts of specialization are then mirrored at the level of application. Hence the emergence not only of cardiologists, nephrologists, and neurosurgeons, but of pediatric cardiologists and hematologists with a sub-specialty in leukemia—sharpening the mastery ever more finely by limiting the focus. What is more, medical knowledge is developing at such a rapid pace that many medical options are experimental, involving increasingly higher risk, which further increases the requirements of the limited focus. Thus today, pharmacologists must try to keep physicians' informed (at Stanford Hospital through a computerized system, at the University of California Hospital, San Francisco, through a periodic bulletin) regarding the harmful interactive effect of the huge number of available drugs.

Although medical specialization is usually singled out in this regard about cost, the nursing profession is also specializing at a tremendous pace—again in response to the clinical expertise demanded by specialized equipment and more problematic trajectories. There are now numerous special-interest nursing groups for nephrology, neurosurgery, emergency room, infectious-disease control, orthopedics, oncology, rehabilitation, and critical care, to name a few. Combined nursing specialties are mushrooming, again in response to perceived need, as for example the pediatric-dialysis nurse who told us she sees herself as the coordinator whom parents need when dealing with the fragmented care in their child's treatment. This process of professional and occupational specialization is bound not only to continue but to proliferate.

Thus modern technology—heart-lung machines which increase the number of candidates for surgery, hyperalimentation machines which bypass the digestive system, intricate blood chemistry tests which give instant and multiple readings on electrolyte status—has made for a variety of options which did not exist before: What technology is to be used? How? When? Where? Who decides? This intricate technology requires specialized knowledge and has led to a proliferation of experts. They are dealing not only with the uncertainty of the disease trajectory or trajectories of a particular patient, but with the risks of the use of available technology—hence all the balancing and juggling of options and the use of consultations. Often debates are going on among the physicians regarding what is the right option, or about the appropriate sequence of options. Each decision about options can be crucial, with multiple factors being weighted and balanced, often by a multitude of people who may have different perspectives and different stakes in the decision making. All along, technologies are being used to facilitate decision making: such as imaging techniques to visualize internal organs, and monitoring machines and laboratory tests for second-to-second appraisal.

In addition, at each point where options are chosen there is a possibility of a new illness trajectory as a result of the decision to apply a given option: steroid drugs often cause secondary disease in kidney transplant patients, machines and procedures can cause infections. Furthermore, the trajectory stretch-out means that diseases associated with advanced age, like degenerative arthritis and arthosclerosis, are superimposed on the major trajectory. If a patient has multiple diseases or even a major and minor trajectory (e.g., ulcerative colitis plus an allergy to sulfa drugs, or kidney disease requiring five hours of dialysis combined with chronic back problems) the options may be counteractive—increasing the balancing decisions, and increasing the need to employ more technology in the service of those decisions.

This, then, is a brief picture of the changed nature of illness and health care. It is against this backdrop that the debate about the considerable cost of medical technology has evolved.

Impact of Chronic Illness

The reality which must be faced is that:

- Costs are even greater than most estimates, and are going to increase, despite the various assumptions—and policies based on them—about the source of increased cost.
- The impact of specialization is also greater than the most extravagant criticism of it, and this process is bound not only to continue but to proliferate.
- The diffusion of medical technology will continue, and blaming specialization for this diffusion is a distortion of the issue.
- The notion that consensus can be reached regarding the efficacy and use of medical technology is an unreachable objective.

In *Technology in Hospitals: Medical Advances and Their Diffusion,* Louise B. Russell examined available statistics for four industrialized countries—the United States, Sweden, Great Britain, and France—and found they have all assumed, until recently, that technology is beneficial for patients (in some fashion) and therefore worth having. She concludes this may reflect the fact that the problems to be addressed—the rapid growth of costs in general, and the arrival of a number of expensive new technologies in particular—are relatively recent. The third and perhaps more pressing problem is still not faced head-on: the needs of increasing numbers of chronically ill people. There is now, and will continue to be for some time, competition among the various chronic illnesses for priority. The technologies for these illnesses are at varying stages of their development—e.g., hemodialysis well established although still being refined, the artificial pancreas as yet in the development stage. "Overuse" of technology makes a convenient target, but it is much more realistic to acknowledge that costs are bound to increase because of this intertwining of new technologies with new and more problematic illness trajectories.

While it is generally assumed (even by critics of applying cost-benefit analysis to the health arena) that costs are easier to measure than benefits, the costs are even greater than the most dire estimates. A host of organizational costs are omitted from discussion:

- Interdepartmental coordination (time spent working out strategies for coordinating and troubleshooting; since the more options, the more possibilities of coordination breakdown, unexpected contingencies, disrupted schedules, etc.).
- New personnel to handle these contingencies: e.g., unit managers, ward clerks, materiel management experts.
- Body-to-machine transportation, and vice versa, within the hospital.
- Machine purchase, maintenance, repair, monitoring; bioengineers to handle this in large hospitals, outside contracts in smaller hospitals.
- Drug purchase, storage, and handling.
- Auxiliary supplies (throwaway tubes, catheters, connections, needles) and their purchase, storage, and distribution.
- Staff to understand, monitor, and enforce regulatory compliance.
- Safety monitoring, including building and maintaining whole departments of safety engineers.
- Time, effort, and space required for backstopping of machines and drugs.
- Resource building of skills; in-service in every department, time spent working and reworking protocols as technology undergoes rapid change.
- Record keeping and reporting.
- Building and rebuilding space to accommodate continually changing needs of departments and wards.
- Nonroutine trajectory decisions: meetings-debates over options, more monitoring; then the next round per phase, and the coordination of these phased decisions.
- Time spent working out the idiosyncracies of a particular machine, or assessing it for feedback to the manufacturer.
- Continuing care at home—clinic costs, technology and supplies at home, post-hospital home visits, and new personnel to handle this (e.g., discharge nurses and liaison nurses).
- Phone networks from hospital to outlying areas in less populous states.

The diffusion of medical technology will continue to increase, and to target specialization as a scapegoat for medical technology diffusion is a misrepresentation. For instance, critics assert that a technology is more likely to be adopted, or is adopted sooner, by hospitals with residency programs. "Open-heart surgery," according to Russell, "is a striking example: medical school affiliation and an extensive program of residency training raised the probability that a hospital would adopt open-heart

surgery by 0.6 (the maximum value a probability can assume is 1.0)."
Steven Schroeder and Jonathan Showstack, relying on Uwe Reinhardt's
study showing that use of medical technology varies directly with den-
sity of physicians, conclude, in a *New England Journal of Medicine*
article: "Controls will have to contend not only with the reimbursement
system as it now operates, but also with the powerful forces toward medical specialization." The California State Health Plan continues the attack. Quoted in this report is the cycle of specialty certification as
delineated by Robert Chase, former president of the National Board of
Medical Examiners:

1. As a result of advances in the field, a new group develops a special expertise in this area.
2. An organization or society is formed for an exchange of ideas and to
   display advances to one another.
3. Membership in the organization becomes a mark of distinction in the
   field, and, in an effort to externalize that recognition, certification of excellence in the field becomes established.
4. Institutions with responsibility for quality of health care soon accept certification as evidence of competence and limit care within that field to
   those certified.

A fifth step is then offered by the California report, suggesting self-interest as the sole motivating force:

5. The specialty promotes use of its own technologies and the development
   of new ones, thereby starting the cycle again.

Again omitted from the cycle by these critics are the needs (and demands) of the chronically ill. At a recent meeting in a metropolitan hospital, a physician reflected this as he struggled for clues in the referral
process: "People are already going to the high-volume hospitals. So if
we could find out why referrals are happening we could perfect the system." People go, or are referred, to oncologists because they are better at
treating cancer; to pediatric cardiologists because they are more skilled
at treating heart disease in children. The incidence of open-heart surgery
is higher in large medical centers with medical-school affiliation, because both patients and their referring physicians know that is where the
most skilled cardiologists, the best equipment and supporting staff, are
to be found. True, graduates of these large research and training centers
then seek opportunities to practice their skills. True also that competition

among hospitals forces equipment requirements upon them. But the assumption that supply is affecting demand ignores the evidence that there is a chronically ill population "out there" on whom these skills are being practiced. Blaming specialization itself for the diffusion of medical technology is like blaming the cure for the disease.

The vision of consensus regarding the efficacy and use of medical technologies is an unattainable goal, as Russell's caveat, in "Making Rational Decisions about Medical Technology," hints:

> Finally, if the process of testing, weighing, and deciding is not to be an empty charade, the final decision must apply to all technology, not to specific institutions, and must be supported by all elements of the medical care sector. It is a waste of time to produce, after consideration of national tests, a regulation against the adoption of a technology by hospitals, only to have a financing program continue to pay for the use of that technology when it is owned by a physician as part of his office equipment or by a contractor who provides services to hospitals.

Others in this arena, such as Schroeder and Showstack, are even more ambitious, calling the decisions about what medical services we need and can afford "social decisions," requiring "political consensus." The debate takes notice of the formidable obstacle of professional stakes biasing the outcome of evaluation studies. But the discussion tends to soft-pedal the genuine diversity in assessment. Procedures such as gastrointestinal endoscopy and respiratory therapy are held up as examples of questionable use, supported by papers or discussions from professional meetings. However, these citations from the American Society of Gastrointestinal Endoscopy or a Conference on the Scientific Basis of Respiratory Therapy reflect more the internal debates than the agreement within a particular specialty, and only serve to illustrate how much more difficult it will be to get political consensus in the larger community.

A look at governmental regulatory attempts is illuminating. Although the Comprehensive Health Planning and Public Health Services Amendments of 1966 did not really get off the ground due to meager funding and unclear direction, many of the state and area agencies set up under this law evolved into the present "health systems agencies" (HSAs) mandated by the National Health Planning and Resources Development Act of 1974. There are now some two hundred health-systems agencies in the country, attempting to rationalize health care and to serve as a restraining hand on profligate spending. The principal legacy of the 1966 act is the enactment of state certificate-of-need laws, which require that the state agency review and approve investments in new health facilities (except doctors' offices), services, and expensive equipment. Not surprisingly, composed as they are of providers of care (i.e., physicians and hospital administrators) and consumers of health care (defined as citizens of the area who are not providers), HSAs are controversial forums, described by Ann Lennarson Greer as "targets of attempted suasion by those who would expand and those who would contain the particular area's health institutions," in other words, "political hotbeds." As to certificate-of-need control, Thomas Moloney and David Rogers conclude in "Medical Technology—A Different View of the Contentious Debate Over Costs":

> At present this strategy is in great jeopardy because it was simply too costly to obtain creditable information with which to limit the distribution of big new technologies. Information about the supply, use, and costs of special equipment and services was reported as sketchy, and consistent review standards were viewed as virtually nonexistent. Thus, the goal of direct technology control is being dropped in several states in which it was attempted.

Another attempt at governmental control of costs is the establishment of Professional Standards Review Organizations (PSROs), as part of the Social Security amendments of 1972. PSROs, composed of local physicians, are mandated to determine whether care is medically necessary, of recognized quality, and provided in the proper facility or level of care. To date, the operational definition of medical necessity and recognized quality has been based on "community standards" or "current practice," and PSROs have tended to place their emphasis on assessing appropriate length of hospital stay. In fact, the hiring of PSROs by private corporations to review employees' utilization and thereby decrease average hospital stay seems to be the trend. Obviously, utilization review is a far less controversial road to follow than the thicket of peer assessment of quality care.

Yes, But

The debate about cost as it pertains to medical technology misses the mark by not focusing on the very real and central problem of an increased number of people with chronic illnesses. However, since on first consideration many of the proposals in this debate appear reasonable, it is important to emphasize just where our quarrel with them lies, by offering a series of "yes...but" qualifications.

Yes, inequities have evolved in the reimbursement system, suggesting that panels might be able to adjust rates of payment to provide more incentive for nontechnical services. Although this will arouse opposition from some quarters, presumably a committee representative of the medical and insurance worlds could surmount the obstacles. *But,* it should not be assumed that this will meet the problem of "overspecialization" and diffusion of medical technologies. Nor will legislative interventions designed to create a better balance of primary-care physicians and specialists and a better geographic distribution of physicians alleviate this situation. Such measures have in the past "either failed to demonstrate the desired impact or have created secondary, almost intolerable, side effects," according to Charles Lewis, Rashi Fein, and David Mechanic in *A Right to Health.* Furthermore, the geographical distribution of physicians is not the prime condition explaining the use of medical technology.

Yes, offering alternative health plans is desirable in that competition might force more comprehensive coverage. *But,* it should not be assumed that this will deal with either equality or quality of care. Although data released to the public from the Health Maintenance Organization (HMO) experience is sparse, indications are that the principal cost-control mechanism is not decreased hospital stay, but decreased number of hospital admissions—the supposition being that these people are being treated on an ambulatory basis. And yet it is common knowledge that those who get quality care in an HMO are those who know how to manipulate the system (such as how to find a trustworthy doctor and ensure assignment to him/her, and how to circumvent the administrative barriers to ambulatory care). Furthermore, that the consumer can make an enlightened choice among health plan options is a questionable assumption; buying a health plan, unlike buying a television set, does not lend itself to consumer cost-benefit analysis.

Yes, assessing "appropriate use" of medical technology and achieving consensus on that assessment sounds like a reasonable expectation. *But,* given all the barriers to evaluate (the inconclusiveness of evidence, the lack of uniform values in medical practice, the constant modification which characterizes new technologies, the variation of use from setting to setting, the long period needed for assessment, the fiscal disincentives for those doing the evaluation, and the ambiguity in the relationship between processes of care and outcomes), assessment in the aggregate is an impossible goal. This is not to say that studies confined to single hospitals or single areas would not be helpful. For example, a study by the San Francisco PSRO verified the high use of emergency room facilities at San Francisco General Hospital by patients who came there because their doctor was unavailable, or because the emergency room is open twenty-four hours a day, admission is quick, and specialists are on call—indicating the need for alternative, less expensive facilities.

Yes, building in early prevention (one of the major arguments in this arena) may reduce eventual costs. But, it will be a long time before the results of prevention programs become evident. In the meantime, HMOs as presently constituted sell themselves on the basis of prevention but are still based on an acute-care model: patients learn that the best way to get prompt attention is on an acute or emergency basis. Worthwhile attempts are being made to provide outpatients with testing and services that were previously available only to inpatients. A prototype is VITAL Physical and Fitness Examination Center at St. Francis Memorial Hospital in San Francisco, which offers pap smears and breast examinations for women; urethral smears, genital-urinary examinations, and tests for prostate cancer for men; procto-sigmoidoscopy to test for rectal cancer; treadmill test for heart function; and an analysis of dietary habits and a personality profile to determine stress factors. Thus far, this program is concentrating on industrial packages for the employed population. Enlarged to wider coverage, such a prevention concept is worthy of support. But it should not be presented as a "cure" for current health costs.

Yes, the cost of medical technology can be reduced through rationing devices such as prospective reimbursement, administrative barriers to treatment, explicit criteria for allocation of new techniques. But, such proposals fly in the face of equality of care, for it is the poor who will suffer most from rationing. Medical servicing of the lower-income groups still exhibits considerable deficiencies. And yet it is lower-income people who have the most chronic illness, who need the support and preventive work, who get cheated out of the best technology. Rationing will only mean, as it has in England, that the elite get better care—they are able to go around the system because they want and can afford the state-of-the-art. Discussion of distribution of medical technology as it pertains to cost is based on the assumption that if you decrease the supply you decrease the demand. In contrast, we are saying that the distribution should be *more* extensive—that most poor diabetics cannot afford a correct diet, often do not have the family structure to help them maintain a regimen, and delay diagnosis and treatment because of their focus on "the deadly earnest present." Far from cost containment, what are needed are additional services which *may* in the end reduce total costs. It is to this that we turn next.

Looking at Patient Work

Those who argue that the present reimbursement system encourages overuse of medical technology claim that a more discriminating use would result if the patient were forced into partnership (for instance, through copayment insurance). A more sensible variant of this argument would be to encourage "patient partnership" by recognizing and assisting the work already being done by patients. In the hospital, patients do subtle work that is taken for granted by staff (lying still, moving one's body, hearing, seeing); they are also doing considerable decision making—small, operational choices as well as major choices between preferred therapies. In some situations, too, patients connect, disconnect, position, and monitor their own machines; in a spatially controlled situation such as on a dialysis unit, they monitor not only their own physical symptoms and their own machines but also each other and each other's machines. Staff seldom think of this as "work," more often making assessment of patients as "cooperative" or "uncooperative." Even more glaring is the inattention of the health system to patient work that goes on at home. When disease was of an infectious kind, the patient was sent home after the danger period ended. The advent of widespread chronic disease, however, makes the sharp division between home and health facility far too simple a solution to the problems faced by the chronically ill. Much of chronic illness has to do with the patient taking care of his/her own body—there is a thin line between therapy and ordinary living. And yet professionals still think predominantly in terms of "adherence" and "compliance," either abjuring virtually all responsibility in guiding or even looking into the patient work that goes on at home, or expressing annoyance with patients who do not follow prescribed regimens.

Gradual recognition of the need for personnel to aid sick people and their families to cope with problems attendant on chronicity can be discerned. The California Plan calls for revision of Medicare and Medicaid to create uniform home health benefits; relaxed restrictions that permit only skilled nursing services in certain situations; permission for non-medical personal care and support services to the chronically ill and disabled at home; the inclusion of day health care and hospice care. More attention is being addressed to the expansion of "non-physician-provided services," in the realization that while diagnosis and prescription are medical responsibilities, prevention and support activities for the chronically ill are not exclusively so. Indeed, while the extension of time allotted to each hypertension patient, for example, is attributable to the many treatment options which must be weighed by the physician, it is also attributable to the intertwining of hypertension with ordinary living and body-care habits. A properly trained home health aide can guide, monitor, correct misinformation, and could offer *phased teaching,* by which we mean teaching appropriate to the present chronic illness phase. Clinics which do not treat but teach, such as the Multipurpose Arthritis Clinic at the University of California, San Francisco, where patients gather to discuss treatment options and their side effects, can be staffed by nurses and a variety of health workers.

A 1979 *Social Policy* editorial called for an expansion of new forms of services—forms which add the health consumer to the existing means for the production of health care: "With some 50 percent of health care directed to chronic illness and about 70 percent of doctors' visits for the maintenance of chronics, support function can be readily, and best, served by self-help/self-care systems." The editorial added that self-care and mutual support as a national program must be developed in concert with the professional services which complement them, and with the financial support and planning of government. Borrowing ideas from groups like Alcoholics Anonymous and Weight Watchers, health self-help groups are expanding: I Can Cope for cancer patients, Mended Hearts for heart patients, Parent to Parent for parents of intensive care nursery graduates. Aside from the valuable contribution these groups make in terms of mutual support and exchange of information, they are performing a reverse service: teaching health professionals what it means to "live with" chronic disease—knowledge the professionals can impart to future patients. Insofar as there could be a greatly supplemented guidance of patient work in the home, and greater support of self-help groups, the health consumer would be provided with enhanced ability to read signs that portend a crisis of his/her disease, improved skill in responding to the crisis of the moment, and greater motivation to establish and maintain a regimen. Certainly the health-sciences—medical, nursing, etc.—schools and professional associations could accord greater weight to the potential of self-care in chronic disease management, and the training of students and practitioners to teach patients to use self-care. Such proposals in the end could reduce total cost: by freeing the physicians from work that other health professionals can do, by slowing up the rate of return to hospitals, by reducing the severity of disease in the population. Not insignificantly, such a course might break the vicious cycle that characterizes health care for lower-income patients—patients who delay too long in seeking treatment for themselves and their children, do not follow regimens, come back in worse condition, and are then further alienated by professionals who have not been trained with the special skills necessary to deliver quality care to these people.

Perhaps the most fruitful aspect of the consumer movement in the health field is its potential for demonstrating the force that the concept of patient work can be in increasing productivity of service. Alan Gartner and Frank Riessman make the point, in *The Service Society and the Consumer Vanguard,* that consumers are workers: they already contribute heavily to the human services through the less obvious ways in which they assist practitioners in getting "their" work done. The tie-in of health services to other service industries has been underscored by Victor Fuchs in *The Service Economy:*

> In the supermarket, laundromat, the consumer actually works, and in the doctor's office the quality of medical history the patients gives might influence significantly the productivity of the doctor. Productivity in banking is affected by whether the clerk or the customer makes out the deposit slip—and whether it is made out correctly or not.... Thus we see that productivity in many service industries is dependent in part on the knowledge, experience and motivation of the customer.

Modern medical care is far too complicated to allow *equal* partnership between patients and physicians in the decision making over treatment options. Both health professionals and patients could benefit, however, from a realization on the part of consumers that good medical care is not, as Norman Cousins has commented wryly, just a matter of shoving one's body onto the doctor's table.

The value of a consumer movement notwithstanding, there is always the danger of any movement being used to counter the good intentions of its designers. Berenice Fisher has warned of the danger in "The Work of Helping Others":

> Since this movement itself takes place in a context in which resources are still limited and directed by those in power, it runs the risk of being coopted by them, of doing the society's dirty work by getting the poorest and most disadvantaged people to serve themselves—to fulfill the old bourgeois admonition that they ought to be taking care of themselves anyway.

Illustrative of a variation of this risk, Under Secretary of Health, Education and Welfare Nathan J. Stark in 1980 suggested a "keep the change" approach as part of the governmment drive for a system in which customers—individual patients and employers who pay for health plans—use price as a major factor in choosing among doctors and hospitals. If a worker chose an HMO whose premium is less than the reimbursement for such plans offered by the government, he would either get the whole saving as a cash award, or split it with the employer—a sterling example of subverting the intent of the consumer movement and engaging the employee in self-discrimination.

Changing Perspectives

A cruel distortion of the consumer movement would be to use it as a wedge in the argument for decreasing health dollar outlay. For in the foreseeable future, despite consumer mobilization, self-help, and prevention through health screening, there will remain a need for expert professional help and massive technological resources at great financial cost. Eradication of diphtheria, smallpox, tuberculosis; control of pneumonia and bacterial infection; improved diet and sanitation—all of these together have given us more people with chronic illnesses who live longer, require medical assistance, and need support services. Americans are thus faced with the following options: we can let more people die faster, or let many people be very sick. As in most industrialized countries, we do not choose to do either of those things, for our health priorities are fairly high. There is yet another option: we can give health care even higher priority—we can make people less sick for a longer time (perhaps by building fewer bombers or nuclear submarines).

Experiments in putting hospitals and private practitioners together in more efficient ways (such as Health Maintenance Organizations and Individual Practice Associations) are all to the good, as are voluntary efforts by hospitals to produce savings through administrative decisions (e.g., group purchasing arrangements, more efficient inventory management). Likewise, studies which demonstrate the need to reorganize hospitals to include physicians in purchase decisions (and responsibility) and pleas for economic "risk-sharing" on the part of physicians should be heeded.

Withal, medical care will continue to be motivated by the "technologic imperative" which has been paraphrased by David Mechanic in *Future Issues in Health Care* as "a tendency to take action, whatever the cost, if it offers even a slight possibility of utility." As an issue of *UCSF Magazine* published in 1980 demonstrates with great force, much of the controversy over high technology in health care revolves around the premise that diagnosis has far outstripped therapy, that we are able to detect at a highly sophisticated level diseases we are still unable to treat. Yet sometimes it is impossible to distinguish where diagnosis ends and therapy begins. Ironically, endoscopy, a procedure which has come under frequent attack for diagnostic overuse, has developed into a procedure called endoscopic sphincterotomy, which is a nonsurgical alternative for removing gallstones. Following the characteristic pattern in such development, the physician who is presently using this technique at the University of California San Francisco, Dr. Howard Shapiro, worked with the manufacturer to refine the prototype. His comments are relevant to this discussion: "We are just beginning to realize the therapeutic potential. With 20 million Americans suffering from gallbladder diseases, the eventual application and cost savings could be enormous." Sometimes it is equally difficult to distinguish where research ends and therapy begins. A machine called the biostandard, which contributed to research on the still-developing artificial pancreas, is currently being used to take care of diabetics undergoing surgery (for reasons unrelated to their diabetes), since it both monitors blood sugar and injects insulin. While use of this machine involves add-on costs, other developments promise decreased costs—for instance, the wider distribution of continual ambulatory peritoneal dialysis, which (for appropriate patients) is expected to cut costs to half that of hemodialysis. These illustrations simply underscore the rapidly moving nature of medical technology and the impossibility of a rigid cost-benefit approach in this arena.

Physicians could, and should, be taught more about not only the value but the limitations of particular tests. Similarly, the public could, and should, be exposed to the ambiguity surrounding many technologies and procedures, rather than mostly to the glamour of technology like the CAT scanner. Without question, there are careless and greedy doctors, duplicate procedures, industries that want to make money—of course, there should be prohibitions to stop abuses of practice and the spending of too much money at inappropriate times. Nevertheless, the real Faustian bargain would be to have the chronically ill bear the cost (in terms of unnecessary suffering or earlier deaths) for the devilment of those who are guilty of excesses (whether in medical practice or in industrial promotion).

It is generally forgotten that the term "halfway technologies" appeared originally in a 1972 report of the Panel on Biological and Medical Science of the President's Science Advisory Committee. This report stressed the difference between *definitive technologies* for the prevention, cure, and control of disease, and *halfway technologies,* described as techniques for palliation or repair. Not only are these distinctions increasingly blurred, but as Dianne Hales has aptly put it, in *UCSF Magazine,* "in the fight against disease, halfway can be a long way to go."

The inability to cope with this issue stems, in part, from the standard categorical-disease perspective taken toward chronic disease in the United States, where medical and public attention and support have been directed to specific illness such as heart disease, cancer, and muscular dystrophy. Indeed, the American health structure—with its governmental health commissions and institutes, its privately funded disease-oriented associations and institutes—supports a categorical-disease approach. Certainly, this approach does stimulate public interest and support, as well as major scientific breakthroughs. The final question we raise here is whether this competition among health specialists and specialties for research funds and resources detracts from the resolution of, or at least the focusing on, the larger issue of the organization of care around a more general perspective on the major health issue in all industrialized countries: chronic illness.

The Price of Survival for Cancer Victims

Morton Bard

Why is a previously dynamic corporation president confined to a wheelchair, with nurse in attendance—ten years after successful cancer surgery?

Why is a fifty-year-old woman "a prisoner in my bathroom," compulsively (and unnecessarily) irrigating a colostomy for twelve hours every other day—six years after successful cancer surgery?

Why does a thirty-five-year-old mother with three children remain a virtual recluse—five years after the loss of a breast in a successful battle against cancer?

Why did a productive businessman sell his business at a loss, become a nonfunctioning invalid, and settle down to await death—after successful cancer surgery eleven years earlier?

Tragic stories like these are dramatic evidence of the gap between today's remarkable advances in medical technology and the unpredictable paradoxes of human emotions and behavior. Such stories of "death expectancy" reveal untold suffering for people whose lives have been saved, and for their families. They suggest a disturbing thought—more and more lives are being saved, but *for what?*

Why should the gift of life become so bitter to the survivors of major illnesses who, only a few years ago, would have invariably died?

To find answers to this paradoxical question, a clinical and research team of psychiatrists, psychologists, and psychiatric social workers was organized at Memorial Hospital and Sloan-Kettering Institute for Cancer Research in New York City, several years ago. The group explored the vastly complex interplay of mind and body in the struggle with cancer—a disease which, throughout the history of man, has carried with it a burden of frightening, superstitious, moral, and even demonic implications. Through repeated interviews with patients we probed into their deepest fantasies and feelings to assemble the disheartening picture that follows.

Cancer patients must be regarded as people under a special and severe form of stress. Cancer is commonly perceived as an always-fatal and particularly loathsome disease, not "clean" and uncomplicated like, for example, the frequently more fatal heart disease. In addition to the expectation of prolonged and intense pain, it carries the threat of disability and, even more frighteningly, recurrence and the repeated threat of death. Thus cancer becomes an unusually stressful experience which disrupts the most important lifelong patterns of behavior.

Every individual, throughout his life, develops a system of beliefs and behavior designed to bring his physical and emotional needs into harmony with the demands of his environment. When these patterns of adaptation are threatened or disrupted anxiety is generated, and the individual believes himself unable to engage in the customary activities which have always fulfilled his emotional needs. Each cancer patient's behavior is designed to prevent, avoid, minimize, or repair injury—not merely to a part of the body, or to the psyche, but also to his basic adaptive patterns and all their social implications.

Reactions to cancer and its therapy, then, must be seen as a sequence of related events which proceeds from the first perception of a sign of illness, to the climax of hospitalization and treatment, and then to convalescence and cure, or to recurrence and death. Any behavior or emotional reaction in the sequence can only be understood in terms of reactions earlier in the sequence, and in relation to lifelong adaptive patterns.

For example, one of our patients was an attractive thirty-four-year-old married woman; when admitted to the hospital for a breast amputation (radical mastectomy) she was in a state of agitated depression. During an interview, she hesitatingly revealed the highly charged circumstances of her admission. For about a year before she noticed any disease symptoms, she had been having an affair with the husband of her best friend. They were also next-door neighbors. Burdened by guilt and self-contempt, she felt that her expectation of punishment for wrong-doing had become a dreadful reality with the onset of cancer. Furthermore, the other couple had driven her to the hospital on the day of admission. Being brought to the place of retribution by the objects of her guilt—for a disease and operation directly threatening to her feminine sexuality—proved to be too much for her.

Her reactions are paralleled in other patients through a wide variety of personal, often unconscious, factors: interference with previously important activities; the threat to one's capacity to be loved; conflicts over the dependency imposed by illness; tensions over the handling of hostility; mistrust of medical authority; sexual difficulties; competitiveness; feelings of inadequacy.

How do most people organize their defenses when they first perceive the symptoms of a breakdown in health? Nearly everyone delays taking any action for at least a short time. This period of delay permits adaptation to the threat and a realignment of defenses for coping with it. If the threat is too overwhelming, the period of delay may be so long that the patient's survival is actually endangered. Such cases are a victory for irrational expectation over both intelligence and the normal process of self-preservation. This self-defeating, but emotionally understandable, delay mechanism may go to the extreme of denying the existence of the physical symptom. Such denial, which occurs most dramatically and with great frequency among cancer patients, must be understood in terms of the magnitude of the threat to the individual, and the emotional danger he faces if he admits the reality of the threat.

As one of our studies showed, when first confronted by serious illness, most people establish some sort of belief in order to explain what has happened, even if this belief is not expressed directly. This is an effort to diminish primitive anxiety aroused by a threat of unknown origin. It is an attempt to find meaning and maintain mastery of an otherwise disordered, chaotic situation.

Out of 100 patients with serious illness in our study, forty-eight spontaneously expressed one or more beliefs about the cause of their illness. The beliefs were classified in terms of assigning culpability for the illness. Beliefs were either *self-blaming* (some real or imagined act of omission or of commission by the patient caused the disease), or *projective* (disease was caused by the action of an external agent, human or not). Typical of self-blame were such comments as, "thinking evil," "didn't take care of myself," or having "pent-up" emotions. Projective beliefs ranged from the capricious act of a malevolent God to the concept of the "evil eye." One striking finding was that a high percentage (37 percent) expressed the deep conviction that interpersonal relations were stressful enough to cause serious physical illness.

There is no specific psychology of cancer patients; there is only the psychology of individuals caught in a special and severe stress situation. The real problems of the cancer patient begin early in his experience with the disease, and a variety of emotional reactions remain associated with them over its entire course. The emotional reactions vary in time and in intensity as the "real" (physiological) events progress. The "reality sequence" consists of four stages: the onset of symptoms; the diagnosis; the hospitalization; and the convalescence. Each stage of this sequence contributes to the patient's ability to integrate the total experience, and, modified by his lifelong adaptive patterns, sets the tone of ultimate post-cancer behavior.

When the first symptom is recognized, the patient immediately begins to anticipate what he thinks will happen to him during treatment. This anticipation is based on the generally frightening ideas most people have about cancer. Often, the very recognition of the symptom can produce such acute anxiety that the patient delays going to a doctor; sometimes, even if medical help is sought, a series of defensive maneuvers follows in order to avoid the inevitable therapy. Fortunately, most people are able to seek medical care and carry through the necessary treatment. Highly individual fears and anticipations develop early and crystallize throughout treatment. For example, patients may project into the future their concern about recurrence; or anticipate social rejection if mutilating surgery is necessary; or develop feelings of unacceptability.

When the diagnosis has been made and the need for therapy established, many of these anticipatory fears acquire a sense of reality. Hospitalization engenders feelings of helplessness. Subjected to awesome and impersonal hospital routines, cut off from the usual sources of emotional gratification, and placed in a dependent, powerless situation, the patient finds his anticipations solidifying.

Some patients interviewed on the day of admission to the hospital express feelings of being trapped and helpless. Some actually telephone their families and ask to be taken home. If they are ward patients, they observe the experience of other patients in a highly selective way to corroborate their fears. The importance of the day of admission cannot be over-emphasized. His very presence in the hospital reinforces for the patient all the fears and anticipations which first occurred at the onset of symptoms and continued through the period of diagnosis.

If surgery is the treatment chosen, as it is for most cancer patients, specific fears concerning anesthesia. are expressed immediately before the operation. Most patients state that total anesthesia must be induced before they could possibly submit to surgery. Some ask that they be completely "out" even before leaving their beds for the trip to the operating room. Conversely, others fear a loss of consciousness through anesthetics.

Signs of tension or panic occur immediately after admission to the hospital. Eating patterns are usually disturbed. Even with sedation, sleep becomes impossible for most. Pre-operative dreams, if they are reported, are usually nightmares; they often directly reflect the patient's anticipations. For example, one patient dreamed she was in a butcher shop with female breasts extended from meat hooks all around her, although in the dream her own breasts were still intact.

Post-operative reactions are sometimes even more severe. Horror dreams, excessive perspiration, and rapidly pounding heartbeat are frequent. Most patients have difficulty in eating; they are unable to swallow food or they lose their appetites. Again there are a variety of sleep disturbances: inability to fall asleep, early waking, fitful and restless sleep, and fatigue on rising in the morning. During the day some patients sit quietly, sometimes crying, without participating in any ward activities; others are overactive.

These reactions, with their marked individual variations. may be understood as a watchful mobilization of inner resources to prevent still further injury. They comprise a response to an environment which to the patient seems hostile and injurious. The patient may believe himself to be overwhelmed by the threat to his safety, or be unable to make decisions; he may show signs of actual disorganization. This state of mind is usually accompanied by profound feelings of dejection, a sense of helplessness, a retreat from function, and possibly even suicidal thoughts. When the patient is in this anxiety-ridden state, he tends to turn to other people for help, seeking advice, consolation, and reassurance.

It is important to remember that, although they are commonly regarded as regressive reactions, depression and dependence are both appropriate and temporary for most patients. Often they can be regarded as a prelude to the process of emotional repair. To what extent these feelings persist depends a great deal on the amount of help the patient gets in solving his problems. Unless he has adequate help, the patient may not be able to solve them, and chronic depression, restriction of function, and pathological dependence may persist long after hospitalization.

On the other hand, some people attempt to master their difficulties by sheer force of will. This is, in effect, a form of denial of the limitations of their own power. When left unguided, it may result in inappropriate solutions which can be bizarre and ineffective, or even result in total failure with subsequent feelings of defeat. Often these enthusiastic attempts to master the situation are closely akin to elation, and are actually a thin veneer for profound depression.

The end of hospitalization heralds the beginning of convalescence. "Going home" is viewed with widely varying feelings. Some patients are eager to see their children and families again and feel that only at home will they be able to recuperate properly. For these patients, family and friends represent the support and warmth they miss in the sterile and symbolically mutilative atmosphere of the hospital. Others, however, are not eager to return home, either because of feelings of weakness or because they feel unable to face people. They are relating the results of their therapy to a social context, and to them the impersonal hospital environment is less threatening than their fears of social inacceptability.

Although the actual surgical experience is over, the feelings it aroused remain. Many patients complain that their families and friends refuse to let them discuss their hospital experiences. These patients are usually resentful; they feel they would be relieved if people would accept the fact that they had cancer, and refer to it as they would to other diseases. However, there are other patients who never want to discuss their experience, fearing they might become depressed. These tend to become hyperactive, doing everything to keep from thinking about it and "feeling blue."

Understanding and support by the patient's family plays an enormously significant part in helping him to resolve his feelings about the whole experience. One woman, who was able to resume full functioning very early, reported that she had never realized how important her family was to her and how deeply they loved her until she became ill.

Of course, the patient's relationship to his family during his illness depends on the nature of the relationship before he became ill. A warm and supportive marriage relationship, with good communication and sexual adjustment between husband and wife, will weather the stormy periods of adaptation. A marriage full of tension, distrust, rejection, and sexual incompatibility will usually deteriorate further under these new stresses.

Cancer presents repeated emotional crises to even a good marriage. A husband may be repelled by the removal of his wife's breast not because of her new physical state, but because of his own unrecognized, long-dormant fears of illness and injury. His uncontrollable withdrawal does not reflect a change in his love for her, but it may nevertheless provoke feelings of rejection in her. Another woman who underwent the same operation may withdraw from her husband because of her feeling that she is no longer acceptable to him.

Not only the family, but the social, economic, and ethnic group to which the patient belongs will influence his view of threatening experiences, determining the confidence he feels in doctors, and defining acceptable ways for him to express his emotional reactions in situations that induce fear and anxiety.

What about the perennial dilemma of "telling the truth"? Nowhere is the anxiety about cancer clearer than in the constantly repeated question, "Should the doctor tell the patient *the truth?*" Plagued by the guilt of bringing bad news, feeling ill-equipped to handle the threatened emotional consequences of the information, burdened by his own confusions about life and death, and often feeling pessimistic even when pessimism is unwarranted, most physicians work out highly personal solutions to this question. The solutions are seldom based on rationality and logic.

As a matter of fact, we have found that in cases where the patient truly trusts the physician's benevolence and skill, the question of "the truth" rarely arises. As for the physician, his decision about what to tell the patient should be determined only by what will help the patient to cooperate in his treatment with a minimum of anxiety. Any other consideration is superfluous. In any case, it seems to me that the question of "truth telling" rests on some highly questionable assumptions—that there is a single disease called "cancer" (that rubric has subsumed under it upwards of 350 diseases); that there is a uniform patient; and that there is a uniform physician. In the absence of such constants, the search for a formula is nonsense.

Nowhere is the power of a good relationship between physician and patient more apparent than in those cases where death is imminent. The most frequent problem here is the physician's withdrawal—reluctant to face what he conceives of as his own failure to prevent the inevitable, he finds himself "too busy" to visit the dying patient. Such behavior on the part of doctors or other hospital personnel is *always* interpreted by the patient as an abandonment. This experience is psychologically very painful to the patient, often interacting with the physiological pain of the terminal period, and he tends to become increasingly demanding, querulous, and hostile, or slips deeper and deeper into depressive despair.

At no other time in life is the need for human contact greater than it is as death approaches. Helpless and dependent, the dying patient experiences a reawakening of the feelings experienced in infancy, when he was also helpless and dependent. Often patients would like to speak frankly about their feelings regarding death, but find themselves either alone or with people who refuse to talk with them (usually family members engaged in self-protective evasion). In no other situation is the inherent difficulty of *listening* clearer than it is in communicating with the dying.

On the other hand, no greater evidence of love exists than in the enactment of the "denial charade." Here the patient and his family all behave as if death were not imminent, but the situation is totally different from the self-serving withdrawal from the dying.

In general, then, the problem of emotional adaptation to cancer and its treatment is inseparable from the larger problems of human communication. Anxiety, present in every cancer patient, is a formidable barrier between him and those around him. It causes distortions, shifts in emphasis, indeed, inability to comprehend, to remember, or even to hear. If one wants to be sure communication is successful, efforts must be made to allay disruptive anxiety. More often than not, allaying anxiety rests more on nonverbal than on verbal means: the "how" of communicating is infinitely more important than the "what" communicated.

Finally, it appears that many of the lives saved by advances in medical science and technology are doomed to psychological invalidism—which could be minimized by sound psychological preparation during illness and hospitalization. Perhaps the time is ripe for the introduction of research programs to develop and refine such techniques in order to bring them into line with the advanced technology of the operating room, of radiation therapy, or of medical diagnostics. Psychological preparation units might be established, to prepare the patient emotionally for procedures which might alter his physical state to the point of disrupting his overall adaptation. Is this any less reasonable than the improvements in techniques which have reduced operative deaths? Is it any less reasonable than the remarkable development of recovery units, or intensive care units?

It seems logical to devote as much energy to preserving psychic integrity as we now devote to preserving physiologic integrity. The patient saved from a serious illness should be enabled to live with dignity and self-respect—not merely to exist. We must eliminate the price of survival—the price of misery and unhappiness for those who are saved from death or physical incapacitation by medical progress.

AIDS and Health Care Deficiencies

Anselm L. Strauss, Shizuko Fagerhaugh,
Barbara Suczek, and Carolyn L. Wiener

AIDS is having a substantial impact on health services. The increasing number of those suffering from Acquired Immune Deficiency Syndrome (AIDS) is greatly taxing the capacities of public hospitals and clinics, especially in cities like New York and San Francisco. AIDS has even affected traditional procedures in medical science. The normal sequence of steps through which treatment drugs reach the public-screening by the Federal Drug Administration (FDA) and then carefully controlled clinical trials—has partly been altered by AIDS activists, who have created a powerful national lobby bent on changing certain features of the health care system. AIDS has heightened tensions around certain moral dilemmas associated with current health care policy by raising issues of personal responsibility for illness and public responsibility for preventing and treating certain illnesses. AIDS also highlights several grave deficiencies in the health care system.

This essay will explore both the moral issues and the preventive/treatment ones, as well as the systemic deficiencies beginning with a discussion of the implications of chronic illness—for AIDS is now recognized as a chronic illness, although still a deadly one. Then the discussion will turn to AIDS in relation to broader health issues. AIDS needs to be thought of not as a uniquely different, late-twentieth century disease, but as a belonging to a broader category. Activists recognize this in part when they talk about the usefulness or political necessity for "mainstreaming" (getting AIDS into political alignment with health issues in general). We offer here a more comprehensive framework for understanding AIDS in relation to several important health issues.

Chronic illnesses are the prevalent contemporary type of disease. The prevalence of this type of illness is due partly to antibiotics that have greatly decreased the rate of acute illness, and partly to Americans' improved nutrition and to medical treatments that have resulted in longer lives (though ones prone to more chronicity in the later years). Some chronic illnesses (cardiac disease, lung cancer) are also associated with certain life-styles; while still others are known or suspected to be associated with inadequate regulation of substances (like some conditions of industrial work and urban air pollution).

Moral and Economic Issues

Moral and economic debates swirl around all of these sources of long-term illness. Our aging population, for example, raises the costs of medical care, especially when the ill are in their last months and years, for then frequent and intensive hospital care is added to other costs of treatment. This being so, the argument has been made that limits be placed on spending for the very old or the hopelessly ill—the money would be better spent on lowering the nation's deplorable rate of infant mortality or at least spent on improving the health of younger citizens. Not so long ago, when the matter of rationing medical treatment for the very old was broached publicly by a governor of Colorado, it roused highly indignant responses on humanitarian moral grounds. There are also the moral issues that have come in the train of medical technology's ability to keep brain-damaged individuals alive. The costs of maintaining these socially dead, but biologically alive, people are frightful, but so are the ethical dilemmas of such situations. Increasing numbers of middle-aged children, especially the daughters, of the very old are faced with giving domestic and nursing care to their sick and sometimes senile or Alzheimer-stricken parents, while forced to expend sorely needed personal resources.

All of this is accompanied by considerable feelings of guilt and moral anguish when it finally becomes necessary to resort to nursing home placement. (In fact, it is entirely possible that a generation or two from now these same children will elect not to live so long, so sick, but be part of a general movement to extend a growing custom of requesting "no heroics during my last days or hours.") If the elderly are able to fend for themselves, they may have to use up all their savings before they die or until the government finally picks up payment for nursing home care. At the opposite end of the age scale, some premature children, who are saved in intensive care nursery units, will suffer from long-term disabilities incurring familial costs for corrective care; but also because "worst case" infants are often not allowed to die, moral dilemmas are created for hospital staffs, parents, and society at large.

Aside from the moral issues resulting from improved medical technology and care, there are also the issues associated with personal and societal responsibility. Passionate arguments have been made for holding individuals responsible for their own condition since life-styles contribute to such illnesses as heart disease and lung cancer, and to the worsening of illnesses such as diabetes and asthma. This version of ethics is countered by, or supplemented with, pointing a finger at a society that has not instituted adequate preventive measures, including extensive and determined educational efforts.

Another line of moral argument faults society for actually causing or increasing the rate of certain illnesses. The state of air pollution in many cities is not only disgraceful but physically harmful; industrial accidents that result in disabilities could be avoided or their numbers lessened by stricter regulation. Lack of access to quality medical care, or any care at all, for many Americans, especially the poor, reflects upon the country's social system and its skewed values. So does the relatively low rate of medical insurance that contributes to lack of access. Personal responsibility, it is argued, is an absurd and ethically dishonest concept to apply to economically deprived Americans. Should the nation's terrible record for child mortality be attributed to failures of personal responsibility? And what about the homeless—at least the involuntarily homeless—are they to be held responsible for their all too evident sicknesses?

The moral issues and dilemmas associated with contemporary (mostly chronic) illness are complex and varied. Bioethicists address mostly the more obvious pertaining to matters of death that have come in the train of effective medical technology and have yet to plumb the depths of their subject by looking at the entire trajectory of chronic illness, the living with it as well as the dying from it. Consider pain for instance. The conflicts between patients and hospital staffs over what constitutes pain relief reflect not just differences over medical care but they raise questions that are deeply moral. One sees this in extremis when dying patients are denied sufficient pain medication because of staff ideologies about addiction ("They will become addicted").

Deficiencies in Health Care

There are several grave deficiencies in the American health care system. Not all are evident enough to attract much attention or public debate, but all are associated with the prevalence of chronic illness. Areas of deficiency include: (1) home care; (2) difficulties of managing new phases of illness (brought about through increased medical knowledge and improved technology); and (3) inequities in gaining access to health care. The third, well recognized and debated, issue will be discussed specifically in connection with two sub-issues concerning discrimination in our health care system against the homeless and against drug addicts (AIDS aside).

These deficiencies in the health care system are largely due to traditional assumptions about what kinds of illnesses are most important to manage. The evolution of our hospitals and clinics was for many years tied to problems posed by infectious and parasitic diseases. The prevalence of chronic illnesses has only recently been recognized and our health facilities are now overwhelmingly in the business of managing chronic illness. The management of crisis, emergency, and acute phases of chronic illness ("acute care" in professional jargon) takes place largely in hospitals. Clinics and private physicians are involved with post-hospital care, minor acute problems, and long-term maintenance of the chronically ill. Hospitals and clinics are fundamentally still organized along lines of acuity. Major resources for clinical care flow to these facilities, with home care and "prevention" (of chronic illness) constituting the elements of the health care system with the least resource support.

Home Care

Critics of the health care system have long pointed to the extraordinary amount of resources directed at acute care. Experts in long-term care, rehabilitation, and gerontology have been particularly vocal and their criticism especially astute with respect to long-term care. They point to failure to provide continuity, flexibility, and responsiveness to and respectfulness for the patients. Strauss and Corbin have recently suggested a model for organizing management of long-term illnesses, with home care at the center of such care. Their argument is based on these points:

- Home is the central site—the major work place where lifelong illness is managed on a daily basis.
- The major concern of the ill and their families is neither merely, nor primarily, managing an illness, but maintaining the quality of life, as defined specifically by them, despite the illness.

Lifelong illness requires lifelong work to control its course, manage its symptoms, and live with its disability. At home, the work is principally done by the indigent themselves, if possible, and by family members, abetted perhaps by agency or purchased services. The health facilities supplement this home management: the physicians and clinics for long-term maintenance and the hospitals for acute phases of the chronic illness.

Effectiveness of care given at health facilities in relation to long-term management depends not only on its technical efficiency and quality, but on how well it supplements and is incorporated into the ongoing management work of the ill and their families.

Home care is very much part of today's health politics. Private medical corporations and companies are much interested in the potential profits of home care; businesses are interested in the potential savings of care given at home rather than in hospitals and clinics; while both the American Hospital Association and the National League for Nursing—and perhaps others—are vying for a share of regulatory power over home care. The danger is that regulation will be minimal and aimed at a relatively low level of quality care, with profits the predominant motive.

New Phases of Illness

In our study of medical work in hospitals we were struck by a new phenomenon: the effectiveness of contemporary medical technology and medical/nursing procedures in making it possible for people to live with chronic illnesses from which they would previously have died. This does not mean that the survivors are always physically comfortable or without grave symptomatology. The more usual pattern is that new developments in the illness, as well as new symptoms, appear. With time, clinicians learn to handle these new symptoms by using, for example, new drugs that were developed for this purpose. Alas, these too may produce "side effects" that perhaps will require additional drugs or other technologies to manage, and so on. Such new phases of illness frequently call for multiple therapies (cancer therapies are an example). And then, the chronically ill often have multiple illnesses—each illness perhaps moving into previously unknown phases.

These ill persons, even if likeable and cooperative, can sufficiently discombobulate the usual organization of hospital care in ways that can be described as producing a "cumulative mess." The mess is clinical and organizational. Some of the difficulties of coordinating care arise when an illness moves into one or more unfamiliar phases then new diagnostic tests will be run, additional treatments will be tried, all of which must be integrated into the stream of staff work. Over the staff's novel work of rearticulation there hangs the dust of battle—battle with the patient but frequently also among the staff members as they debate what to do next. Patients may refuse to go along with additional tests and treatments. Staff members eventually feel a loss of control and inability to keep their work coordinated, what with all the tests, treatments, consultants streaming in and out—minor and major interferences with their medical and nursing plans, and the obvious disintegration of interactional and work relationships.

Such cases of cumulative mess, when we studied them a decade ago, were an aggregate phenomenon. That is, care for individual patients could develop into cumulative mess patterns, but only on an individual basis. Extreme disruptions, though not rare, only happened from time to time. Nevertheless, the organizational fabric of the hospitals is being stressed by these disruptions that have their sources in new and difficult phases of illness. Hospitals, and perhaps clinics too, will eventually, if not sooner, be at hazard. They will need to reorganize themselves, and retrain their staffs for this new kind of organizational danger.

We only add that this development is not at all simply due to increasing numbers of patients, but derives from an increasing number of very sick people with new and particularly difficult kinds of previously unencountered physiological and behavioral developments. (Picture, for example, a long-standing agency, geared to providing services to the blind, suddenly faced with a new group of patients suffering from AIDS-related blindness and needing death and dying support services from a staff unfamiliar with those particular procedures.) Americans who are concerned with health care policy would be wise to think about this particular deficiency in our health system too. It will not be eased by thinking only of how to improve acute care. Surely the system must—must it not?—incorporate a much broadened conception of chronic illness and how best to manage it, in and out of the health care facilities.

The general aspects of inequity are well recognized as well as hotly debated in the public arena. Since early in this century, both professional and lay critics have written about the unequal access to health facilities as well as to "quality care" by sectors of our population. Some of this inequity is the consequence of regional differences but much of it, of course, is because of income differences (and illness or "disability" producing work) between social classes and between various ethnic groups.

Medical inequity is just part of the larger national pattern of economic deprivation, poor housing, inadequate diet, and so on, suffered by certain segments of our population. As one research report put it: "Most of the factors influencing the health of a people lie outside what is conventionally defined as the responsibility of...'health care'." Yet this does not exonerate the nation for its markedly differential treatment of poorer citizens, with consequently differential rates of mortality, well being and health care.

The United States has essentially a two-class system of health care, one for the very poor and one for its other citizens. Many critics have noted this, among them one of the authors of this paper who published "Medical Ghettos" in *Society* in the late 1960s. The intervening years have not radically changed this situation.

Most Americans now recognize "homelessness" as one of the major social problems of our time. Besides people who are without any housing, there are countless others who live in inadequate housing, including tiny rooms in skid-row hotels and overcrowded small apartments in the ethnic and black ghettos of our cities. Add to this the numbers of people who live alone, even if they live in "family" houses, especially the elderly and the aged. In this context, health care is not only a matter of how to deliver care to those populations (mostly ill with multiple chronic illnesses) but how to devise ways to improve their health despite the many environmental and health system obstacles that currently block improvement.

Inequity of Care

The problem is twofold. In the first place, health facilities, primarily centered in hospitals and clinics, are not organized to reach out to where these people live and die. Institutional outreach, it is true, has strikingly, but still insufficiently, increased in the last decade due largely to shrinking hospital and clinic finances and to intense competition for customers.

It falls far short of supplying adequate health care to poorer populations at whom the marketing efforts are not at all directed.

Conversely, institutionalized or systematic ways of getting emergency or acutely ill poor people to the facilities are manifestly lacking. If indeed these patients do get there, they are treated by staff members who have little knowledge or interest in conditions that interfere with their patients' carrying out necessary regimens after leaving the facilities—regimens that are crucial for maintaining the stability of their chronic illnesses. These populations are widely regarded by personnel at hospitals and clinics to be irresponsible about their regimens or intellectually incapable of carrying them out properly—"non-compliance" is the term directed at this woeful behavior.

The first step in reorganizing health care for the homeless is for professionals and government officials to understand that new kinds of health care arrangements are necessary in order to service the great numbers of those Americans who now receive very little or ineffective care. What is needed is bi-directional coordination guiding clients through the health care maze, and making providers give appropriate service to clients rather than, as so often now, acting toward them with animosity, ignorance, or indifference. Personnel who work within the facilities are very often overworked, have few resources, have to compete with other health facilities or with other departments within their own facility. Also they are unaccustomed to working with the special problems of the homeless, including those with AIDS, many of whom are also suffering from drug addiction. Moreover, as is usual, there is little or no follow-up after care for patients at facilities; and of course the homeless ordinarily do not go to private physicians for this care.

Addiction and Health Care

It has been observed, by us and others, that drug and alcohol addicts are far from welcome at clinics and hospital. Of course, they too are patients: so, staffs are either obligated or committed to giving them adequate care. Nevertheless, the common practice of using terminology that refers to patients as "good" or "bad," "cooperative," or "uncooperative," heard so often in these facilities extends also to addicts. To the staff's frequent perception of them as truculent or uncooperative or irresponsible or unpleasant, even violent—as well as their actual behavior—add the evident lower socioeconomic status of some addicts and it becomes clear why the social value of these particular patients is especially low. "Uncooperative" ones tend to get even less attention, all the more so because the personnel "know"—sometimes from sound experience—that these patients will soon be back because they will not follow their regimens.

What this means is that a considerable, and seemingly increasing, proportion of the ill is getting less than adequate care. But why? The answer cannot simply be found in staff attitudes but must be sought in the way facilities are organized—including how their personnel are, or are not, trained to work with addicts as well as in the low value placed on working with this population. After all, these organizations are focused on giving acute care, not on managing the addiction related problems of these particular patients. In the case of minority drug addicts, this is partly a matter of poverty-generating national conditions and partly a national obsession with the evil character of drug addiction, derived from many years of media blowup and propaganda efforts by government agencies. However, even middle-class, educated white patients, who are addicts, may present many of the same problems to personnel at the facilities.

To grasp the organizational, psychological and clinical aspects of drug addiction and hospital care (whether the patients have AIDS or not), consider these points. Customarily the patients are not allowed to keep their own drugs, including aspirin, and clinical justification is given for this rule. Drug addicts are as dependent as other chronically ill on their drugs for physical and psychological comfort, if not for life itself, but their persistent requests for pain medication or complaints about receiving insufficient medication are met with denigration and they are labelled as "addicts" and as "manipulative." It is true that addicts are more likely to complain since they are accustomed to dealing with psychological pain through use of drugs; but hospital personnel generally either do not know this or are unsympathetic. Personnel will also ordinarily not address or discuss addictive problems with the patients, because these are not perceived as relevant to clinical care.

Not surprisingly then, these patients may leave the hospital against medical advice because tagged and treated as "junkies." Also, the emergency rooms tend to function as screening agents for hospitals, often by either giving poorer addicts relatively cursory care or by referring them to clinics. At emergency rooms, particular addicts may get labelled as "repeaters" and be viewed as nondesirables. Not infrequently, however, addicts will go to the emergency room anyhow because they know from experience or hearsay that they are likely to get more satisfaction there than in the hospitals. Besides to be admitted to a hospital takes organizational skills they often do not have. They are also unlikely to possess health insurance. Meanwhile, as funding is cut back, services at drug treatment centers (for many the only site where HIV testing is sought) are likely to be cut back or eliminated also.

Characteristics of AIDS

The AIDS epidemic highlights all of these health care issues. When AIDS was first recognized as a threat, the focus was all on an infectious disease that could or would quickly lead to high mortality rates. Prevention and care of the dying were primary public health and clinical concerns.

Yet it did not take much prescience to foresee that with improved treatment, people with AIDS would be living longer, and like other chronically ill would have to be treated and cared for both at home and in the health facilities. At the same time, the number of those needing care was likely to increase because of the extent of the epidemic. AIDS, as a chronic illness, greatly taxes the capacities of health care facilities and health practitioners. Because of its clinical characteristics and the populations susceptible to it, AIDS highlights specific directions in which health care "delivery" needs to be reorganized. Although one may presume general familiarity with the disease, it will be useful to state briefly a few characteristics that are particularly relevant to the issues addressed here.

AIDS was recognized in the United States only a few years ago. Since it has been affecting only certain segments of the population and has many symptomatic manifestations, it is not always diagnosed quickly or correctly. Much uncertainty remains about how long a period transpires before the HIV virus develops into AIDS, and indeed whether it always does so, to which populations it will spread, what treatments will turn out to be most effective, and with whom.

Sexual practices and intravenous drug use are the two principal modes of transmission. This makes prevention as well as treatment difficult. Health professionals, whether in the Public Health Service or in the various health facilities, have been relatively unsuccessful in combatting either sexually transmitted diseases or drug addiction. Issues of morality and privacy intrude on what might otherwise be purely public health or medical problems.

Health professionals confront another difficulty: dealing with recalcitrant populations that need to change their behavior. Combatting HIV/AIDS is comparable to persuading alcoholics or cigarette addicts to abandon their habits—but possibly even more difficult. Even if someone is well aware of the dangers of AIDS and educated in how to prevent it—or to spread it if one already has it—only one "slip," one incautious sexual encounter or contaminated needle can be disastrous. Besides, each new generation needs to be educated about HIV/AIDS and persuaded to act sensibly or responsibly. These obstacles are exacerbated by the possibility of a long asymptomatic incubation period during which innocents may spread the virus.

Concerning treatment, rather than prevention: AIDS affects the total body system. So there is an array of management problems, including those derived from medication as well as from the great diversity of body symptoms, ranging from diarrhea to dementia. It is not always clear whether particular problems have their source in the illness or in the treatments.

While a person suffering from this disease may pass through several phases, from emergency periods to deterioration and to dying, there may also be relatively stable periods. Yet, aside from the problems of dying or being close to death, those suffering from AIDS are very often prone to unstable physical states. Various symptoms will appear and then perhaps vanish, ordinarily leaving the sick person in a generally precarious physical state during which symptoms are unpredictable. Performance of paid work, and even sociability, become particularly difficult during these periods of uncertainty.

AIDS and the Health Care System

AIDS has thrust the lack of home care provisions in the American health care system increasingly into the daily newspapers. Without going into the details of American governmental policy on handling AIDS, suffice it to say that the burden of caring for AIDS sufferers has rested primarily on voluntary and community agencies. In San Francisco, for example, a middle-class gay community is widely recognized to have cared for the very sick and dying in their own homes. They have been able to do this because of personal and community commitment (including that of gay physicians).

A few organizations, like Hospice, which have been able to muster volunteers for service to people with AIDS at their homes have found their resources strained because of the great demand for their services. Also, there are long waiting lists. For the most part, voluntary services reach only a small segment of the population: white, educated, and homosexual. So, even in San Francisco (but nowhere else in the Bay Area), which possesses probably the most successful "model" for managing the AIDS epidemic of any American city, the burden of care is still on the ill themselves and on their committed friends and kin.

These voluntary, but overall restricted and insufficient, services highlight the glaring deficiencies in America's health care system with regard to the financing and servicing of both the dying and chronically ill when they wish or must be cared for at home. It can be anticipated that, as the numbers of chronically ill people with AIDS grow and are seen to, or actually do, overwhelm the hospitals and clinics, the health care system will be forced to incorporate much more home care.

AIDS also highlights the organizational abyss that yawns between managing chronic illness in the health facilities and at home, insofar as it makes clear how ill equipped our health care system is to coordinate services for the care of people who suffer from multiple chronic illnesses that necessitate multiple regimens, multiple specialists, multiple visits even to different facilities for different chronic illnesses. This particular problem is especially acute in AIDS since those stricken with the disease are likely to circulate between home and hospital because of new and little understood developments of their diseases. AIDS is likely to produce collective rather than merely aggregate disruptions for two reasons. First, as with other chronic illnesses, AIDS therapies produce untoward side effects that need to be controlled with still more therapeutic actions. This will happen simultaneously to many people hospitalized with AIDS. Second, AIDS produces multiple physiological breakdowns. Symptoms and associated therapies are also multiple, but both contingencies will increasingly affect hospital wards where many AIDS patients are housed together. The cumulative organizational strain will have its source in large numbers of physiologically and interactionally difficult patients, rather than deriving from an occasional such patient.

Just recently it has been reported that the number of elderly AIDS patients much exceed anticipated rates; they are at further at risk because they are often already on various medications for other diseases. Imagine the difficulties on geriatric wards before long.

Inequity of Treatment

Although many people who are dying from AIDS wish to die at home, they end their days in hospitals adding to organizational disruption. This is so because care at home often becomes very difficult or impossible since potential caretakers may also be debilitated by AIDS, are dying or are already dead. Even if hospitalized only for treatment, AIDS patients will increasingly precipitate organizational problems for hospitals, just because they are living longer and so will be hospitalized more frequently. This is especially so, given the deficiencies in America's home care services.

Furthermore, the instability characteristic of the course of the illness, combined with developments in treatment technology, inevitably lead to comparable instability in managing health facilities and in their staffs' clinical work. Each advance in technology, especially if major, is likely to destabilize the organization, the work, and the course of the illness itself. An instance of this was recently observed in connection with organizing special hospital treatments around aerosol pentamidine. During the initial use of this drug, it was found that treating patients in a confined area put health workers at risk from the aerosol. Later, with new funding, space was reorganized for the treatments, and a treatment team was recruited and trained. Still later, pentamidine was recognized to lower blood sugar to dangerous levels; this resulted in a reduction in the ward's eligible patients and a reassignment of staff and space.

In short, the combination of disease, medical technology, organization and clinical work—all beset with uncertainty and instability-makes management of this particular chronic illness very difficult. The magnitude of the difficulties, quite aside from the steadily growing numbers of people with HIV and AIDS, is sure to raise general awareness of the deficiencies in American health care.

AIDS has contributed to the impoverishment of many of those who are affected. In this regard, AIDS is much like other chronic illnesses that eat up individual and family savings, while reducing rates of employment. AIDS characteristics complicate the equity issue. As remarked earlier, this illness produces a variable number of symptoms, making steady employment often difficult. The side effects of AIDS medication may also lead to salary reduction through the loss of days of work. The drugs for combatting AIDS are expensive and the treatments at this point are lifelong. In addition there are expenses for subsidiary medications and care. People with AIDS may find that their health insurance does not—or no longer will—cover them. Indeed this is a major issue in the AIDS arena. Poorer Americans who contract AIDS often do not have health insurance anyway. With the growth of clinical and technological knowledge and skills, more and more AIDS sufferers live longer and, of course, need treatment. Some, though no longer fearing death, may eventually become unemployed. Others who have been diagnosed with HIV but have no symptoms are taking the drug AZT, recommended as delaying the onset of AIDS. Where, as has happened so often in San Francisco, two gay partners become ill from AIDS, one or both may be unable to work; so even relatively affluent white, middle-class Americans may run through their savings before one or both die—or may just remain chronically debilitated and unable to pay for care. The very poor and the homeless have a heavy personal responsibilities; of getting to the health facilities and finding their way through what is widely known, even among health personnel, as "the medical (or bureaucratic) maze." Although AIDS in this country is primarily an illness of gay men, it increasingly affects poorer people in black and certain ethnic communities, whether gay or straight. It is these poorer Americans who will die in great numbers from AIDS, victims of our health care system's basic inequities.

Homelessness and AIDS

AIDS is just beginning to highlight the issue of homelessness as a deficiency in our health care system too. We say "just" because until very recently this was not so. But as the homeless and other poverty stricken people are infected with HIV and AIDS, they too come to professional and public notice. Yet since they count for very little in the American hierarchy of issues, and since servicing them adequately would call for considerable reorganization of health care arrangements—if not the facilities themselves—recognition and action are still rudimentary. Besides, they are scarcely, if at all, represented in AIDS lobbying activities. These activities are understandably powered by middle-class AIDS sufferers and their friends and legislators are primarily moved to action by active and well represented constituencies. Many urban homeless are on addictive drugs and this too adds to the problem of "delivering" adequate health care to them.

In San Francisco, AIDS outreach programs do not include many, if indeed any, health components. Most AIDS outreach programs in the United States were funded as projects to discover and demonstrate ways of preventing AIDS, not as projects to handle the actual health aspects after AIDS has been contracted or HIV has been diagnosed. San Francisco has no effective plan to deliver adequate services to the homeless with AIDS. There is only one known health outreach team in this city that diagnoses the illness, visits the ill in their lodging and on the street, persuades them or makes arrangements for them to be seen at health facilities, steers them through the institutional maze once there, and does follow up work too. In short, this team operates effectively on a case management basis. The team's social worker contributes time voluntarily and the nurse receives a salary as an "AIDS Liaison Public Health Nurse" with the Department of Public Health, although he has never really had full departmental backing. Neither the city nor any government agency would fund their work directly, although some officials in the local Department of Public Health apparently respect this team's work—yet they are, in a real sense, outside "the system." This health outreach team underscores the difficulties of operating outside the established health care system (local in this case), both in the funding and organization.

What the situation of the AIDS homeless makes manifest is the need for coordinated case management—into and through the facilities, and also encompassing preventive work and follow-up care with the chronically ill. So, in the end, AIDS may turn out to be the experimental ground for such necessary new arrangements for managing illness among the homeless. Without this reorganization, the health care system will continue to fail most of our less fortunate citizens.

Addiction and AIDS

An addict who has AIDS bears an added burden, especially, but not necessarily only, if homeless or poor. As noted earlier, fatigue or diarrhea are symptoms that loom large in AIDS for which the emergency room is not very helpful. Neither do these symptoms warrant referral to the hospital. Fatigue and diarrhea also mitigate against a patient's keeping clinic appointments. (What does one do about diarrhea during a long bus ride to the clinic?)

The increasing number of addicts of any socioeconomic strata who have AIDS and exhibit multiple symptoms of multiple chronic illnesses points to the need for follow-up care after treatment at a hospital or clinic. If hospital personnel are to give adequate care to those AIDS patients who are also drug addicted, then it is incumbent on them to discuss openly the implications of addiction with their patients. As for the homeless, in San Francisco as probably in many other cities, with or without AIDS these people cannot even get access to public housing unless they can prove that they are off drugs. Although welfare services should go hand in hand with effective health care, social welfare agencies are quick to refer addicts elsewhere or may give them short shrift. AIDS will probably make this common practice more publicly visible.

Here are two additional points relevant to the impact of AIDS on health care for addicts. The first pertains to the prevention of AIDS versus its treatment as a chronic illness. Outreach projects apparently have been successful in some major cities, like San Francisco, Chicago, and Boston, in making lower class addicts aware of AIDS, persuading them to use condoms and bleach and to participate in needle exchange. Yet the realization is gradually spreading that such preventive programs are not sufficient for meeting the health needs of addicts, including those posed by AIDS as a long-term illness.

The second point is that the unstable nature of the illness itself, along with the diverse pharmaceutical treatments and their side effects, have had a major impact on drug treatment centers. It is at these centers that addicts may also receive some primary medical care. In the major cities, many different agencies are likely to be involved with drug abuse (over seventy in San Francisco). These agencies are generally structured according to, or "specialized" by, different criteria: type of addiction, phase of addiction, limits on days of treatment, treatment modality, treatment ideology, but also by number and age of clients accepted, their gender, whether gay or not, religious or ethnic affiliation, geographical location of the center, whether community based or not, and so forth. To this organizational heterogeneity, AIDS and HIV effect further fragmentation as well as reorganization of services, as the centers struggle with the additional problems represented by the combination of addictive and medical treatment drugs and the cumulative symptomatology of both.

A somewhat ironic, if small, change in the clinical research aspects of our health care system is this: though known addicts have always been eliminated from clinical trials (of treatment drugs), very recently researchers have been attempting to recruit them into the trials of AIDS drugs. (At least this is happening in San Francisco.) It is unlikely that this can be done successfully with poorer addicts unless they find bridging agents who already have the confidence of these addicts. Presumably they will be found or will volunteer, and thus AIDS will have made one more contribution toward highlighting a small hole in the health care system.

Apropos of AIDS and clinical trials that are indirectly, if negatively, pertinent to poor addicts: The AIDS activists, who are having such an impact on the clinical trials sequence by their pressuring of the Federal Drug Administration and by their own parallel trials of possibly effective treatment drugs, are mainly middle-class, gay, educated, white men. It is they who will benefit directly if the trials prove successful and the drugs become more readily available. The poorer AIDS sufferers— whether addicts or not, whether men or women—will probably not be much affected, or at least not very soon, by this change in the health care system, since they are relatively marginal to it. But it is true that they may benefit from some of the more far-reaching changes in the drug production to distribution patterns.

Economic and Moral Issues

As with chronic illness in general, moral and economic dilemmas abound in the case of AIDS. They are essentially the same as those discussed earlier, but their specifics highlight, again, deeply problematic features of health care in the United States.

When first noted, AIDS was accurately classified as an infectious disease, though little was known then about its transmission mechanisms or vectors and rates of distribution. That AIDS is sexually transmitted became quickly apparent, and was seemingly confined primarily to gay men; although some hemophiliacs also contracted the virus through infected blood supplies. Intravenous drug use was soon added to the list of transmission routes, as was heterosexual intercourse involving addicts or bisexual men. The women would then transmit the disease to their babies. Gays and addicts were of low social value on the American scene, both because of what they stood for and the specifics of their behavior. Not surprisingly, they were openly blamed for their own misfortunes, and increased antagonism was felt, often accurately, by gays.

Widespread belief in personal responsibility for personal woes—even to death—turned what ordinarily would be a purely public health issue into a major policy debate. As in all such debates, profound disagreement existed over the degree of risk to the nation and its population, over allocation of resources, over proper means of action, and ultimately over deeply held values. Consider degree of risk: Estimates of risk run from the most dire predictions to beliefs that it is all a CIA plot to make us believe in a nonexistent disease. Concerning resources: Urgent voices created a now powerful AIDS lobby press for increased funding for prevention, treatment and research; but they are meeting with great resistance from competing proponents of funding for other chronic illnesses, and other audiences who believe AIDS funding should be curtailed in favor of other demands. The proper means of combatting AIDS is also a matter of bitter dispute. These disputes are reaching even, and perhaps especially into the gay communities. They are reflected in disagreements among government officials who put their faith in treatment versus prevention efforts. Disagreements also exist over how to reach, say, black intravenous drug users—whether through outreach workers (and need they be black?) or through needle exchange ("This will increase addiction among us").

At the bottom of these arguments, not always fully explicit but sometimes brutally so, are clashes over moral values. Senator Jesse Helms, standing like a rock against any preventive or treatment action with regard to AIDS, is a visible and hated symbol to those who see people dying in pain and discomfort, in poverty, and perhaps needlessly because deprived of drugs and other medical care and insufficient research efforts. Economic considerations (resources need reasonable and efficient distribution), are pitched against moral fervor and anger (resources should be distributed equitably to all Americans, and certainly people should not be just left to die without resources).

Early on, blood banks had insisted their products were absolutely free from AIDS contamination until the lobbying of outraged hemophiliacs and their supporters brought reforms. Values are balanced against values within ethnic communities whose leaders or activists must decide which values are most pressing. Will it be AIDS prevention or drug prevention or crime control or religious values (versus sex education and sexual immorality) or struggling for more funding to combat poverty among blacks?

Values are balanced against values in constitutional rights cases, otherwise organizations like the American Civil Liberties Union (ACLU) and anti-discrimination units of local governments would not be so deeply involved in defending AIDS sufferers in discrimination cases. Even health professionals have to make moral decisions, sometimes with anguish. Do surgeons, for instance, have an obligation to operate on patients known to have AIDS or to refuse such cases in favor of their own life chances and the good of their families? Nor have scientists escaped criticism, since they too are part of this embattled arena.

The latest in a long string of incidents is the accusation that release of a National Institutes of Health (NIH) commission report was delayed by several months because some members did not want their publications in medical journals upstaged by an early release. By contrast, some months before, urgent pressure to save lives had led some scientists to release their research reports to physicians months prior to publication, ethical considerations winning over personal ones.

Having noted these specifics of the AIDS arena, we repeat that AIDS basically highlights many of the economic and moral issues attending chronic illness in general. What weight to give personal responsibility? Societal responsibility? Central too are questions of expenditures and cost containment. Also, on whom should limited health dollars be spent? - which involves also balancing questions of equity against national efficiency and rewards for individual attainment in a relatively open society.

Health Care Management

Some policy implications can be derived from the foregoing discussion. These implications pertain not only to deficiencies in the American health care system and the impact of AIDS, but to deeper issues regarding the rationing of health care for chronic illness.

A highly industrialized nation faces the problem of how to manage—financially as well as medically and humanly—the increasing rate of chronic disabilities. These are being generated both by conditions of life in contemporary societies and by the dramatically increasing longevity of its citizens. Our own population has opted for high-tech medicine, combined with a patchwork (Gary Albrecht calls it a "tattered umbrella") of health service varieties.

In recent years, these have developed largely in response to chronic disabilities and the entire system has increasingly come to be dominated by business concerns (pharmaceutical companies, medical supply and equipment firms, hospital and nursing home corporations). In the health market economy, companies aim at those areas where profits are to be made, leaving government—federal; state and county and city—to deal with the relatively unprofitable sectors of the health market.

In effect, our health care system embodies an implicit rationing of health care: both in quantity and quality. (Perhaps this is the only principle on which there is a consensus within the health arena.) This has been the American way. The attempts in other countries to manage the chronic illnesses of their citizens are different. But everywhere the management is done in conjunction with two major and difficult issues: the costs of health care and how funds are spent—that is, who gets the care, what kind, and how much. In the United States, among the counterbalancing forces during the last two decades has been an increasingly health-oriented (anxious?) and educated (often skeptical) population ("health consumers").

The rise of activists—environmental, feminist, AIDS, and the like—also has had a countervailing effect on the heavily business tilt of health services. Yet both sets of influences are largely middle class in perspective and participation. They are likely to affect the current rationing of health care only indirectly. This is not their participants' central issue; it is peripheral at best. The implicit rationing of health care raises the larger issue of how health dollars might best be spent in preventing and managing chronic illness. In the fiercely waged national debate over the direction of health care, voices reflecting cost accounting and technological efficiency have tended to dominate, drowning out the moral and humanitarian ones, though AIDS has brought the latter set very much to the fore. The implications for a reassessment of the health care system, in terms of rationing considerations and rationing options, can be summed up this way: The policy of inequitably rationing health care, albeit implicitly, is probably in accordance with what most Americans believe is only just and proper. Health care is assigned in terms of social worth; those who deserve less, get less.

Why should addicts and the homeless get more care if this costs us citizens more money? Why should those who are economically worthless, or contribute far less to the economy, get equal treatment? As for AIDS and homosexuals, this is, of course, a strongly felt moral argument, not simply an apparently rational economic one. An alternative to social worth, or social value, is to direct major services toward those who are medically most salvageable, and let those who are minimally salvageable go.

Another rationing option is to insist on the value of human life per se, and to avoid both implicit and explicit rationing as much as possible. The objections to this option are obvious: they are either economic or moral. The economic comes down to this: There are not enough resources to cover everybody adequately, so some of the sick inevitably will get less or very little care. The moral objection adds up to: Some people deserve less or very little or none; that is, they are less deserving, as producers, as citizens, as human beings, as not even fully human though they have human bodies.

Moral objections are difficult to make effectively, dominant American beliefs being what they are. The economic objection is countered—and we are not at all the first to say so—by the suggestion that Americans rethink what portion of the GNP they wish to assign to health as opposed to the many other competing pressing claims. If the proportion that flows to health services does not increase, then the current system of implicit rationing will be what Americans genuinely want to continue.

The major phenomenon to be considered is the relationship of health rationing to the increasing chronic disabilities. (If not thought about with wisdom, the consequences will surely continue to haunt the next generations. Historically this is a quite recent phenomenon.) A major policy issue therefore concerns how to handle this phenomenon. To state the matter this way leads inexorably to the proposition that a concerted drive to decrease both the amount of disability and the chronic illness itself should be mounted. This means producing conditions (as through effective and widely distributed health care) that slow up the evolution of a chronic illness as well as conditions that prevent a chronic illness in the first place (prevention, environmental, economic, and behavioral). In either case, high-tech, acute care medicine would not be eliminated, but certainly would be reassessed and reassigned in light of the prevalence of chronic illness.

Planning to Die

Jeanne Guillemin

Thirty years ago, in *The American Way of Dying,* Jessica Mitford roundly criticized Americans for their obsessive denial of death and their equally obsessive fixation on immortality. To the puritanical American sensibility, a miasma of shame surrounds the event of death. The quicker one died and the less the family and community were troubled, the better. Funeral directors, a uniquely American profession, assumed all responsibility for the corpse, including its embalmed, cosmetic display and its rapid dispatch to the cemetery or to the crematorium. Denial of death was also the theme of Philippe Ariès' work *Western Attitudes Toward Death* (1974). He credits early twentieth-century America with the invention of the modern attitude toward mortality. Death, once so banal a presence that Renaissance markets were held in graveyards and so communal that relatives and friends crowded the bedchambers of the dying, lost its tame aspect. Under the influence of urban industrialization, it became detached from domestic traditions, not the least of which was a religious understanding of the appropriateness and even the banality of the self's demise. In our times, Ariès argues, death became wild and obscene because we cherish an individualism that cannot be relinquished without extreme anguish. As with sex, death was not to be talked about in front of children or in polite company.

Today the American public is confronting mortality in ways that were unthinkable when Mitford was writing and improbable even to Ariès. The emphasis now is on rational planning for one's death that goes far beyond buying a burial plot. Topics such as traversing the emotional stages of dying, how to compose a living will to instruct final medical decisions, and the merits of rational suicide are ordinary fare on television and radio talk shows and in popular magazines. The head of the Hemlock Society, Derek Humphry, has a bestseller in *Final Exit,* a how-

73

to book on happy death. Jack Kevorkian, another book author, has gained notoriety for his "mercitron" devices, recently used by three women to end their lives. Despite his subsequent indictment for homicide, the public is far from outraged by the idea of physician-assisted suicide. In 1991, the state of Washington gained national attention with a popular referendum on the issue. The voting public there ultimately balked at granting it legal status, but polls had already revealed widespread support for the option of medically supervised suicide. In 1992, the state of New Hampshire initiated the nation's first legislation that would authorize physicians to write prescriptions to hasten the death of terminally ill patients.

This new frankness concerning death is due in part to changing demographics. The population of the United States has aged, with more people than ever living out a seventy-two year life span. Many are surviving decades beyond it. Perhaps aging alone would shift any society's focus to the end of life. Yet death itself has become unexpectedly familiar because of the AIDS epidemic, which has brought grief to hundreds of thousands of young victims, their families, and friends. Add to this the fact that the United States has the highest homicide rate of any industrialized country, with a disproportionate number of casualties among young minority males, and the difficulties of denying death and its repercussions become clear. Old or young, one thinks, "This could be me."

Still, death is far from tamed; it is now newly wild and familiar. The current discussion of how to die gives evidence of terrible fears that those final circumstances are beyond one's control. In a culture that prizes individual autonomy, there is a no more degrading scenario than the gradual diminution of physical and mental powers, the prolonged and painful helplessness, with mental lapses preceding and even obscuring the experience of dying. American anxiety about dying centers on how the individual can avoid dependence. Unfortunately, the two environments where death is likely to happen are poorly prepared to reduce this anxiety and are, in fact, increasing it. Neither the hospital, where 80 percent of Americans die, nor the home, where growing numbers of patients are being cared for, can be counted on to alleviate fears about death as a scenario of degradation.

Hospital Care and Uncare

In pondering the phenomenon of shameful death ("la mort inversée"), Ariès sees the modern hospital as the environment where depersonalized efficiency and order quell the fears of the dying. As a cultural instrument of repression, the hospital guarantees that the graceless, physically repulsive facts of expiration are hidden from view and that the emotional climate at the bedside is restrained. The sheets are clean, the meals regular, and the staff professional. Replacing family and friends is the hospital team, led by the physician. "They are," wrote Ariès, "the masters of death—of the moment as well as of the circumstances...."

In the last two decades, hospital-based medicine has undergone radical changes and Americans have largely lost confidence in its protective guarantees, as chill and repressive as they have been. Hospital organization, once able to guarantee benign order for both birth and death, has been altered not with reference to the social or spiritual needs of patients, but in reaction to market incentives that favor large hospitals selling progressive medicine. The hospitals that survived the fierce competition of the 1980s did so by heavy investment in new and experimental technologies and by the build-up of centralized facilities offering a profitable mixture of specialized and acute care services. Small community hospitals closed by the hundreds. Public hospitals, burdened with welfare patients, are foundering. Private mega-hospital chains, like Humana, thrive because they serve only privately insured patients.

Far from being beneficent institutions, most hospitals today are businesses that serve clients. Linked to proliferating technological options and required to support high-priced professionals, their main incentive is to maximize returns on their investments. They are only unlucky if they do not. Cost control measures to cap procedure charges, such as Diagnostic Related Groups (DRGs), have merely succeeded in moving patients more quickly out of their hospital beds to make room for more. Costs for hospital medicine and services continue to rise and inflate health insurance coverage, which growing numbers of Americans cannot afford.

The progressive technologies being marketed through American hospitals fall into two categories. Both affect how we die. One kind addresses the diseases of the growing numbers of patients fortunate enough to survive past youth, at which point they become vulnerable to cardiac disease, cancer, stroke, kidney and liver failure. When Aaron Wildavsky coined the phrase, "doing better and feeling worse," in reference to modern American health care, he aptly summarized its major problem. The important determinants of health and illness—life-style, genetics, and the environment—are outside the scope of medicine. Its principal technologies, geared toward an aging clientèle, must be of the patch-and-mend variety, lacking the "magic bullet" efficiency of penicillin and sulfa drugs. Success with these "half-way technologies," as Lewis Thomas called them, is difficult and uncertain. Very sick patients do much more than lose faith in medicine. They take it on, they wrestle with it, and often they feel defeated by it. They are not just disappointed consumers. They engage their bodies and souls in a battle for life.

The role of the physician in treating the very sick patient is problematic, in part because doctors are only apparently disinterested in advising about medical treatment options. Many patients fail to understand that physicians like car dealers, will promote their products, if asked. Not that physicians are necessarily driven by profit motives, but they are integrated into the hospital reward system, now heavily invested in high-technology resources—machines, laboratories, consultants—that must be used to get a return. Perhaps unwittingly, physicians often inform seriously ill patients about therapy in ways that encourages it. The use of statistical odds, for example, is a commonplace, as when a doctor refers to scientific studies to inform a patient about survival rates for cancer, using surgery or drugs or some combination of both. When cancer or any other disease is in an advanced stage, this tactic is little better than offering a lottery ticket to someone who is destitute. What even educated patients often do not know is that many clinical studies are poorly executed—without controls and on small samples—and yield only the most tentative results. Or, if they are well-conceived and implemented, the patients researched may share none or few of the characteristics—age, gender, medical history, and so on—of the patient being informed. There is little or nothing in their training that prepares physicians to develop a posture of integrity and more genuine disinterest or new words of counsel for the seriously ill who should perhaps not venture any therapeutic course.

For a very sick patient, surgery, chemotherapy, or organ transplant might work. Then again, it might not. It will certainly be a physical and emotional ordeal, causing pain that is especially alienating because it is impossible to know whether it is part of recuperation or a sign of further degeneration. The patient cannot know, nor can the therapist, until test results come back. Even then, many therapies require years of monitoring, especially in the case of cancer, during which one simply does not know if a true cure has been effected. Starting with Susan Sontag's *Illness As Metaphor* to the essay on resisting chemotherapy

by the anthropologist Susan DiGiacomo, the patient-as-survivor literature constitutes a searing criticism of how physicians mishandle patients confronting death.

The really bad news is that medical technology can offer multiple
sequential therapeutic options for the same fatal disease. This creates
uncertainty and uncertainty in medicine, as Wildavsky and others have
noted, is often resolved by doing more. If drugs and surgery fail, other
drugs or more surgery are substituted. The more advanced the disease,
the more the desperate patient will value inclusion in an experimental
trial of some new therapy, whereby she or he is diminished to a statistic
and risks more physical devastation. This way of progressing toward
death—by hopes raised and dashed, by technological assaults on the
body, followed by periods of incomplete and uncertain recuperation—is,
of course, not the road traversed by people who are cured. Many people
overcome blocked arteries, for example, or cancer because the therapy
works. But subjection to experimental medicine is the pathway of
everyone's last cure. No matter what the patient's age or how advanced
the disease, or even if it is considered incurable, the options for more
tests and treatment exist, in refined or experimental form, appropriate or
inappropriate, as the physician advises.

The intensive care unit is the other important kind of technology that
hospitals market. It has revolutionized the way Americans die, but not
for the better. The concept of high-technology life support took hold in
the early 1970s in response to a perceived need, public and professional,
for emergency medical services. The argument for emergency medical
units was and is based on the reduction of waste in human lives. Immediate aggressive intervention, not unlike that of a M.A.S.H. unit, would
save victims of accidents, of heart attack and stroke, as well as premature infants, and post-operative patients. The key was vigorously sustained intervention with the maximum resources of a large central hospital.
Emergency and intensive care facilities, costing billions of dollars, became part of the expansion of central hospitals throughout the 1970s and
1980s. Patients *in extremis* are always in good supply and treating them
quickly in high-use beds has often helped hospitals underwrite less profitable services. Such heavy investment in acute care emphatically denied
a preventive and more cost-efficient approach to health problems and to
the general social problem of death by violence. Nor did emergency care
enthusiasts predict that many whose lives were saved would not be able

to resume normal lives or even a conscious existence, and would be passed off to chronic care facilities or to their families.

Even less concern is being expressed for the I.C.U. patient's experience of having to live attached to machines or dying that way. From the perspective of the conscious patient, experiencing what it means to be "worked on" by teams of strangers, to be coded for resuscitation (or not), to lie among others near death or already dead, to be dependent on and surrounded by wires and machines, intensive care imposes the most feared scenario: prolonged helplessness, often in pain. For years, hospital staff have known about "I.C.U. psychosis," the severe and not uncommon disorientation of patients reacting to the windowless, mechanical environment. For years, the only remedy has been to set a clock where the patient could see it.

The impact of the intensive care unit on the American way of dying has been profound, for it is there that contemporary medicine routinely eliminates the primary actor, the patient, from the ritual of dying. This is done by first selecting uncommonly passive patients in crisis. Medicine then perfected the way of artificially sustaining the clinically (if not legally) dead patient and replacing the old rituals of professional-patient interaction with emergency medical intervention, that is, professional team management of machines and bodies. Dying in this context is not something the individual patient, potentially a living corpse, really does, since it is a matter of the staff's withdrawing life supports. It has also become increasingly unclear what responsibility the once "masters of death" assume in hospital death scenarios. With few exceptions, modern physicians are revolted by death, leaving to nurses the "dirty work" of interacting with grieving families, the actual release of the patient from support machines, and ministering to the dead body.

Dying at Home

Recalling a time, long gone, when people died at home, Michel Foucault describes the family's gaze fixed on the sick person as full of "the vital force of benevolence and the discretion of hope." The contemporary alternative of dying at home guarantees no such comfort. Yet many households, prepared or not, must accept the prospect of such caretaking, even though the patient's death at the last minute takes place in the hospital.

Since the introduction of DRGs in 1983, the allowable length of hospital stay for Medicare patients has been sharply decreased. Growing numbers of chronically ill and elderly people are being cared for by relatives. But the family context has its problems: emotional ambivalence, instability, isolation from the larger community, and even violence. Hospice care, once hailed as the humane alternative to dying in the hospital, provides only minor support in terms of supplies and service. Family members, especially women, are left with the daily responsibility for patient care, which now often includes complex regimens of infusion drugs, intravenous feeding, oxygen support, and physical therapy. For most of the elderly, long-term nursing home care is economically not feasible. Hospitals have no room for those who are dying slowly—but then who does?

The toll of rejection may be seen in the increasing rate of suicide among the elderly. Between 1981 and 1986, suicides among people over sixty-five rose sharply, from 12.6 per 100,000 to 21.8. Starvation, refusal of medication, and guns were the principal means. How such private decisions are reached or even if they can count as rational, we do not know, although fear of being a burden is frequently reported in anecdotes. Such a fear itself is not irrational. Government and professional support for home care is minimal. Home-care providers receive scant training for the technical tasks they perform, no provision for relief, and no credit for the round-the-clock time they give. Having little or no reimbursement incentives, physicians generally ignore patients cared for at home. Cost coverage for home care varies with the insurance carrier. Even under private insurance plans, many items must be paid for out-of-pocket. In the last ten years, unregulated commercial agencies have taken over the growing, multi-billion dollar home-care industry and have inflated the retail cost of everything—needles, gauze, plastic tubing, rubber sheets, bed rentals, and drugs—in ways that parallel hospital charges for aspirin and the price of Pentagon coffee pots.

As death re-enters the American household, it is tamed only by the resources a family or perhaps only a single relative or friend can muster. Maybe the community has a free slot in the hospice program, maybe the physician will do more than telephone, maybe a member of the clergy will visit. But there are no guarantees. If the scenario of hospital death is daunting, so too is the vision of a drawn-out, painful expiration, resented and uncomforted by those intimates or the intimate to whom one is a burden. The choice to refuse medication or even food may be rational, if one truly believes it is time to die. But the rationale "I am only a burden" threatens all of us, for we are all at some time in our lives completely dependent on others.

Confronting Death

The present controversy surrounding physician-assisted suicide and rational suicide in general may be all to the good, if it promotes change in our institutions. How many people would be interested in a quick (six minutes), painless death in a parked van (the scenario for Janet Adkins, the first user of Kevorkian's mercitron machine) if hospitals and homes provided a more humane context for dying? Or is it that Americans, Puritans still, ask for nothing more than clean sheets and a morphine drip? This may be true. The rational suicides reported in the media all have a tidy, pain-free aura about them.

Critics, such as Mitford and Ariès, accurately identified our cultural denial of death as a serious aberration. We want death to never happen, to be a nonexperience, or an event that cannot threaten our dignity. Yet, as the philosopher Paul Ramsey used to say, there is nothing at all digni-fied about dying—one might add, nor happy either. Death must be seen for what it is—cruelly inevitable, a painful rendering, our finitude if we are to understand the human condition and even begin to ask about the meaning of life. Death is momentous, in the general and in the specific. For the dying person, spirit and body are inescapably involved in a final reckoning. No witness can be untouched, except by a distortion of the most fundamental truth, that we are mortal. The distance between us and the dying person is only an accident of time.

It is this sense of mortality we try to hide from and the reason we have created institutions of denial. Oddly enough, we even deny the extent to which these institutions contribute to our problems. In the innumerable debates and discussions about death, the focus remains on individual strategies, as if, for example, one person's choice of suicide over pro-tracted terminal illness constituted a justification in itself, prompted by psychology, legitimated by one's will, and with no social consequences or meaning. Yet our hospitals are strange and alienating environments to the extent that they obfuscate this truth of mortality by therapeutic ex-perimentalism, intensive care, and also the "harvesting" of organs from living corpses. Our homes are threatening to the extent that people are left in isolation to deal with life as a burden and death as an obscenity. The quick-fix suicide machine or the plastic bag method described in *Final Exit* might relieve the individual of woe and suffering, but what about the rest of us, who will dutifully attend to our living wills and then await the worst? We know that death is not obscene; it cannot by itself deprave us. But it is frightening in its familiarity and cannot be simply planned away. Rather, we should envision institutional reforms. We need physicians educated to say more to the dying patient than "Have a nice rip" (Kevorkian's farewell to Janet Adkins). We need hospitals with staff motivated to give humane attention, not overtreatment, to the dying. We need compensation for families that give home care so that they can afford to be kind and old people can die in relative peace. Death is indeed a wild beast of sorts. These are ways to tame it.

Moral Dilemmas

Elizabeth W. Markson

With technological change, norms about how and when to die are in flux. Popular support for "death with dignity" is growing. A recent *New York Times*-CBS poll reported that 53 percent of the respondents agree that doctors should be allowed to assist a severely ill person to commit suicide. The American Hospital Association has recognized that many of the approximately 6,000 hospital deaths per day are in some way planned by patients, their families, or physicians. Other estimates suggest that as many as 70 percent of all deaths in hospitals, where most mortality in the United States occurs, are preceded by *ad hoc,* often *sub rosa,* decisions to withdraw care. The high cost of medical care for the terminally ill in a nation where health care costs are the most rapidly rising portion of the consumer price index, where Medicare expenses are the highest in the last year of life, and where an estimated 35 million people remain uninsured, all this makes euthanasia an increasingly salient social policy issue. Faced with great pain and the emotional and financial burden on one's family that accompanies the prolonging of life during terminal illness, the decision to take one's life is not necessarily irrational, psychotic, or delusional, but pragmatic. The mode of suicide advanced by the Hemlock Society—self-administration of barbiturates (if one can obtain them) coupled with a plastic bag over one's head to ensure successful death—highlights the grotesqueness of the means available for the final exit.

Proponents of euthanasia demand that patients should be allowed to choose the time and method of their death. A 1991 referendum in Washington State, for example, if passed would have permitted physicians to bring about death through administration of intravenous or oral medication to a patient who: (1) makes such a request in a written document witnessed by two independent witnesses; and (2) has been examined by two physicians who certify in writing that the patient has a terminal illness likely to result in death within six months. Other states have introduced similar referenda that were defeated at the polls. Less extreme is the Patient Self-Determination Act passed by Congress in 1990, requiring that, as of December 1991, health care facilities inform patients about their right to prepare advance directives or "living wills."

Enter physician-pathologist Jack Kevorkian with a new solution. In *Prescription Medicide: The Goodness of Planned Death*, Kevorkian extends the concept of euthanasia (literally, good death) to medicide or planned death, described as "a rational system that honors self-determination and extracts from a purposeful, unavoidable death the maximum benefit for the subject, subject's next of kin, and for all humanity." That Kevorkian's "mercitron," or suicide machine, has received so much publicity reflects both the horror and fascination with which Americans regard death.

Four interwoven values in American society shape our contemporary attitudes toward death. First, work and activity are valued as ends in themselves so that death is the apotheosis of cessation of productivity. Second, self-determination and individual responsibility are highly prized. Third, technology and its ability to modify or control the environment—and life itself with the advent of genetic engineering—is esteemed (death too should lend itself to active manipulation, if not actual conquest). Lastly, as Richard Kalish pointed out over two decades ago, if the United States can be said to have a common religion, it is human health with physicians as its high priests. Death is a disruptive factor in a technological, activity-oriented society and it is best handled by medical personnel in specialized facilities.

That death should be perceived to be the purview of physicians—as Kevorkian states, a medical, not a human, problem best handled by technical experts in specialized facilities—absolutely separate from law, politics, religion, and the judiciary, is thus not surprising. Kevorkian's view of "planned death is a system for making death, euthanasia, and suicide positive instead of negative" proposes the harnessing death to benefit life—an activist, technological solution in the hands of a new specialty of medical experts created to control and administer planned death.

But what is this "goodness of planned death?" It is neither relief from pain for the terminally ill patient nor alleviation of the psychological distress of family members. Nor is it reduction of the heavy financial burden for family or patient, depletion of assets, or waste of societal resources. As Kevorkian stated in an interview in *Free Inquiry:*

> These minor benefits do not counterbalance the loss of a human life. But if the patient opts for euthanasia, or if someone is to be executed, and at the same time opts to donate organs, he or she can save anywhere from five to ten lives. Now the death becomes definitely, incalculably positive. The patient may opt to undergo experimentation under anesthesia, from which he or she won't awaken. This could affect millions of lives now and in the future.... For example, if a patient is dying of Lou Gehrig's disease, he can stipulate that the experiment must deal with that affliction.... Another suboption would be to allow the doctor to do any experiment.

A truly technological solution to dying, with a new specialty of medical experts (medicidians??) created to administer death, enabling both acquisition of body organs and medical experimentation for the good of society! Whether there is a moral distinction between killing patients upon request, or allowing them to die by withholding "heroics," continues to be debated by ethicists and physicians alike, reflecting confusion about appropriate norms for dying in the United States and much of Europe. In Britain, although the British Medical Association has firmly rejected the attempt "by anybody to terminate another person's life" and euthanasia is regarded as attempted murder, a brother and sister were conditionally discharged in 1990 by the court for attempting to kill their terminally ill mother. In the Netherlands, the only nation in Europe where euthanasia is openly practiced, ending life, even at a person's request, remains technically a crime, punishable by up to twelve years. Since the 1970s, however, many Dutch physicians have violated the ban on euthanasia, and courts have set forth conditions that excuse the act. Dutch patients whose lives will be medically ended must be rational, request death repeatedly, such requests to be certified by two physicians as reasonable, and must be suffering from unbearable pain without hope of relief although not necessarily terminal illness—"psychic suffering," "potential disfigurement of personality," and "necessity" have also been noted as sufficient grounds.

As Robert K. Merton noted some years ago, every act has more than one outcome with unforeseen consequences that may undermine the goals of policy. What may we learn about the latent functions of euthanasia from the Netherlands experience to clarify the moral dilemma of when and how to die? Although only about 150 cases of euthanasia are reported annually to government officials, unofficial estimates range from

2,000 to 6,000 physician-aided deaths per year or 1 percent to 15 percent of all deaths, typically recorded officially as cardiac arrest. The equivocal status of euthanasia in the Netherlands makes systematic analysis of the incidence, prevalence, and characteristics of those patients who opt to have their lives ended impossible. Critics of the Dutch system, such as cardiologist Richard Fenigsen, have argued that euthanasia is being differentially applied and is not always voluntary; rather, physician-implemented "crypthanasia" (literally, secret death) takes place, making many infirm and elderly afraid to seek medical attention when ill. Although this charge has been hotly disputed by other physicians and ethicists, the point is clear: without formal social control, the potential for murder of those judged to be mentally or physically inferior and a social burden, even in a society with universal health care such as the Netherlands, is strong.

As health care costs escalate and rationing of health care becomes increasingly likely in the United States, medicide may enhance the winnowing process. But at what social costs? If the way in which a society handles its sick and infirm indeed reflects the regard in which human life itself held, what does the proposal to create a new specialty to control and administer death say about basic values? Does any one profession have the right to decide who should live or die without checks and balances?

Here one descends a slippery slope. Killing patients for their own good is not a new concept; it is the fundamental theme a work by Binding and Roche, *Release to Destroy Life Unworthy of Life,* published in Germany in 1920. Nor is killing patients for the perceived greater good of society a new notion, as the death camps and many experiments by Nazi physicians have shown. Although Americans treasure their self-determination and the right to "do it my way," these beliefs are at best half-truths. As solo practitioners or small group practice physicians are gradually being replaced by profit-making companies that own chains of hospitals, nursing homes, medical office centers, and walk-in clinics, a two-class system—private and profitable for those who can pay, public and underfunded for the poor—is increasingly evident. Research has already shown that social class determines not only how we live but how we die. A public official or popular culture figure will receive more attention than a drunken derelict, an elderly person, a woman, or other person considered to be of low social worth. Self-determination can all too easily turn into differential application. The powerless, poor, or undesirable are at special risk of being "encouraged" to choose assisted death.

Nor is it impossible that an additional, unanticipated consequence of death-upon-demand may be an increase in "altruistic" suicide. Those sixty-five and over spend about three and a half times as much per person on medical care as do younger people. For the elderly, for AIDS victims, and others who require long-term care, the cost of hospital or nursing home care rapidly depletes personal savings. It is not only in science fiction scenarios that chronically or terminally ill people may feel obliged to commit suicide in order to spare their families anguish and to avoid financial expense, whether or not they themselves wish to die.

But perhaps in the debate about euthanasia, and its extension, medicide, the wrong question is being asked. The question is not "should we help people to die?" but rather "what can we do to make living more positive for the chronically or terminally ill?" American health care costs are higher than those of several other nations, and with poorer results. The United States is one of the few industrialized nations where health care costs are either borne by the people themselves or administered by the private sector. Without national health insurance, existing class differences in health services cannot be narrowed. A national health plan should include both preventive and palliative treatment not covered by most insurance plans. The hospice movement illustrates that pain can be minimized or eliminated if sufficient medication is given. Dying can be dignified at relatively low cost. Although diseases such as Alzheimer's (still only definitively diagnosed upon autopsy) do not readily lend themselves to hospice care, would Janet Adkins have chosen the mercitron if good, affordable care had been available? One wonders.

Turf Battles on Medicine Avenue

Mark G. Field

In a letter to the editor of the *New York Times,* on August 6, 1977, Charles Harris. M.D., laments the recommendation of the New York Board of Regents that doctors and other professionals be allowed to advertise in the press and on television. Recounting that his father, also a doctor and dental surgeon, had spent a great amount of energy in eliminating dental parlors in New York and the advertising that enabled them to exist, he bemoaned that measures were being taken "permitting some among us to optimize their talents as entrepreneurs, rather than physicians." That recommendation was not an arbitrary decision: it was in compliance with the law of the land, the result of a Supreme Court decision in 1977 to the effect that professional associations—in this case, the American Medical Association (AMA) and its affiliated state and local societies—were not exempt from antitrust regulations. This meant that these associations did not have the right to prohibit their members from advertising their services, that is from soliciting business, because to do so constituted an illegal restraint of trade, inhibiting competition, driving prices up or fixing them, and depriving the public of information (including the cost of services) needed to select a physician. The Court decision itself upheld an earlier charge made by the Federal Trade Commission (FTC) in 1975 that the AMA inhibited competition through ethical restraints on advertising and solicitation, a ruling the AMA had appealed and eventually lost. This decision did not apply to medicine only: in its recommendations, the New York Board of Regents specifically listed twenty-nine professions including medicine. Each state makes its own rules regarding professional advertising, although the Court ruled that the AMA may regulate advertising that is false and misleading.

The Supreme Court decision, as regrettable as some see it, goes to the core of the concept of "profession," particularly because it tends to blur the traditional (and. to many, hallowed) distinction between a profession and business, between an "ethical" service and a "self-serving" trade. Are doctors, for example, to be considered from now on purveyors of services, commercial entrepreneurs as Dr. Harris complains? Is there no difference, any more, between an occupation that has certain aspects of a calling and the crass pursuit of self-interest at the expense of the patient or the consumer? This issue has divided the medical profession between the "traditionals" and the "moderns." The traditionals contend that advertising per se is bad or evil. It reduces the practitioner to the level of a purveyor of services or a tradesman. It leaves the burden of choice to the consumer who is held not able to judge the quality of medical services, only the price. In many instances, the consumer (patient) is in pain or unconscious and must "trust" the physician to do the best to "serve" the individual. Doctors have long nurtured the image that they are "a breed apart." That special quality will disappear under the onslaught of entrepreneurship and commercialization, and in the final analysis it is the individual patient who will lose. As one traditional physician put it: "The net effect will be a Gresham's law as bad care drives out good because it's cheaper." He added that it has always been true that "some doctors have exploited patients by ordering unnecessary procedures for monetary gains, but it is unlikely that advertising will control bad practice. Rather, it is likely to force more and more doctors to become businessmen in the competition to survive." The moderns, on the other hand, may not be upset by the Court decision: quite the contrary, they seem to have welcomed it. They see nothing wrong with advertising their services as long as it is true and not deceptive. As a dermatologist in Toms River, New Jersey said to the *New York Times: "I* have no shame about advertising. I am a guy who provides a service just like other merchants, even if it did take me longer to get here."

The moderns, indeed, see themselves as purveyors of services, competing for market shares. They face a situation different from that confronted by their elders, most of whom are traditionals. Society and medicine have changed dramatically in the last few decades (after World War II), and some of these changes are, indeed, painful to those who started their professional life in an earlier, perhaps less turbulent atmosphere.

A profession is an occupation. It is part of the division of labor and the exchange of goods and services without which our type of society would not function. Physicians (or lawyers, professors, architects. or clergy) provide specialized services, usually on a full-time basis. As such, they do not have time to attend to their own needs, such as raising their own food, building their own houses or offices, educating their own children, or making their own clothes or equipment. The time of the professional must be exchanged for the time of others in the form of goods, services, and commodities produced by these others. The exchange is mediated usually through money, but need not be: it could be eggs and chickens, or the provision of room and board; or it can be in the form of a fixed salary. Thus, the professional is, by necessity, involved in an economic network. Although we may quibble to the end of time about the fairness of the remuneration or incomes of physicians, nurses, clergy, lawyers, and Indian chiefs, this exchange must proceed. A breakdown in that process would almost immediately affect professionals and others in their work. (A starving physician is unlikely to give the best professional attention.) Even those who provide "free" services must eat with some regularity.

Although professionals must be concerned with their income, the ideology of the profession has been to decouple remuneration from service. This is, according to professional ideology, what distinguishes it from business. If the patient dies, or if the case is lost in court, the physician and the lawyer will still send their bills for services rendered. The assumption is that the professional did the best professional job, regardless of anticipated reward. On the other hand, one does not pay a plumber who has botched the job. The profession claims it is so special because of its orientation to service, particularly service that allegedly the patient or client is not qualified to judge or to compare. The relationship between professional and client must include a fiduciary component. Professionals claim to be different because they are expected, in all instances, to place the interests of the client before their own. A surgeon should be able to tell a patient he or she does not need an operation, although surgery might yield a sizable fee. A salesman is not expected to tell a prospective customer that he or she does not need a new Cadillac, that the customer had better go across the street and buy a more reasonably priced Ford. In a business-oriented society like ours, this claim (as long as it is believed by the population) places the professional in a highly respected position; it is why the professions in any popular poll of prestige rankings are at the top, surpassing business occupations. This view that the professional is a cut above other mortals tends to become a judgment of the personal character of professionals: that they are basically altruists because they tend to behave like altruists.

Sociological analysis, particularly role theory, provides us with a more sophisticated view of the physician's comportment: it is in the nature of the social prescription, and for good functional reasons, that the professional is expected, indeed enjoined, to act unselfishly. In one sense. this altruistic behavior not only serves the patient or client well and protects him or her from exploitation by the professional, but this is the best way for professionals to maximize their own egotistical aspirations for success. recognition, and prestige. Physicians or lawyers who consistently abused the trust placed in them for personal gains would benefit in the short run but would eventually suffer; after a while no patients or cases would be referred to them in light of their tainted reputation. But the same physician in other roles (for example, that of a consumer) would behave like any other person. No physician to my knowledge has ever sold a house below market price because a would-be buyer was not able to afford the price. We are therefore dealing with a sociological, rather than a psychological, variable when we examine the behavior of professionals in their occupational roles and in their other roles.

What then of advertising and its commercial implications and associations? What may be even more interesting and intriguing than the fact that professionals are now allowed to advertise is that for about six decades, in a society that calls itself capitalistic—a society in which the business of America is business, a society in which commercial interests predominate—physicians did not advertise, indeed were enjoined by their codes of ethics from soliciting patients, or engaging in any form of advertisement, except the mildest and most discreet announcements that they were in practice or had opened an office. There was almost a conspiracy of silence on the part of the courts which did not invoke antitrust laws in the case of the professions. The situation was different in the nineteenth century, particularly in the second half and the beginning of the twentieth century. Physicians did not shy away from advertisement and shameless self-promotion.

In the nineteenth century, medicine was more of a trade than a profession. Physicians advertised their services in newspapers, in bills they passed on, in large sized promotional cards that bore their photographic likeness on one side and a "commercial" message on the other. Thus, Dr. W. H. Long had cards printed with his photograph. seated in his frock coat, a flower in his lapel. a top hat on his knee, and what looked like a gold-headed cane. Under his name there was, in parentheses, "Diamond Jack" followed on the next line with the title "The Great Disease Detective," and then his Philadelphia address and the information "Bell and Keystone Phones." Robie Blake. M.D., of Cornish, Maine, the "Originator of Eucalyptus Compound," described himself as a druggist and chemist and proprietor of the compound "The Great Blood Purifier and Kidney Regulator." In addition, Dr. Blake dealt in drugs, medicines. chemicals, paints and oils, watches, jewelry and silver-plated ware, fancy and toilet articles, millinery, etc., and the list goes on including tobacco and cigars, all grades of corsets, trusses, shoulder braces, supporters, and even musical instruments. Dr. J. E. Briggs of New York City advertised he had the "Gift of Magnetic Healing" in addition to being a "Practical Physician" with the M.D. degree, and he added the testimonials of three satisfied former patients. It might be surmised that this unabashed self-promotion, the variety of different medical doctrines, the herbalists, Thompsonianists, the quacks, the frauds, and snake-oil salesmen did not lend medicine an aura of great dignity and respect. The unregulated nature of advertisement, the wilds exaggerated, and patently false claims for cures" by frauds, as well as doctors, associated advertising with quackery and deception and gave it a bad name. On the other hand, as Paul Starr has noted in *The Transformation of American Medicine*, medical practitioners of the nineteenth century did pretty well by themselves. They did not need access to hospital facilities, since little medical care took place there. They advertised themselves either by their manner, or in the press, or through what economists call "product differentiation," that is, by offering a different brand of medicine. The orientation of the profession was competitive rather than corporate.

The situation changed radically by the beginning of the twentieth century. The biological and chemical revolution of the latter part of the nineteenth century, the advances in scientific medicine dramatically changed the nature of medical practice. By 1910 or 1912, as L. J. Henderson wrote, for the first time a random patient with a random illness consulting a physician at random had more than one chance in two of benefiting from the encounter. The increased effectiveness of medicine as an applied science led to a radical transformation of American medicine. This was the result, among others, of the Flexner Report, commissioned by the Carnegie Foundation in 1910, which critically surveyed the state of

American and Canadian medical education. Gradually, marginal medical schools (similar, perhaps, to the "schools" that today teach television repairing) disappeared, and the pattern that is still in force emerged: medical schools were to require a completed college education; students must take at least two years of basic sciences in their preclinical years, to be followed by an internship in a hospital; medical schools must affiliate with a university and indeed become part of the faculty of that university in order to lend scientific credibility to their training and subsequent practices.

At the same time, the American Medical Association intensified a campaign to transform medicine into a "respectable" occupation, that is, a profession, to change it from a group of individuals hustling for clients into a corporate and solidary group that came to be called the organized voice of American medicine. The association managed to establish a quasi-monopoly for allopathic medicine—which it maintained was scientific and thus effective—and to drive away other approaches (including medical cults) from the pantheon of approved medical practices. By tightening standards of medical education, by restricting or controlling access to medical schools, by insisting on the licensing of practitioners. the AMA succeeded in turning American medical practitioners into "professionals." The association became a strong political power, particularly in the thirties and in the immediate post-World War II years when membership in the AMA was practically mandatory for physicians to practice (for example, to obtain staff or admitting privileges in hospitals). One of the important criteria that characterized a gentlemanly occupation was that its practitioners do not solicit clients or patients: advertising became taboo precisely because of its symbolic association with business. with commerce, with trade, with competition and, as we have seen, with fraud and deception.

In the seventies, once again the ground began to shift under physicians. This time it was not so much a scientific revolution (it was more of a technological one) but a series of changes taking place in American society and medicine in general. As a result, the corporate nature and the unity of medicine (so painstakingly forged by the AMA over several decades) has begun to erode. For example. because of court decisions, the association and state societies were no longer able to force physicians to join it if they wanted staff appointments or to restrain them from accepting salaried positions (a salary was held by the association to be indicative of the subordination of the physician to an organization and incompatible with professional autonomy). The opposition of the profession to the passage of Medicare (an admirable example of ideological consistency but suicidal from a public relations point of view) further weakened the association. The proportion of physicians who are members of the AMA has, as a result, considerably decreased over time. The unity of the profession has been further weakened or splintered because of the trend toward specialization and the growing diversity of work settings, so that the practitioners face different situations and different problems, and cannot easily constitute a unified and solidary interest group. In fact, a battle for turf is also taking place between specialty associations. Thus, the American Academy of Family Physicians is now in the middle of a three-year, $5.1 million public relations campaign to enhance the image of today's family doctor. One of the full-page ads asks: "Ever wish you had a doctor who specialized in you?" At the same time, the American Society of Internal Medicine has been conducting its own public education campaign. There are areas of overlap between what these practitioners do, and these involve market shares and competition.

A further weakening of the role of the physician has resulted from the technological changes that have taken place primarily in the hospital. Medical technology is both labor and capital intensive. It thus contributes to increasing the costs of medical care and to the growing complexity of the contemporary hospital. Power in the hospital, which in the past rested squarely with the doctors, is slowly passing to the managers and administrators. Technological changes plus an increasing surplus capacity (both in personnel and in facilities) as well as increasing costs are some of the factors that are altering the ground on which physicians stand. Advertising by some doctors may be but a symptom, a reflection of these major changes.

There are other forces at work in American society that further contribute to the changing atmosphere in which physicians and other professionals provide their services: one is an ideological shift toward less government, more deregulation and competition (to stem inflation and reduce costs). This reflects disappointment with what government (or "big government") can accomplish and reflects a belief in the power of market mechanisms and free enterprise to resolve many problems. The FTC ruling of 1975 and the confirmation of its constitutionality in 1977 were in line with such ideological shifts. The FTC ruling, as might be expected, was vigorously attacked by the AMA. which argued at the time that it would lead to the destruction of professionalism and would reduce medicine to a "non-ethically oriented, non-concerned pure trade activity." This is not, by far, the entire story: a second force is the growing surplus of physicians and hospital beds. In the early post-World War II years and until the mid-sixties, the conventional wisdom was that there were not enough physicians (partly as a result of the restrictions successfully imposed by the AMA on medical school admissions). This also accounted for the fact that American medicine, in those years, had to rely to an important degree on foreign medical graduates. Gradually, American medical schools increased their enrollments, and the number of medical schools also grew. The net result was that an increasing number (almost twice as many as in the past) of young physicians and foreign medical graduates came on the market. In earlier years, in a country hungry for physicians. they could pretty much settle where they wanted and dictate their own terms. As the supply caught up with the demand, and a surplus began to appear, the old nemesis of the medical profession reemerged: the fear of a glut of physicians, the specter of underemployment, or even unemployment, of physicians.

The AMA is now quietly studying ways to again curb the supply of physicians. This would take place through a decrease in admissions to the medical schools and further restriction on foreign medical graduates. The association is being very cautious on this because it does not want to run afoul of the restraint of trade provision and because it is reconsidering its assumption that market forces, rather than regulation, should control the supply of physicians. The association depicts this as an issue concerning quality, arguing that physicians who are underemployed cannot maintain a high level of skill. The other and more traditional issue for the association is the economic impact of a highly competitive and surplus situation in terms of physicians' incomes which are already slowly declining. In the past, a doctor could hang a shingle, discreetly announce the opening of a practice, and very soon the office appointment book would fill up (often to the point of overflow). Not any more. Physicians—particularly newly minted ones, and among these those in the specialties—increasingly have to fight for their turf by attracting clients and keeping the ones they already have

The ban on advertising before the Supreme Court decision had not always been observed when doctors faced a critical threat to their livelihood. Thus. the growth of the Kaiser-Permanente Health Plan in the West and HIP (the Health Insurance Plan) in the East in the fifties, as Starr pointed out, aroused deep anxieties among private practitioners because these plans attracted middle-income patients—their bread and butter. Doctors organized their own plans and advertised them in newspapers and on highway billboards and passed pamphlets to Kaiser workers when they had to choose between Kaiser and a new "Doctors' Plan." There are limitations on professional advertising and each state regulatory agency is free to outline these limitations. "False, fraudulent, misleading or deceptive" ads are out. The New York State Board of Medical Examiners, for instance, can require doctors to substantiate their advertising statements, but it has no control over public relations campaigns or press releases. Also prohibited are: claims of superiority, promotion of a service a practitioner is not licensed to perform, offering free or discounted services, testimonials. and computer advertising by telephone. Ads should be, "presented in a dignified manner without the use of drawing, animation dramatization, music, lyrics or clinical photographs."

It is not possible. at least at this time, to determine the extent of advertising by professionals (in this case, physicians) nationwide. Practices vary from state to state and take different forms. Even the term "advertising" does not convey the range of activities in this sphere: one reads of announcements, marketing, merchandising, public relations, image polishing, promotion, packaging. and patient/public education and other euphemisms coined by the perpetrators of hard sell. In 1983, health-care professionals, according to the Television Bureau of Advertising, spent $41 million on television spots alone, compared with just $3.7 million in 1977. This figure excludes newspaper and radio advertising and all promotional activities. Although I do not have aggregate figures on such expenses, a few illustrations might be instructive. A New Jersey obstetrician recently spent $4,000 on T-shirts, baby bibs and waterproof tote bags sporting his name and a stork. A Monmouth County, New Jersey ophthalmologist pays $15,000 a year to a public relations firm "in part to counteract the image of doctors as entrepreneurs, an image he believes has been conveyed by recent ads." Another physician launched a newspaper and magazine advertisement campaign to promote his liposuction surgery, a technique for removing fat. The cost of the campaign is $25,000 per year.

What then are the implications? For one thing, some loss of professional dignity that may lower the standing of the professions: the distinction between a professional and a commercial occupation becomes blurred, to the chagrin of the traditionals the profession becomes an enterprise, the doctor an entrepreneur. This promotes a certain level of hucksterism and, as most advertising does, sometimes tends to create a need when there was none before. As one traditional physician wrote to me on this subject: "Those of us who regard advertising as evil regard what has happened since it became permissible as proof of the correctness of our judgment. One now sees plastic surgeons soliciting customers for face lifts, ophthalmologists soliciting the nearsighted for radical keratotomies [a hazardous procedure of dubious value] and a thriving business on the West Coast among surgeons who tattoo pigment into the eyelid for permanent 'eyeliner'"; as professionals scramble for their share of the "business." Corporate solidarity begins to vanish in the advertising slipstream; the costs of advertising must inevitably be passed on to the clients or patients in the same way as the costs of car advertisements are, in the final analysis, passed on to the buyer. The awe and respect in which the profession was held by the clients (because people expected members of it to be more oriented to clients' needs and interests than to their own) may well decline as will trust: the caveat emptor of the marketplace may replace the caveat vendor philosophy of an earlier time.

So far, the manifest trend has not been catastrophic, although latent aspects of it may well lead to fundamental changes in the ways in which professional services are regarded by American society. It may possibly downgrade the legitimacy of the professions as special kinds of occupations entitled to certain considerations by the public and the law. For the time being, professionals who advertise justify the practice by saying that they want a piece of the pie. They want their market shares in the face of competition by their colleagues or peers, and because of the increasingly aggressive campaigns waged by institutions that have many more resources and clout than individual practitioners and do not shy away from trumpeting their wares to the public—the hospitals. surgical day-care centers. standing clinics in shopping malls. the so-called emergency "docs on the box," the health maintenance organizations, and so on, that now crowd the medical marketplace.

Some hospitals even go beyond the bounds of acceptable practice in their desperate efforts to fill empty beds. In one such hospital (in Tonawanda in upstate New York) physicians were offered bonuses (in fact, bounties) for referring patients for admission. These ranged from a cash allowance (more for inpatient admissions. less for outpatient treatment) or a dinner for two or a round of golf at the Buffalo Country Club. These may be good examples of acceptable marketing practices, but they are dubious practices in the medical field. Both physicians and the hospital were cited by the state Department of Health for violating the state public health law and unprofessional conduct (the incentives were considered fee-splitting). Health Maintenance Organizations (HMOs) have been put on notice in New Jersey because of dubious advertising directed at the more than 50,000 state, county, and municipal employees they are competing to serve. Similarly, physicians have been reprimanded for making exaggerated or inaccurate claims and have been forced to retract such claims. Thus, Dr. Terrance David Lesko of San Francisco had advertisements printed for hair implants, claiming they were safe and effective. The Federal Trade Commission ordered him to buy $8,000 worth of newspaper ads to warn readers that "implants are likely to promote infection and may cause a patient to lose his or her hair."

Although there is a fair amount of self-serving sanctimony in the traditional professional stance, there is also a certain amount of dignity conferred on occupations that deal with human life and health and, in the case of law, with property and freedom and justice. I can sympathize with the sadness of the traditionals as they see the marketplace mentality invade the professions, when they see what has been variously described as the commercialization, the monetization, or the commodification of services that deal in areas of great emotional and functional significance to human beings, as they see the jargon and the practices of Madison Avenue used to sell professional services. As Paul Starr remarked to a class of graduating physicians, "negotiating the conflict between the medical and the business aspects will become a significant preoccupation of professional life in medicine."

Because of my own interest in medicine in the Soviet Union, and because of the elimination of the professions as corporate bodies in that country, I became curious about the practices in a society where all physicians are state employees working for a fixed state salary. Even before *glasnost*, or openness, became the order of the day in Gorbachev's Russia, corruption, the taking of bribes, the exacting of money or "gifts" by health personnel (who are notoriously badly paid even by Soviet standards) had become common practice. In a long article "On Compassion," recently published in *Literaturnaia Gazeta,* Daniel Granin complains that kindness and mercy seem to have disappeared from the Soviet scene. He recounts the case of a friend of his whose mother became ill and needed an operation. His friend, a shy, decent engineer, had heard that one must "give" to the physician. Because of his concern for his mother, he overcame his reticence and, using the pretext that certain medications would be needed for her (and pharmaceuticals are perennially in short supply), offered the physician twenty-five rubles, ostensibly to pay for the medicines, but in reality a bribe for the doctor. The physician replied: "I do not take such money." "And how much is needed?" Granin's friend asked. "Ten times more." The engineer was not a rich person. Two hundred and fifty rubles is more than the average monthly salary; but he managed to get the money, and with some embarrassment gave it to the physician in an envelope. The doctor had no compunctions: he quietly took the cash out and counted the bills. After the operation, the mother died. The physician explained to her son: "I checked up, and your mother did not die as a result of the operation. Her heart simply could not take it. And, therefore, I am keeping the money." The author adds that the physician was convinced of his own decency; if the woman had died as a result of the surgery, he would have returned the money—just like any decent plumber. The writer adds that he told that story not because it is exceptional, but because it is not considered exceptional: it is a common occurrence. It occurred in a noncapitalist society, where the physician working in a state clinic was paid a salary and where advertising is rare and unheard of among medical practitioners. This was simply "commercial" behavior. Clearly, practices other than advertising that may corrupt medical practitioners.

Those who defend advertising see positive aspects: it builds awareness among patients, it educates consumers, it keeps fees in line and fair. Patients may thus benefit from competition, although the risks posed by hucksterism represent a difficult trade-off to negotiate. The fact that eyeglasses are much cheaper nowadays is also considered a result of increasing competition and the breaking of the monopoly of ophthalmologists in prescribing and optometrists in selling glasses. Patients now have more choices, and they can go "doctor shopping."

The nagging questions remain: Is the market interested in those who cannot pay? Shall we soon see ads that promise "twice your money back if I fail to cure you" and will "decent" physicians not bill you or return the money if you die on the operating table? When will the ads appear urging people to come and get their red-hot cataract or hernia operation? Or any two specified surgical procedures for only one additional dollar? Are we really more comfortable, and do we sleep better now that the New Jersey Board of Medical Examiners not only allows doctors to promote their services on radio and television. as well as in newspapers and magazines, but also on billboards, fliers, and even matchbook covers?

Regulating Commerce in Fetal Tissue

Emanuel D. Thorne

Doctors are fairly confident that within the next few years we will be able to transplant brain tissue from aborted human fetuses to alleviate, perhaps cure, several crippling diseases of the brain and central nervous system, such as Parkinson's disease. Physicians have already transplanted kidneys and a heart from a fetus, and clinical trials are taking place in which fetal pancreatic cells are transplanted into adult diabetics.

As many as 5 million Americans suffering from Parkinson's disease (1 million), Alzheimer's disease (2.5 to 3 million), Huntington's disease (25,000), type 1 diabetes (600,000), stroke (400,000) and spinal-cord injuries (several hundred thousand) may be helped if these treatments prove successful. Present organ-transplant activity, which helps about 11,500 Americans each year, is a cottage industry compared with the fetal-tissue transplant industry that is likely to emerge.

Current state and federal regulations were enacted principally to prevent exploitation of the fetus in biomedical research. At the time, therapeutic transplants of fetal tissue were the stuff of science fiction. We can expect that the profound moral dilemmas inherent in the use of human organs may be exacerbated by the potential large-scale therapeutic use of fetal tissue. Commercialization of fetal tissue could lead transplant agencies to offer the poor material incentives for abortion. It could lead physicians to manipulate the timing and method of abortion to suit the transplant recipient. It might also provide incentives to conceive with the intent to abort.

A debate on the proper uses of fetal tissue is taking shape, and several states have already proposed regulatory initiatives. At present, the debate is being waged primarily between abortion opponents, who fear that the medical use of fetal tissue will legitimate what to them is an abhorrent practice, and those in the pro-choice community who oppose any

103

restraint on a woman's rights regarding her body. Some pro-choice supporters resist this technology out of fear that some women might be willing, or coerced for economic reasons, to lease their wombs for the production of fetal tissue. When interest groups representing those who will benefit from fetal transplants (such as the Parkinson's disease and diabetes lobbies) weigh in with their views, the politics of the debate will change significantly.

Anticipating dilemmas and possible abuses in this area and seeking to avert them, Congress in 1985 enacted legislation establishing a Biomedical Ethics Board. The board has been slow to get started, apparently because of controversy and stalemate regarding the composition of the board's advisory panel and its mission. In April 1988, the Reagan administration placed a moratorium on funding by the National Institutes of Health of any research using fetal tissue for transplantation until an advisory panel that is currently meeting reports on proposed guidelines. Clearly, there is, at the highest levels of the United States government, uncertainty as to how to proceed and an impulse to the slow development of this technology until debate produces a consensus on appropriate guiding principles.

The ethical and economic issues associated with regulating human tissue are inextricably enmeshed, yet the economic issues draw little attention. This is not surprising. The primary urge to regulate trade in human tissue derives not from a failure of markets to provide the necessary tissue but, rather, from a moral revulsion at the commodification of human beings. However repugnant the idea, the human body now has value that cannot be wished away or ignored. Simply legislating sentiment about commercialization will not be enough. Regrettably, there is a lot of unclear thinking about how to regulate transfers of human tissue. What lessons can we draw for regulating fetal tissue from our attempts to regulate other human tissue?

Moral repugnance at commercial exploitation of human body parts has led all fifty states and Congress to adopt legislation limiting property rights to human tissue. The most important is the 1984 National Organ Transplant Act, which barred all sales of human organs. Thus, while people cannot sell their organs, they retain the right to donate; and nobody has the right to take their organs from them.

Revulsion at commercialization is the primary motivation for limiting property rights to human tissue, but other moral reasons have been offered. For example. commercial developers of the human body, such as pharmaceutical companies, argue that a person has no right to the value of his tissue since he did nothing to create or add to its value. This argument has been advanced in a case pending in California. A patient there is suing his physician for the economic value of his spleen, which was removed in the course of his treatment for leukemia, and from which the physician developed a patentable cancer-fighting product.

The physician argued, and most researchers agree, that the patient has no moral right to the value of the spleen since it was worth nothing to him. In fact, the spleen was worth less than nothing to the patient since he was willing to pay the physician to remove it. Now, after the physician has applied his education, experience, and talent to saving the patient's life and, incidentally, to developing the spleen, is it not outrageous for the patient to ask for royalties?

Consider a farmer who hires a specialist to rid his land of a brown substance that is bubbling up, destroying his ability to grow corn. Upon investigation, the specialist discovers that the brown substance is oil. Is there any doubt as to whether the value of the oil should belong to the farmer or the specialist? Even if the specialist were to do more than discover oil, say, invent the refining process and the machinery that would use the refined oil, would not the farmer still be entitled to the value of the resource? Out of ignorance the farmer might pay the specialist to remove the oil, but when other farmers realized that the oil had value, they could, under our system of property rights, command the oil's market price, even though they had contributed nothing to its value.

We insist on limiting donors' rights to their tissue, but they are the only participants in the production process expected to be altruistic. Neither doctors, pharmaceutical companies, nor test-tube makers offer their services for free. What happens to the economic value of the donated tissue? Does it pass to the transplant beneficiaries, as the law intends? Or, by allowing physicians or test-tube makers to charge more, is the value appropriated by the other factors of production?

The current organ-procurement system is a poor model for the regulation of fetal tissue, because it fails to control adequately the economic value of the organ. The 1984 act prohibiting sales of organs did not make them valueless. It made them free goods that can be used by anyone who can establish a claim to them.

To understand how the intent of the 1984 act might be subverted, imagine that a market for transplantable kidneys exists. Imagine there are three parties to a transaction—the donor, a surgical and hospital team, and the recipient—and they are able to carry out the transaction at prices agreeable to all. Let us assume that the amount required by the owner of the kidney to provide the kidney is $20,000, the amount for the team's services is $30,000, and the recipient is willing to pay the total sum of $50,000. Suppose that a law like the 1984 act is passed requiring all transplants to be gifts. Who will reap the $20,000 value of the kidney? Undoubtedly, the intent of the law was to treat the kidney as a gift to the recipient so that he might pay $30,000 rather than $50,000. However, nothing in the law assures this outcome. The medical team could reap the entire value of the kidney by charging the recipient $50,000.

A Pulitzer Prize winning series of articles in the Pittsburgh Press in 1985 reported that in 1984–85, while nationwide 10,000 Americans waited for transplants, at several hospitals nearly 30 percent of kidney transplants were performed on foreigners allowed to bypass the queue of Americans. Surgeons' fees were as much as four times and hospital charges almost twice as high for foreigners as for Americans. An August 1986 report by the Department of Health and Human Services confirmed that a high percentage of American kidneys were being transplanted into foreigners who were being charged fees several times those charged Americans.

By denying the donor the organ's economic value, Congress wanted to remove human organs from the realm of the market. Lamentably, human beings have in many respects become commodities, and Congress did not succeed in removing notions of economic value from the organ-procurement system. More troublesome perhaps, Congress also failed to specify who owns the property rights to the organ.

In the process, Congress not only caused an ethically questionable result—the transfer of economic value from the donor to the doctors and hospitals—it also created a situation in which government intervened inequitably and inefficiently in the supply and demand for organs. Whether or not paying donors for their organs would yield a greater supply and reduce current shortages is an unsettled empirical question. There can be little doubt, however, that the already short supply of organs would shrink if potential donors became aware that the current system leaves the value of their organs up for grabs.

How should we organize transplant services that depend on altruistic donations of human tissue? Of the three parties involved in tissue transfer—donor, intermediary, and transplant recipient—markets in human tissue would in theory give the tissue's economic value to the donor. By prohibiting markets and insisting on altruism, our laws favor the intermediary, which, given the twin goals of equity and efficiency, is the least desirable result.

Both for-profit and nonprofit organizations are involved in delivering transplant services. Nonprofit entities such as the American Red Cross collect and distribute human tissue. Except for nonprofit hospitals, almost all the other participants are profit-making. In fact, there already are publicly held for-profit companies that use fetal tissue. One company is attempting to grow insulin-producing pancreatic cells from fetal cells, and has led in developing techniques for treating Parkinson's disease with transplanted fetal neural tissue. Should its technique prove successful, it stands to profit considerably.

For the end-user (either the transplant recipient or purchaser of a product developed from donated human tissue) to benefit from the donation by paying less, some special market conditions must obtain, such as considerable competition at each stage in the production of transplanted tissue. But health care is not a competitive industry.

Neither the government, which pays for kidney transplants through the Medicare program, nor the nonprofit organizations that collect the tissue, exercise sufficient control to ensure that the economic value of the tissue does not end up with for-profit intermediaries. The government could arrange for the transplant recipient to receive the value by controlling the entire process; however, the government has thus far been reluctant to intervene extensively, and that is not likely to change.

There may be no practical way to ensure that the value of the donated tissue is passed on to the end user. We might consider schemes that would socialize the value of the tissue. For example, the government could auction licenses to private firms, allowing them to collect donated tissue. The licensed firms could charge market prices for the tissue, and the government would extract the firm's excess profits (that is, the value of the tissue) through its licensing fees. A favorite of economists, it is doubtful that this arrangement would succeed; people are unlikely to donate to private firms.

Alternatively, we might encourage nonprofit organizations to charge the profit-making intermediaries the market value of the tissue, and to use these earnings to finance other worthy activities. The reason nonprofit organizations are successful at soliciting donations is that the donor needs a trustworthy agent in lieu of knowing or being in contact with the transplant recipient. This can be seen in the example of food assistance in which people who wish to provide support to impoverished persons overseas donate money to CARE rather than engage the services of an experienced and efficient organization already in the food business, such as Safeway. According to Henry Hansmann, in the 1980 *Yale Law Journal,* "consumers may be unable to evaluate with any accuracy whether the promised good or service has been delivered. In such circumstances the market may well provide insufficient discipline for a profit-seeking producer." Because the donor would have great difficulty verifying that Safeway had fulfilled its part of the agreement, he "needs an organization that he can trust, and the nonprofit, because of the legal constraints under which it must operate, is likely to serve in that role better than its for-profit counterpart."

We may need to rely on nonprofit organizations, but. for several reasons, they may not solve the problem of decommercializing trade in human tissue. First, many nonprofit organizations consider it unethical to charge a market price for tissue donated to them. Consequently, most charge a price based solely on their administrative costs, leaving others to pick up the extra value. A recent study by the Office of Technology Assessment reported that in 1980 the average cost of a unit of red blood cells distributed to hospitals was thirty-two dollars, while the average hospital charge to a patient for that unit was about eighty-nine dollars. Second, even if nonprofit organizations wanted to charge a price reflecting the value of the tissue, market conditions might not allow them to. For example, if there were considerable competition among the nonprofit organizations, buyers, such as hospitals, could potentially bid the price of tissue down to the nonprofit organization's cost of processing it. This would give the tissue's value to the buyer. Third, there is the well-known potential for abuse and inefficiency in the nonprofit form of organization.

Despite their deficiencies, properly organized nonprofit organizations offer the best means for achieving an equitable and efficient human tissue procurement and distribution system. Indeed, if we succeed in getting nonprofit organizations to assume responsibility for carrying out the wishes of the donor, we may not need to trade off equity for efficiency; instead, by promoting one, we may enhance the other.

Donating human tissue to strangers may be one of the purest forms of altruism; no exchange, direct or implied, takes place. Consider that the

American Red Cross would like to recruit 100,000 persons to be standby donors of bone marrow. This registry of donors is needed because a bone marrow transplant between unrelated persons whose tissue is not closely matched is rarely successful. To furnish bone marrow, the donor is made unconscious with a general anesthetic, 100-to-200 holes are punched in his or her hips to extract the bone marrow through 5-to-6 skin punctures, and the donor may require a transfusion of one-to-two pints of blood. Not only is the procedure unpleasant, it is painful and not without real risk. Nonetheless, 15,000 donors in the United States have already pledged to undergo this operation should any person, even a complete stranger, need their bone marrow. The American Red Cross will charge hospitals and physicians a fee for this bone marrow based solely on its administrative costs—not a market price—and the hospitals and physicians, in turn, could charge their patients several times what they pay the Red Cross.

The abdication by the government and nonprofit organizations of the responsibility to see that the donor's altruism is not abused will not do—not for bone marrow, fetal tissue, or any other donated human tissue. Our system must be worthy of the donors' gift and must honor their values. The compassion displayed by bone marrow donors is not common, it is noble and precious. If we do not control cynical exploitation by intermediaries, we endanger more than the *supply* of donations. We put at risk a fundamental human virtue: the impulse to give.

The Health of Haight-Ashbury

David E. Smith, John Luce, and Ernest Dernburg

Conventional middle-class populations receive the best care our present conventional medical institutions can supply. Middle-class people pay their bills on time or have health insurance, which does it for them. They trust the doctor to do what is best for them. They have diseases that go with respectability, and the doctor who treats them need not feel tainted by associating with people whose medical problems arise from activities that are illegal or immoral.

People who do not measure up to middle-class standards pose a problem for organized medicine. They require medical care no less than others, but the profession does not do well in providing it. People who have no money or insurance, who mistrust doctors, who seem to the physician to be immoral criminals, find it difficult to get care. Doctors don't like them; they don't like the doctors. The profession, used to providing medical care in a style that suits it, and supplied with plenty of middle-class patients who like that style, has never bothered to figure out how to deliver medical care in a way that suits other populations who live differently.

San Francisco's hippie invasion of 1967 created an acute problem of this kind. The city's officialdom made no adequate response to the medical and public health problems it produced, but a number of volunteers founded the Haight-Ashbury Free Medical Clinic, a unique experiment in providing medical care to a deviant population on terms it would accept. The story of the clinic—the problems of staffing, supplies, finances and the changing population needs it encountered—suggests some of the difficulties and some of the possibilities involved in such an innovation.

Three years ago *Time* magazine called San Francisco's Haight-Ashbury "the vibrant epicenter of America's hippie movement." Today the Haight-Ashbury District looks like a disaster area. Some of the frame Victorian houses, flats and apartment buildings lying between the Panhandle of

111

Golden Gate Park and the slope of Mount Sutro have deteriorated beyond repair, and many property owners have boarded over their windows or blocked their doorways with heavy iron bars. Hiding in their self imposed internment, the original residents of the area seem emotionally exhausted and too terrified to leave their homes. "We're all frightened," says one 60-year-old member of the Haight-Ashbury Neighborhood Council. "The Haight has become a drug ghetto, a teenage slum. The streets aren't safe; rats romp in the Panhandle; the neighborhood gets more run down every day. The only thing that'll save this place now is a massive dose of federal aid."

Nowhere is the aid more needed than on Haight Street, the strip of stores that runs east to west through the Flatlands. Once a prosperous shopping area, Haight Street has so degenerated by this time that the storefronts are covered with steel grates and sheets of plywood, while the sidewalks are littered with dog droppings, cigarette butts, garbage and broken glass. According to Henry Sands, the owner of a small realty agency on the corner of Haight and Stanyan streets, over 50 grocers, florists, druggists, haberdashers and other merchants have moved off the street since the 1967 Summer of Love; property values have fallen 20 percent in the same period, but none of the remaining businessmen can find buyers for their stores. The Safeway Supermarket at Haight and Schrader streets has closed, Sands reports, after being shoplifted out of $10,000 worth of merchandise in three months. The one shop owner to open since, stocks padlocks and shatterproof window glass. "The only people making money on Haight Street now sell dope or cheap wine," the realtor claims. "Our former customers are all gone. There's nothing left of the old community anymore."

Nothing is left of the Haight-Ashbury's new hippie community today either. There are no paisley-painted buses on Haight Street, no "flower children" parading the sidewalks, no tribal gatherings, no HIP (Haight Independent Proprietor) stores. Almost all the longhaired proprietors have followed the original merchants out of the district; the Psychedelic Shop at Haight and Clayton stands vacant; the Print Mint across the street and the Straight Theatre down the block are both closed. Allen Ginsberg, Timothy Leary, Ken Kesey and their contemporaries no longer visit the communal mecca they helped establish here in the mid-1960s. Nor do the rock musicians, poster artists and spiritual gurus who brought it international fame. And although a few young people calling themselves Diggers still operate a free bakery and housing office out of the basement of All Saints Episcopal Church on Waller Street, Father Leon Harris there considers them a small and insignificant minority. "For all intents and purposes," he says, "the peaceful hippies we once knew have disappeared."

They started disappearing almost three years ago, when worldwide publicity brought a different and more disturbed population to the Haight and the city escalated its undeclared war on the new community. Today, most of the long-haired adolescents the public considers hip have left Haight Street to hang out on Telegraph Avenue in Berkeley or on Grant Avenue in San Francisco's North Beach District. Some of the "active" or "summer" hippies who once played in the Haight-Ashbury have either returned home or re-enrolled in school. Others have moved to the Mission District and other parts of the city, to Sausalito and Mill Valley in Marin County, to Berkeley and Big Sur or to the rural communes operating throughout northern California.

A few are still trapped in the Haight, but they take mescaline, LSD and other hallucinogenic drugs indoors and stay as far away from Haight Street as possible. When they must go there, to cash welfare checks or to shop at the one remaining supermarket, they never go at night or walk alone. "It's too dangerous for me," says one 19-year-old unwed mother who ran away from a middle-class home in Detroit during the summer of 1967. "Haight Street used to be so groovy I could get high just being there. But I don't know anybody on the street today. Since I've been here, it's become the roughest part of town."

A new population has moved into the district and taken over Haight Street like an occupying army. Transient and diverse, its members now number several thousand persons. Included are a few tourists, weekend visitors and young runaways who still regard the Haight-Ashbury as a refuge for the alienated. There are also older white, black and Indian alcoholics from the city's Skid Row; black delinquents who live in the Flatlands or the Fillmore ghetto; Hell's Angels and other "bikers" who roar through the area on their Harley Davidsons. Finally there are the overtly psychotic young people who abuse any and all kinds of drugs, and psychopathic white adolescents with criminal records in San Francisco and other cities who come from lower-class homes or no homes at all.

Uneducated and lacking any mystical or spiritual interest, many of these young people have traveled from across the country to find money, stimulation and easy sex in the Haight and to exploit the flower children they assume are still living here. Some have grown long hair and assimilated the hip jargon in the process, but they resemble true hippies in no real way. "Street wise" and relatively aggressive in spite of the passive longings which prompt their drug abuse, they have little love for one another and no respect for the law or for themselves. Instead of beads and bright costumes they wear leather jackets and coarse, heavy clothes. Instead of ornate buses they drive beat-up motorcycles and hot rods. Although they smoke marijuana incessantly and drop acid on occasion, they generally dismiss these chemicals as child's play and prefer to intoxicate themselves with opiates, barbiturates and amphetamines.

Their individual tastes may vary, but most of the adolescents share a dreary, drug-based life-style. Few have any legal means of support, and since many are addicted to heroin, they must peddle chemicals, steal groceries and hustle spare change to stay alive. Even this is difficult, for there is very little money on Haight Street and a great deal of fear. Indeed, the possibility of being "burned," raped or "ripped off" is so omnipresent that most of the young people stay by themselves and try to numb their anxiety and depression under a toxic fog. By day they sit and slouch separately against the boarded-up storefronts in a drug-induced somnolescence. At night they lock themselves indoors, inject heroin and plan what houses in the district they will subsequently rob.

Although the results of this living pattern are amply reflected in the statistics available from Park Police Station at Stanyan and Waller streets, the 106 patrolmen there are apparently unable to curb the Haight-Ashbury's crime. Their job has been made easier by the relative decrease in amphetamine consumption and the disappearance of many speed freaks from the district over the past few months, but the rate of robbery and other acts associated with heroin continues to rise. Making regular sweeps of Haight Street in patrol cars and paddy wagons, the police also threaten to plant drugs on known dealers if they will not voluntarily leave town. Yet these and other extreme measures seem only to act like a negative filter in the Haight, screening out the more cunning abusers and leaving their inept counterparts behind.

Furthermore, the narcotics agents responsible for the Haight-Ashbury cannot begin to regulate its drug flow. According to one agent of the State Narcotics Bureau, "The Haight is still the national spawning ground for multiple drug abuse. The adolescents there have caused one of the toughest law enforcement problems we've ever known."

They have also created one of the most serious health problems in all of San Francisco. Many of the young people who hang out on Haight Street are not only overtly or potentially psychotic, but also physically ravaged by one another as well. Although murder is not particularly popular with the new population, some of its members seem to spend their lives in plaster casts. Others frequently exhibit suppurating abrasions, knife and razor slashes damaged genitalia and other types of traumatic injuries—injuries all caused by violence.

Even more visible is the violence they do to themselves. Continually stoned on drugs, the adolescents often overexert and fail to notice as they infect and mangle their feet by wading through the droppings and broken glass. Furthermore, although some of the heroin addicts lead a comparatively stabilized existence, others overlook the physiological deterioration which results from their self-destructive lives. The eating habits of these young people are so poor that they are often malnourished and inordinately susceptible to infectious disease. In fact, a few of them suffer from protein and vitamin deficiencies that are usually found only in chronic alcoholics three times their age.

With gums bleeding from pyorrhea and rotting teeth, some also have abscesses and a diffuse tissue infection called cellulitis, both caused by using dirty needles. Others miss their veins while shooting up or rupture them by injecting impure and insoluble chemicals. And since most sleep, take drugs and have sex in unsanitary environments, they constantly expose themselves to upper respiratory tract infections, skin rashes, bronchitis, tonsillitis, influenza, dysentery, urinary and genital tract infections, hepatitis and venereal disease.

In addition to these and other chronic illnesses, the young people also suffer from a wide range of drug problems. Some have acute difficulties, such as those individuals who oversedate themselves with barbiturates or "overamp" with amphetamines. Others have chronic complaints, long-term "speed"-precipitated psychoses and paranoid, schizophrenic reactions. Many require physiological and psychological withdrawal from barbiturates and heroin. In fact, heroin addiction and its attendant symptoms have reached epidemic proportions in the Haight-Ashbury, and the few doctors at Park Emergency Hospital cannot check the spread of disease and drug abuse through the district any better than the police can control its crime.

To make matters worse, these physicians appear unwilling to attempt to solve the local health problems. Like many policemen, the public health representatives seem to look on young drug-abusers as subhuman. When adolescents come to Park Emergency for help the doctors frequently assault them with sermons, report them to the police or submit them to complicated and drawn-out referral procedures that only intensify their agony. The nurses sometimes tell prospective patients to take their problems elsewhere. The ambulance drivers simply "forget" calls for emergency assistance. They and the other staff members apparently believe that the best way to stamp out sickness in the Haight is to let its younger residents destroy themselves.

Given this attitude, it is hardly surprising that the adolescents are as frightened of public health officials as they are of policemen. Some would sooner risk death than seek aid at Park Emergency and are equally unwilling to go to San Francisco General Hospital, the city's central receiving unit, two miles away. Many merely live with their symptoms, doctor themselves with home remedies or narcotize themselves to relieve their pain. These young people do not trust "straight" private physicians, who they assume will overcharge them and hand them over to the law. Uneducated about medical matters, they too often listen only to the "witch doctors" and drug-dealers who prowl the Haight-Ashbury, prescribing their own products for practically every physiological and psychological ill.

A few are receptive to responsible opinion and anxious to be properly treated, particularly those individuals who want to kick heroin and those younger adolescents who have just made the Haight their home. Unfortunately, however, they have nowhere to go for help. Huckleberry's for Runaways and almost all the other service agencies created to assist the hippies in 1967 have suspended operations in the area. Although Father Harris and several other neighborhood ministers offer free advice at their respective churches, they can hardly deal with all the young people who come their way. Indeed, the only major organization that can reach the new population is the Haight-Ashbury Free Medical Clinic. But today, the first privately operated facility in America to employ community volunteers in providing free and nonpunitive treatment of adolescent drug and health difficulties has serious problems of its own.

This is ironic, for although it is still somewhat at odds with the local medical establishment, the clinic is better staffed and funded than at any point in its 2½-year history. It is also more decentralized, with several facilities in and outside of the Haight-Ashbury. Its oldest operation, a Medical Section located on the second floor of a faded yellow building at the corner of Haight and Clayton streets, is now open from 6 p.m. until 10 p.m. five evenings a week. Over 40 dedicated volunteers are on hand in the 14-room former dentist's office, so that 558 Clayton Street can accommodate more than 50 patients a day.

Of the young people who use the facility, only half live in the immediate area. The rest are hippies, beats and older people who come with their children from as far away as southern California. Accepting the clinic because it accepts them, the patients are treated by a staff of over 20 volunteer nurses and physicians in an atmosphere brightened by poster art and psychedelic paraphernalia. Some of these health professionals are general practitioners committed to community medicine. Others are specialists hoping to broaden their medical understanding. Many are interns and residents looking for experience or studying the Medical Section as a philosophic alternative to the practices of the Public Health Department and the American Medical Association.

Whatever their motivation, the doctors' primary objectives are diagnosis and detoxification. After examining their patients, they attempt to treat some with donated drugs which are kept under lock and key in the clinic pharmacy. Others require blood, urine and vaginal smear tests that can be performed in the laboratory on equipment furnished by the Medical Logistics Company of San Francisco and its 35-year-old president, Donald Reddick, who serves as the clinic's administrative director. Most of the patients have chronic problems, however, and cannot be treated adequately on the premises. They must therefore be referred and/or physically transported to other facilities, such as Planned Parenthood, the Society for Humane Abortions, the Pediatrics Clinic at the University of California Medical Center on Parnassus Street six blocks south, Children's Hospital, San Francisco General Hospital and the Public Health Department Clinic for VD. The Medical Section maintains a close working relationship with these institutions and can therefore act as a buffer between its hip patients and the straight world.

Although the physicians and nurses contribute to this mediating process, much of the referring, chauffeuring and patient-contacting at 558 Clayton Street is carried out by its staff of clerks, administrative aides and paramedical volunteers. Twenty such young people donate their time and energy to the Medical Section at present, most of them student activists, conscientious objectors fulfilling alternative service requirements and former members of the Haight-Ashbury's new community. Emotionally equipped to handle the demands and the depressing climate of ghetto medicine, several core members of the paramedical staff live together in the Haight as a communal family.

Supervising the volunteers is Dr. Alan Matzger, a 37-year-old general surgeon from San Francisco who developed an interest in community medicine after working at 558 Clayton Street for over a year. The clinic's first full-time resident physician, Dr. Matzger is actually employed by the United States Public Health Service, which has asked him to conduct a long-range investigation of health needs in the Haight-Ashbury. He is now nearing completion of this study and will soon develop an objective and comprehensive plan for community medical care.

Since heroin addiction is such a pressing current problem, Dr. Matzger and an anesthesiologist named Dr. George Gay have recently launched a heroin withdrawal program at the Medical Section. Working there five afternoons a week for the past four months, the two physicians have treated over 200 patients, less than 50 percent of whom consider the Haight their home. "The remainder are adolescents from so-called good families," Dr. Matzger reports, "most of them students at local colleges and high schools. Significantly, they follow the same evolutionary pattern as young people have in this district, progressing from hallucinogenic drug abuse to abuse of amphetamines and then to abuse of barbiturates and opiates. The 'Year of the Middle-Class Junkie' in San Francisco may well be 1970. If it is, we hope to expand our program as addiction problems mount throughout the entire Bay area."

Another expansion being considered at the clinic is a dentistry service. Organized by Dr. Ira Handelsman, a dentist from the University of the Pacific who is paid by a Public Health Service grant to study periodontal disease, this would be the first free program of dentistry in the city outside of the oral surgery unit at San Francisco General Hospital. As such, the service is under fire from the local dental society, which is opposed to this form of free dental care. Nevertheless, Dr. Handelsman is committed to his effort and has recently secured three donated dental chairs.

Although this and other programs at 558 Clayton Street are intended to operate somewhat autonomously, they are closely coordinated with those operated out of the clinic's second center in the Haight-Ashbury. Known as "409 House," it is located in a pale blue Victorian residence at the corner of Clayton and Oak Streets, across from the Panhandle. On

the first floor of this building is a reading and meditation room supervised by Reverend Lyle Grosjean of the Episcopal Peace Fellowship who
counsels some adolescents about spiritual, marital, draft and welfare
problems and offers shelter for others coming in from the cold.

On the third floor at 409 Clayton Street is the clinic publications office, staffed by volunteers who oversee the preparation of the *Journal of
Psychedelic Drugs*, a semiannual compilation of articles and papers presented at the drug symposia sponsored by the clinic and the University of
California Medical Center Psychopharmacology Study Group. Aided by
several health professionals, the volunteers also answer requests for medical information and administer the affairs of the National Free Clinics
Council, an organization created in 1968 for the dozens of free facilities
in Berkeley, Boston, and other cities that modeled their efforts after those
of the Haight-Ashbury Free Medical Clinic programs.

Sandwiched in between the Publications Office and Reverend
Grosjean's sanctuary is the Psychiatric Section. This service, which is
supervised by Stuart Loomis, a 47-year-old associate professor of education at San Francisco State College, provides free counseling and psychiatric aid for over 150 individuals. Roughly one-half of these patients
are hippies and "active hippies" who either live in the district or com-
mute from rural and urban communes where physicians from the Medical Section make house calls. The remaining 50 percent is made up of
young people who suffer from the chronic anxiety and depression common in heroin addicts.

Loomis and the other 30 staff psychologists, psychiatrists and psychiatric social workers at 409 Clayton Street are able to counsel some of these
patients in the Psychiatric Section. They usually refer the more disturbed
multiple drug-abusers and ambulatory schizophrenics now common to the
Haight either to such facilities as the drug program at Mendocino State
Hospital or to the Immediate Psychiatric Aid and Referral Service at San
Francisco General, whose director, Dr. Arthur Carfagni, is on the clinic's
executive committee. When intensive psychiatric intervention is not called
for, however, they frequently send the patients to the clinic's own Drug
Treatment Program in the basement downstairs.

This project, nicknamed the Free Fuse, is led by a Lutheran minister
in his mid-thirties named John Frykman. Financed by personal gifts and
by grants from such private foundations as the Merrill Trust, its goal is
to wean drug-abusers away from their destructive lifestyle. Using meth-

ods developed by Synanon and the Esalen Institute, Frykman and the other Free Fuse counselors have attempted to create a close and productive social unit out of alienated adolescents living together as the clinic's second communal family. They have also provided educational and employment opportunities for more than 500 young people in the past 1½ years.

Since many Free Fuse graduates are still involved in his project, Frykman has also found it possible to expand. Having recently opened an annex in the drug-ridden North Beach District under the supervision of a psychiatric nurse, he has allowed the Drug Treatment Program to geographically qualify for inclusion in the Northeast Mental Health Center, a cachement area encompassing one-quarter of San Francisco. Because of this, the Free Fuse will participate in a substantial grant from the National Institute of Mental Health being administered by Dr. Carfagni. Frykman's Drug Treatment Program has already received some of these funds, and he is therefore making arrangements with the downtown YMCA to open a similar center in the city's Tenderloin area. "We've never gotten a penny from any public agency before," he says, "but the future looks bright from here."

This optimism certainly seems justified, and Frykman is not the only staff member who insists that the clinic is in better shape than at any other point in its history. Yet, as indicated earlier, the facility has problems all the same. In the first place, although the volunteers working at 409 and 558 Clayton Street can point to their share of therapeutic successes, they cannot really help most of the individuals who now live in the Haight-Ashbury. Many of the volunteers are actually former patients; some of them can keep off drugs only if they are kept on the staff.

Second, and most important, is the fact that the Haight continues to deteriorate in spite of the clinic's efforts. Thus, the relatively healthy adolescents tend to abandon the district, leaving behind their more disturbed counterparts, as well as the older individuals who preceded them in the area. Because of this, some staff members at the Medical and Psychological Sections believe that the clinic has outlived its usefulness in its present form. Others argue that the facility should address itself to the problems not only of the new population but of the old community as well. Dr. Matzger will probably have an important voice in this matter, and although his study might prompt the United States Public Health Service to support the work at 409 and 558 Clayton Street, it may mean a radical transformation in these centers as they now stand. This is a distinct possibility, for the clinic's future, like its past, is intimately connected with the district it serves.

To fully appreciate this it is necessary to visualize the Haight in 1960, before its present population arrived. In that year, rising rents, police harassment and the throngs of tourists and thrill-seekers on Grant Avenue squeezed many beatniks out of the North Beach District three miles away. They started looking for space in the Haight-Ashbury, and landlords here saw they could make more money renting their property to young people willing to put up with poor conditions than to black families. For this reason, a small, beat subculture took root in the Flatlands and spread slowly up the slope of Mount Sutro. By 1962 the Haight was the center of a significant but relatively unpublicized bohemian colony.

Although fed by beats and students from San Francisco State, this colony remained unnoticed for several years. One reason was its members' preference for sedating themselves with alcohol and marijuana instead of using drugs that attract more attention. Another was their preoccupation with art and their habit of living as couples or alone. This living pattern was drastically altered in 1964, however, with the popular acceptance of mescaline, LSD and other hallucinogens and the advent of the Ginsberg-Leary-Kesey nomadic, passive, communal electric and acid-oriented life-style. The beats were particularly vulnerable to psychoactive chemicals that they thought enhanced their aesthetic powers and alleviated their isolation. Because of this, hallucinogenic drugs swept the Haight-Ashbury, as rock groups began preparing in the Flatlands what would soon be known as the "San Francisco Sound." On January 1, 1966 the world's first Psychedelic Shop was opened on Haight Street. Two weeks later, Ken Kesey hosted a Trips Festival at Longshoreman's Hall. Fifteen thousand individuals attended, and the word "hippie" was born. A year later, after Diggers and HIP had come to the Haight, the new community held a tribal gathering for 20,000 white counter-culture Indians on the polo fields of Golden Gate Park. At this first Human Be-In, it showed its collective strength to the world.

The community grew immeasurably in size and stature as a result of this venture, but the ensuing publicity brought it problems for which its founders were ill prepared. In particular, the immigration of more young people to the Haight-Ashbury after the Be-In caused a shortage in sleeping space and precipitated the emergence of a new living unit, the crash pad. Adolescents forced to reside in these temporary and overcrowded structures started to experience adverse hallucinogenic drug reactions and psychological problems. The new community began to resemble a gypsy encampment, whose members were exposing themselves to an extreme amount of infectious disease.

Theoretically, the San Francisco Public Health Department should have responded positively to the situation. But instead of trying to educate and treat the hippies, it attempted to isolate and thereby destroy their community. Still convinced that theirs was a therapeutic alternative, the young people packed together in the Haight grew suicidally self-reliant, bought their medications on the black market and stocked cases of the antipsychotic agent Thorazine in their crash pads. Meanwhile, the Diggers announced that 100,000 adolescents dropping acid in Des Moines and Sioux Falls would flock to the Haight-Ashbury when school was out. They then tried to blackmail the city into giving them food, shelter and medical supplies necessary to care for the summer invasion.

Although the Public Health Department remained unmoved by the Diggers' forecast, a number of physicians and other persons associated with the University of California Psychopharmacology Study Group did react to the grisly promise of the Summer of Love. Among them were Robert Conrich, a former private investigator-turned-bohemian; Charles Fischer, a dental student; Dr. Frederick Meyers, internationally respected professor of pharmacology at the Medical Center; and Dr. David Smith, a toxicologist who was then serving as chief of the Alcohol and Drug Abuse Screening Unit at General Hospital. Several of these men lived in or were loyal to the Haight-Ashbury. Many had experience in treating bad LSD trips and felt that a rash of them would soon occur in the district. All had contacts among the new community and were impressed by the hippies' dreams of new social forms. But they also knew that the hippies did not number health among their primary concerns, although they might if they were afforded a free and accepting facility. In April they decided to organize a volunteer-staffed crisis center which might answer the growing medical emergency in the area.

As they expected, the organizers had little difficulty in gathering a number of hip and straight persons for their staff. However, they did face several problems in implementing their plans. First, they were unable to find space in the Haight until Robert Conrich located an abandoned dentist's office and obtained a lease for half of its 14 rooms. Paying the rent then became problematical, but Stuart Loomis and an English professor from State College, Leonard Wolf, offered funds if they could use half the facility for an educational project called Happening House. Finally, the organizers learned that local zoning regulations prohibited the charity operation they envisioned. This obstacle was overcome only after a sympathetic city supervisor, Jack Morrison, suggested that Dr. Smith establish the clinic as his private office so that his personal malpractice insurance could cover its volunteers.

Once this was accomplished, the organizers dredged up an odd assortment of medical equipment from the basements of several local hospitals. Utilizing the University of California Pharmacology Department, they also contacted the "detail men" representing most of America's large pharmaceutical houses and came up with a storeroom full of donated medications, including some vitally needed Thorazine. They then furnished a calm center for treating adverse LSD reactions at the facility.

Next, the organizers told the Public Health Department of their efforts. Its director, Dr. Ellis Sox, indicated that he might reimburse the organizers or open his own medical center if it was required in the Haight-Ashbury. Encouraged by this, the organizers alerted the new community that they would soon be in business. On the morning of June 7, 1967, the door to 558 Clayton Street was painted with the clinic's logo, a blue dove of peace over a white cross. Underneath this was written its slogan, Love Needs Care. The need itself was demonstrated that afternoon when the door was opened and 200 patients pushed their way inside.

Although the organizers anticipated the need for a regional health center in the Haight, they never dreamed that so many adolescents would seek help at the Medical Section. Nor did they suspect that the Diggers would be so close in their estimate of the number of individuals coming to the district that summer. Not all 100,000 showed up at once, but at least that many visitors did pass through the Haight-Ashbury during the next three months, over 20,000 of them stopping off at 558 Clayton Street along the way. A quarter of these persons were found to be beats, hippies and other early residents of the area. A half were "active" or "summer" hippies, comparatively healthy young people who experimented with drugs and might have done so at Fort Lauderdale and other locations had not the media told them to go West. The final quarter were bikers, psychotics and psychopaths of all ages who came to exploit the psychedelic scene.

Most of these individuals differed psychologically, but sickness and drugs were two things they all had in common. Some picked up measles, influenza, streptococcal pharyngitis, hepatitis, urinary and genital tract infections and venereal disease over the summer. Uncontrolled drug experimentation was rampant, so others had bad trips from the black-market acid flooding the area. Many also suffered adverse reactions from other drugs, for the presence of psychopaths and multiple abusers brought changes in psychoactive chemical consumption on the street. This first became obvious at the Summer Solstice Festival, where 5,000 tablets were distributed containing the psychomimetic amphetamine *STP.* Over 150 adolescents were treated for *STP* intoxication at the clinic, and after an educational program was launched, the substance waned in popularity in the district. But many of its younger residents had sampled intensive central nervous system stimulation for the first time during the STP episode. As a result, many were tempted to experiment next with "speed."

Such experimentation increased over the summer, until the Haight became the home of two separate subcultures, the first made up of "acid heads" who preferred hallucinogens, the second consisting of "speed freaks" partial to amphetamines. At the same time, the district saw the emergence of two different life-styles, the first characterized by milder adolescent illnesses, the second marked by malnutrition, cellulitis, tachycardia, overstimulation and the paranoid-schizophrenic reactions associated with "speed." This naturally affected the calm center, where student volunteers were treating more than 50 adverse drug reactions every 24 hours. It also made extreme demands on the doctors in the Medical Section, who were dealing with more than 250 patients a day. Discouraged and exhausted by their efforts, the physicians pleaded with the Public Health Department for assistance. Yet the department refused to help the facility and never attempted to open a crisis center of its own.

Fortunately, this refusal did not pass unnoticed by the local press, and 558 Clayton Street received a great deal of community aid. Shortly after the clinic's plight was reported, the facility was flooded with doctors disappointed by the Public Health Department and with medical students who came from as far as Indiana to volunteer. Several Neighborhood Council members dropped by with food for the workers, while contributions began arriving through the mail. One of us (Dernburg) and more than 30 other psychiatrists arrived at 558 Clayton Street and established a temporary Psychiatric Section on the premises. They were followed by

Donald Reddick and his partners in Medical Logistics, who donated over $20,000 worth of equipment and organized the staff procedures along more efficient lines. The second set of seven rooms was leased; a laboratory, pharmacy and expanded calm center were installed. Then, Dr. William Nesbitt, a general practitioner, invited the organizers to join Youth Projects, an agency he headed, and to use its nonprofit status to accept donations. When all was completed, the clinic was the best-equipped neighborhood center in town.

It was also the most chaotic, of course, a fact that was causing increased friction with the psychiatric staff. Once a Psychiatric Section was furnished at 409 Clayton Street, however, the doctors were able to counsel young people in relative privacy, to segregate the more violent amphetamine abusers and to reduce the traffic in the Medical Section to a more manageable flow.

While this was going on, the clinic was also involving itself in the crumbling new community. *Time* and other publications somehow assumed that the Haight was still full of hippies at this point, but the physicians at 558 Clayton Street knew otherwise. Realizing that the district was becoming even more disorganized, they created an informal council with Huckleberry's for Runaways, All Saints', the Haight-Ashbury Switchboard and other groups trying to prevent its total collapse. They then launched the *Journal of Psychedelic Drugs* to disseminate pharmacological information and started to participate more actively in community town hall meetings at the Straight Theatre. These several activities greatly enhanced the clinic's reputation in and outside of the Haight-Ashbury.

Although this publicity proved helpful to the facility in certain respects, it also caused several new crises. The first occurred two days after the publication of a *Look* magazine article on the clinic, when Dr. Smith was notified that his malpractice insurance was to be cancelled because he was "working with those weirdos in the Haight." This crisis was resolved when Dr. Robert Morris, a pathologist who was then chairman of the executive committee, suggested that he apply for group coverage under the auspices of the San Francisco Medical Society. Dr. Smith doubted that this organization would ever support his advocacy of free medical care. He was therefore delighted when the Medical Society not only granted him membership but also endorsed the programs at 558 and 409 Clayton Street.

His delight did not last long, however, for shortly after the endorsement the clinic had to contend with a number of persons who tried to capitalize on its good name. First were a number of bogus doctors, most of whom worked under stolen or forged medical licenses in the Haight-Ashbury. Then came the Diggers who resented the facility's influence in the community. Finally, the Medical Section was besieged by several older psychopaths, one of whom, a drug-dealer named Al Graham, hoped to turn it into his base of operations in the Haight. "Papa Al" was ultimately exposed and run out of the clinic, but shortly after he left, Robert Conrich, who was close to collapse after serving for two months as administrator, retired.

Although a severe blow in itself, Conrich's departure was also an ill omen. In fact, less than a week after he tendered his resignation, the Medical Section ran out of funds. The volunteers rallied to meet this new crisis; phone calls were made to potential contributors; and several paramedical staff members begged for money on Haight Street. Two dance-concert benefits with local rock groups that used the facility were also held, but only one was successful. In desperation, Peter Schubart called Joan Baez, who helped take patient histories and sang to entertain the lonely youngsters as they sat quietly in the waiting room. Yet even she could not save the clinic. On September 22 the door was locked at 558 Clayton Street. Two weeks later, what was left of the new community held a "Death of Hip" ceremony to bury the term "hippie" and remove the media from its back. "Haight used to be love," a participant wrote on the steps of the Medical Section after the event. "Now, where has all the love gone?"

This question could be easily answered, for by the end of the Summer of Love almost all of the original hippies had moved to urban and rural communes outside of the Haight. Many summer hippies had also left the district, and those who remained either fended for themselves or were assimilated into the new population. Staying in the Haight-Ashbury, they quickly changed from experimental drug-users into multiple abusers and needed even more help. For this reason, the clinic organizers were determined to open the Medical Section again.

At the same time, they had another good reason to renew their efforts in the Haight. With the hippie movement spread across the United States by this point, other cities—Seattle, Boston, Berkeley, Cambridge, even Honolulu—were being swept by drug problems. New clinics were being created in the face of this onslaught, all of them looking to the Haight-

Ashbury for guidance. Although always a confused and crisis-oriented center, the Haight-Ashbury Free Medical Clinic had become the national symbol of a new and successful approach in reaching a deviant population of alienated adolescents. Thus, its organizers had not only their medical practice but also their position of leadership to resume.

However, not all of them could still work in the Haight, a few were turning to other projects, others went back to prior commitments such as teaching.

But in spite of the losses the organizers looked to what was left of the new community for support. Another dance-concert benefit was held, this one under the guidance of Fillmore Auditorium owner Bill Graham, and several thousand dollars was raised. Smaller events were hosted at the Straight Theatre and at the John Bolles Gallery. In addition, a wealthy local artist named Norman Stone stepped forward to finance a substantial part of the Medical Section program. The clinic had still received no private or public grants, but by the end of October it had the funds necessary to open again.

When operations were resumed, however, the staff had a great deal more speed and more violence to contend with. In late February of 1968 a tourist ran over a dog, prompting a large crowd of adolescents to assemble on Haight Street. This in turn allowed Mayor Joseph Alioto to unleash his latest weapon for crime control, the 38-man Tactical Squad. After cleaning the street with tear gas and billies that afternoon, the squad vowed to return and enforce its own type of law and order. It did so four months later, when the district was ripped by three nights of rioting, rock-throwing and fires.

After the flames died down, it became apparent that the disturbance had marked yet another turning point in the history of the clinic. Many of its nurses, doctors and paramedical volunteers interpreted the riot as a sign that the Haight was now hopeless; mail contributions also ceased; and several psychiatrists who felt they could do little with or for the new population resigned from their positions. Low on money at this point, the clinic's business manager decided to host a three-day fund-raising benefit over the Labor Day weekend at the Palace of Fine Arts. The Affair was sabotaged by Mayor Alioto, who denied the cooperation of his Park and Recreation Commission. When the benefit, Festival of Performing Arts, was finally over, the organizers had lost $20,000. Two days later, the Medical Section was once again closed.

But, in spite of these obstacles, some progress was made. First, one of us (Smith) was awarded a grant to study adverse marijuana reactions which could be run in conjunction with the clinic. Stuart Loomis was installed as chief of the Psychiatric Section; Roger Smith raised more money for the Drug Treatment Program. In December the clinic received financial pledges from Norman Stone, the San Francisco Foundation and the Mary Crocker Trust. By January 7, 1969, 558 Clayton Street was in business again.

In contrast to previous years, its business went relatively smoothly in 1969. The amphetamines gradually ran their course in the district, and many of the multiple drug-abusers here switched to opiates, barbiturates and other "downers" after becoming too "strung out" on "speed." This change in chemical consumption naturally affected treatment practices, as heroin addiction increased tenfold and young people suffered even more types of chronic illness as a result of their drug abuse. Yet, in spite of the new population's problems, the year was a productive one for the clinic. Over 20,000 patients were treated at the Medical and Psychiatric Sections; research programs were initiated; efforts were made to reach the hippies in their communes; the volunteers became more experienced, although fewer in number; and several ex-staff members became involved in treatment programs of their own.

This year has also been a period of growth. More grants have been secured, and the inclusion of the Drug Treatment Program in the Northeast Mental Health Center, which provides for 14 new paid staff positions, has meant the facility's first official recognition by a public agency. In sum, the Haight-Ashbury Free Medical Clinic has finally become established—and, some say, part of the Establishment. From its third opening until the present, it has enjoyed a time of expansion, improvement and relative peace.

Whether these conditions continue depends, as always, on the Haight-Ashbury. This is particularly true today because its resident population seems to be changing once again. As some of the drug-abusers drift out of the area, their places are apparently being taken by adventurous college students. More black delinquents from the Fillmore ghetto are also frequenting the district, contributing to its heroin problem, though participating in the Drug Treatment Program for the first time. The Neighborhood Council and Merchants' Association still function, but both are demoralized and at a political impasse. In addition, the area is seeing an increased influx of older black families. Because of this, some staff members are urging changes at the Medical and Psychiatric Sections. One faction sees the clinic evolving into a health center for the entire neighborhood and wants to purchase one of the abandoned buildings on Haight Street so that all future programs can be consolidated under one roof. Another argues for more decentralization, de-emphasis of certain activities and/or increased expansion within and without the Haight.

Dr. Matzger, who knows the district intimately, has not yet decided what policy changes will stem from his United States Public Health Service study. However, he does not feel that both 409 and 558 Clayton Street will be different tomorrow from what they are today. "The clinic is at a crossroads," he says. "It may continue as a screening, diagnosis, detoxification and referral unit. It may become an expanded Drug Treatment Program. It may evolve into a large neighborhood health facility, particularly if we get the required dose of federal aid. On the other hand, it may have to cut back on some of the present programs. But whatever happens, it will continue to be an amalgam of individual efforts and an inspiration to people who seek new approaches in community medicine. Furthermore, no matter how the Haight-Ashbury changes, we are certain that the clinic will never close again."

Editors' note: Dr. Matzger's prophecy held true. Federal aid did arrive as a result of the needs of drug addicted Vietnam veterans, and the Haight Ashbury Free Clinics flourished. The clinics now occupy 22 different sites throughout the San Francisco Bay Area and 50,000 patients are seen every year. The Haight Ashbury Free Clinics are the major outpatient treatment provider to the uninsured outsider in the Bay Area. They have stimulated a national free clinic movement and organizations across the country, responding to the growing number of uninsured outsiders in our society. In fact, the American Medical Association has declared that the free clinic movement is an interim solution for the uninsured until a long-term solution can be found. In the political environment of 1996, no long-term solution is yet on the horizon.

Part II

Compound Fracture:
The American Hospital

Past Is Prologue

Rosemary Stevens

Hospitals for the poor and sick have existed since ancient times; the modern hospital is a relatively recent institution. If two factors can be said to define it, they are the presence of round-the-clock skilled nurses and the ability to undertake major surgery. Neither of these was a general feature of American hospitals until at least the 1880s. The first professional nursing schools, based on Florence Nightingale's precepts, were established in 1873 at Bellevue Hospital in New York, the New Haven Hospital, and the Massachusetts General Hospital. Others followed rapidly in the next decade. Many, if not most, of the new hospitals springing up in the burgeoning towns and cities of the late nineteenth century were predicated from the beginning on the integral development of the nursing schools. Through changes in nursing alone the hospital was transformed from the often filthy, disorganized, and terrifying older institutions of the early 1870s into a monument to hope, science, and efficiency.

Total national expenditures on hospital operations for tax-supported and voluntary hospitals in 1903 were estimated to be at least $28.2 million; of this, 43 percent came from charges made to paying patients, 8 percent from tax funds, and the remainder from charitable donations and endowments. American hospitals were already mixed institutions—only partly charitable, increasingly selling their services for a fee. By the mid-1920s middle class people were using hospitals for obstetrics, tonsillectomies, and appendectomies.

Medical science was transformed through two concurrent movements between 1880 and 1914, with effects lasting to the present. The first was the professionalization of American physicians; the second, the discovery and acceptance of the germ theory, giving medicine the confidence that its major justification as a profession was its scientific base. By the late 1880s, when aseptic techniques were replacing antisepsis in the op-

133

erating rooms and in the dressings used on the wards, the idea that disease was borne by specific microscopic organisms—which could be identified, avoided, and destroyed—and, more generally, that disease could be explained, was on the way to revolutionizing the intellectual outlook and practical applications of modern medicine. Surgeons began to wear white gowns in the 1880s. Nurses and other hospital staff wore uniforms, suggesting not only cleanliness but specialized roles and organizational rituals.

Beds were lined up with military precision, sheets were folded into knife edges. Even before World War I there were complaints that the needs of patients as individuals were being subsumed to the demands of hospital organization, a process that would later be called "depersonalization." Patients were expected to conform cooperatively and passively to the cultural expectations of the institution; they were beneficiaries and prisoners of medical expertise.

Surgery became—and has remained—the heart of the American hospital, the most obvious evidence of medicine's success and an emblem of twentieth century American values: science, know-how, the willingness to take risks (on the part of both doctors and patients), decisiveness, organization, and invention. In the 1883 *Transactions of the American Surgical Association,* Samuel Gross, the famous Philadelphia surgeon, expressed the drama of American surgery in the 1880s in words that could be applied to any decade since:

> Progress stares us everywhere in the face. The surgical profession was never so busy as it is at the present moment; never so fruitful in great and beneficient results, or in bold and daring exploits.... Operative surgery challenges the respect and admiration of the world....

Because American hospitals developed as modern institutions at the time they did—largely between 1870 and 1914—they assumed an unusually important function as the embodiment of cultural aspirations. The hospital served both as a modern and an ideal institution, symbolizing the wealth of the new and expanding American cities, the order and glamour of science, the happy conjunction between humanitarianism and expertise in a society rife with money making. It is not coincidental that American hospitals have been among the most luxurious and costly structures ever built. An observer writing about the New York Hospital for *Harpers Magazine* in 1878 described its elevator, which was larger than those of a fashionable hotel, as so smooth in motion that it was like "a mechanical means of getting to heaven."

Demonstration or show, even conspicuous waste, became a lasting aspect of the American hospital as a symbol—one that has as yet received too little attention by social scientists, and one cause of increasing costs. That the modern American hospital is a monument, symbolizing in its architecture and equipment more than its basic function, is apparent not only in the historical literature, but in the lavish style of buildings erected even in time of depression (including those built by the WPA in the 1930s). Another example can be drawn from the early 1960s, when there was enormous public concern about the poor hospital care available in rundown hospitals in inner-city areas. The solutions sought were for rebuilding and major renovating, rather than for the kind of making do in draughty basements that has been a continuing characteristic of British hospital care. Today's hospitals, despite concern about the massive costs of hospital care, are among the most modern, high technology, costly structures being built in modern America. They continue to speak, subtly, to an implied link between cost and expertise.

The hospital was also to symbolize medicine as a vehicle of precision and control. Mastery of diagnosis (understanding the causes and progression of disease) gives a comforting illusion of control to both doctors and patients, even when little effective treatment is available—and for most nonsurgical conditions there was little effective treatment, except good nursing techniques, until the advent of sulfa drugs in the 1930s and antibiotics after World War II. The promise of surgery and of specific remedies against infectious diseases, inherent in major discoveries before World War I, consolidated the image of the doctor as a hero fighting disease with twentieth century tools. The increasing subdivision of medicine into specialties after World War I carried forward this image by placing the greatest emphasis, in terms of prestige and income, on the most heroic interventions. Thus neurosurgery carried greater prestige than psychiatry: radiotherapy than pediatrics.

As a projection of a profession whose archetypes were control, daring, and entrepreneurship, the twentieth century American hospital (along with the medical schools) was always ill-suited to deal with chronic diseases—of which causes were multifactorial and for which medical success was often problematic—and with the collective realms of public health. Even before World War I, hospitals could be criticized for a tendency to view the hospital merely from the inside; that is, from the self-generated perceptions of its Board of Trustees and its physicians. It followed, as S. Goldstein wrote in the 1907 *Charities and the Commons,* that the hospital did "not feel itself an intimate part of the social order: it stands forbiddingly isolated and aloof." The fact that the potential existed, in theory at least, for the hospital to provide health services to the whole population in a defined service district, to compile epidemiological statistics, offer public health education and maternal and child welfare clinics, and to deal with the patient's family as well as with the patient, was to be a source of irritation to generations of disappointed critics.

The success and visibility of the hospital in providing acute, specialized care obscured its relatively limited role in the overall picture of health and disease. Nevertheless, the hospital could be described by the 1920s, as later, as an expression of pessimism, a "negative instrument of evolution," somewhat akin to refuse and sewage disposal, in that it dealt with problems of society rather than with positive solutions. Departments of social work were started in leading hospitals, following the example at the Massachusetts General Hospital in 1905, with the belief that such facilities would help to eradicate the widely held notion that the hospital was an impersonal institution and would help to elucidate the social causes of disease. Social service failed to become the core of community health care efforts for at least three reasons: the concentration of social service work on the poor, who attended outpatient departments with socially unappealing conditions—including venereal diseases, unwed motherhood, and tuberculosis; the lack of fees for social work, making it dependent on charity and on cost shifting from the hospital's paying patients; and the lack of power and the desire by the social workers themselves to become a clinical profession on the medical model, dealing with the psychosocial symptoms of individual patients rather than with community service needs.

American hospitals became successful at marketing acute services to paying patients. Public relations became an acceptable aspect of hospital management in the 1920s, with hospital fairs, radio spots, and even movies extolling the virtues of hospital care. Even in the depths of the depression of the 1930s—with enormous pressures put on local government hospitals, as the unemployed sought free medical care, together with the closing of hundreds of small institutions—most of the income to the hospital industry came from patient fees. In not-for-profit hospitals, the standard bearers for hospital quality in the United States, 71 percent of hospital income came from patients in 1935. The development of Blue Cross insurance plans in the 1930s, commercial hospital insurance in the 1940s, and Medicare in the mid-1960s buttressed the idea of hospital care as acute services, while increasing hospital income. None of these schemes typically included out-of-hospital diagnosis, preventive services, health education, or social services, whereby hospitals could reach out to the community as comprehensive health care centers. There were no financial incentives to override the heroic, specialized medical model for hospital care.

Community Ties

Besides the emerging character of the American hospital as an acute care facility, thriving in a market for paying patients and oriented to both a broader vision of the medical profession and a money-value nexus, the hospital acquired values whose properties were largely mythological— and no less powerful for that. One of the most potent of these values was (and is) the idea of community. Nonfederal acute care hospitals are termed "community hospitals" by the American Hospital Association, irrespective of their location, size or level of care. The term appears to be idiosyncratically American.

Two initial points can readily be made about the notion of the community hospital. First, since hospitals are not community health centers, the term has an ironic ambiguity. Second, the word "community," like the word "voluntary" (long applied to not-for-profit hospitals) has emotive power in a much larger social and political context than the hospital field. Community flexibility stands in contrast to state or national standard-setting; voluntary activity against the implied rigidity of government intervention. Communities suggest creative, local, private activities in America, such as volunteer fire departments, school boards, or the PTA: they are part of American cultural tradition. Part of the attachment of the word "community" to hospitals reflects vague assumptions about the public good. Yet, in three specific ways American hospitals have traditionally had strong community affiliations. First, hospitals have traditionally served communities of interest within local power structures. Second, hospitals have been an important part of the hierarchical organization of the medical profession. Third, hospitals have provided centers for training, employment, and voluntary work for community residents. The combined effect of these patterns has been to define, further, the American hospital as "American."

As major expressions of charitable, social, and economic interests, the hospitals that developed in the late nineteenth and into the twentieth century reflected the segmentation of American society into diverse ethnic, religious, and occupational groups and into defined social classes. Hospitals were both a concrete expression of solidarity and a means of providing training for nurses and doctors in groups likely to be excluded from other institutions (notably, Jewish and black physicians and black nurses). They represented both community successes and community failures. By 1920 America was dotted with hospitals run by hundreds of different private associations, including Roman Catholics, Lutherans, Methodists, Episcopalians, Southern Baptists, Jews, blacks, Swedes, and Germans, depending on the power structures of local populations. Philadelphia, for example, had seventy-one hospitals in 1923, general and specialized; it now has seventy-two. Most were run by not-for-profit associations. Their varied social origins were apparent in names such as Hospital of the University of Pennsylvania (for teaching), Jewish Hospital of Philadelphia, St. Mary's (Roman Catholic), Methodist Episcopal, Frederick Douglass (founded by the black community), and Lankenau (originally a German hospital, the name being changed because of the German role in World War I).

In many areas local governments developed hospitals out of their poorhouses for the indigent. These hospitals, like hospitals under not-for-profit auspices, ranged from tiny units of 25 or fewer beds to enormous barracks-like institutions (Philadelphia General Hospital, run by the city, reported 2,000 beds in the early 1920s). Railroads, lumber companies, and occasionally other corporations built hospitals for their employees. For example in the first decade of the century, the Sante Fe Railroad, which ranged from Chicago to Houston and Galveston and from Sante Fe to San Francisco, could report emergency hospitals for accidents at all its major maintenance shops. These were supported by monthly contributions from employees.

The federal government operated a string of hospitals in seaports and on the major rivers, to care for sick and injured merchant seamen. and developed veterans hospitals after World War I army hospitals served United States camps and forts. An uncounted army of physicians opened their own small hospitals to serve their paying patients, technically on a profit-making basis. In short American hospitals arose concurrently as diverse and multipurpose institutions, serving different clienteles, with different communities of interest, and with a distinctive set of social meanings.

Reflecting patterns of social stratification and discrimination in their local communities, the new hospitals of the early twentieth century were rarely community hospitals in the sense of serving the entire population on an equal basis, even for inpatient care. The city and county hospitals that developed from the old poorhouses, such as Philadelphia General, Bellevue and Kings County in New York, Cook County in Chicago, or San Francisco General, remained institutions primarily for the very poor. When governmental or voluntary hospitals accepted private patients, they were typically housed in separate buildings, in well-furnished private rooms rather than wards, with better food cooked in separate kitchens, and with less restricted visiting hours. Indigence continued to carry the heavy weight of social stigma. even as hospitals were medicalized around progressive scientific ideas.

Until well after World War II, major differences in the patterns of disease treated by public and not-for-profit city hospitals added to the sense of social distinctions. Cleveland City Hospital (with 785 beds) was excluded from a major survey of hospitals in Cleveland in the early 1920s because it treated large groups of patients with tuberculosis, alcoholism, venereal diseases, and contagious diseases that did not appear (because patients with them were not accepted) at any other hospital in the area. Cook County was criticized in the late 1930s, as it has been since, for its poor physical surroundings, overcrowded waiting rooms, patients lying on stretchers in corridors, machinery that does not work, and shortages of even common equipment. In short, American hospitals have never, as a group, served as egalitarian forces in the culture as a whole.

Mirroring the diversity of community structure across the United States, there have also continued to be enormous variations in the relative roles of tax-supported. voluntary, and profit-making hospitals from place to place. In a settled city such as Philadelphia, class differences could be seen even among the poor patients admitted to the Pennsylvania Hospital ("respectable," "deserving" poor) and the city hospital dumping ground for all the rest. However small, governmental hospitals in counties with only one hospital probably always behaved similarly to not-for-profit or

profit-making institutions in the same circumstances—taking in all social classes, with income from paying patients representing the great
majority of their budgets. Such an observation suggests that control of
the hospital may be less important as a distinguishing factor of American institutions than segmentation of hospital services across diverse
social groups. The important variable, for social policy purposes, is not
stratification by ownership but stratification by clientele, a direct reflection of "community" in the 1980s, as in the 1950s and earlier. Relatively
homogeneous communities (as in rural areas or suburbs) are likely to
produce more homogeneous institutions, with less social distance between patients and between staff and patients than, for example, in a
major city teaching hospital, which may attract two kinds of patients—
the relatively rich (on its boards and committees and as private patients
of leading physicians) and the very poor, the traditional recipients of
charity care. Such differences shape differing institutional personalities
for different hospitals and add to the diversity across hospitals in the
United States. The differences have also been sharpened recently, at least
in perception, by the location of investor-owned hospitals in relatively
homogeneous, middle-class areas—suggesting that ownership and social class are necessarily correlated—and by the lack of funding for indigent patients.

The passage of Medicare (for the elderly and disabled) and Medicaid
(for the indigent) in 1965, in a brief period of egalitarianism, was to
indicate that, at least for a short time, everyone—rich, poor, young, and
old—was to be given similar if not identical hospital treatment. The power
of community patterns, as well as cutbacks in Medicaid, were to prove
such optimism unrealistic and short-lived. In retrospect, the egalitarian
expectations for Medicaid appear as an aberration in a long history of
class discrimination in hospital care in the United States. Financially
tottering city and county hospitals remain the dumping grounds for patients no one else will take.

The focus on competition and managerialism of the 1970s-80s has
added a new dimension to the diversity of hospital care across different
communities and classes by sanctioning, on business grounds, the refusal by hospitals to serve patients who cannot pay (either directly or
through insurance, Medicare, or Medicaid). For example, in Pensacola,
Florida, the city turned over the management of its hospital to a profit-
making organization in the 1970s, closed its emergency room and opened

a fee-paying ambulatory center instead. Hospitals can indeed be seen as community institutions, in the broadest sense, reflecting the patterns and priorities of the societies in which they are based—both at the local and national levels.

At the same time, the community of reference for many hospital purposes has expanded beyond the local area, to national and state programs and national consensus-building. Physicians, through the American College of Surgeons, launched a major movement to standardize hospitals around national norms and expectations in 1917–18: the beginnings of hospital accreditation. As Blue Cross plans developed after the 1930s into statewide programs, the definition of hospital care for reimbursement purposes was extended beyond the town or city. Statewide planning of hospital care was initiated at the time of the Hill-Burton Act in 1946, stimulated by federal construction monies provided to the states under that program and further developed through the federal health planning programs in the 1960s and 1970s, and through state certificate-of-need legislation. Medicare provided the force of national regulation and national expectations, while allowing for substantial local service variations. The diagnosis related group (DRG) program can be seen as an extension of national standard-setting through attempts to define and standardize courses of hospital treatment across the United States, for Medicare patients at least.

The courts have also had a role to play in defining national community norms, whether through asserting hospitals' responsibility for the quality of their medical care, requiring racial desegregation, or providing definitions of life and death. In these examples, the term "community" can be seen as divisible into questions of community service, community control, and community consensus. Community still remains a vague concept at best, a cherished aim with ambiguous meanings, constantly to be sought but never to be fully achieved. Its strength may lie in its idea that something should be done at the local level. In this sense the present development of local health care coalitions (of businesses, other groups, or some combination) can be seen as a continuation of a traditional theme.

The development of competing hospital systems sets up new forms of segmentation of hospital service at the local level, threatening the idea of the hospital as part of its local community power structure, or structures. The visibility of groups other than boards of trustees, physicians, and administrators is changing the broader power structure of hospital care. Stockbrokers, fringe benefit managers, business leaders, self-help groups, and unions also have legitimate, often powerful roles to play in hospital development. A 47-day strike against 30 hospitals and 15 nursing homes in New York City in the summer of 1984 affected 18,000 patients and 52,000 workers. A single bond issue can lock a hospital into a pattern of fiscal operation for 30 years, whatever its pattern of ownership may be. The activity of major purchasers of stocks and bonds, including pension funds and insurance companies, affects the availability of capital for hospital development.

In these and other examples, there is a growing array of new communities—vested interests, with diverse purposes, in constant conflict. The idea of a hospital as the embodiment of medical expertise has given way to the exercise of monopoly power by numerous groups. Hospital management and planning become the outcome of a continuing process of bargaining, negotiation, and consensus-building among differing points of view, both inside and outside the institution.

The relationship of the community of doctors to hospitals has also been marked by ambiguity. In comparison with hospitals in most other countries, American physicians have had, and still largely have, a peculiar relationship to medicine's major institution. The typical American physician remains in private, fee-for-service practice, working independently or as a member of a physician group. When the modern hospital developed in the United States, local fee-for-service practitioners volunteered their services in the hospitals, serving charity patients without charging them a fee. The medical profession became, in effect, a volunteer attending staff, since the doctors who admitted patients (and were thus crucial to the financial viability of the hospital with respect to admitting private paying patients) were not employees of the institution. From the hospital's point of view, the physician could be seen as a guest of the institution. To the physician, the hospital was an extension of his or her private practice of medicine.

American hospitals have also developed in large part as open staff institutions—that is, with the expectation that all qualified physicians in a given field ought to have appointments on the attending staff of local institutions. The great majority of all physicians had some kind of hospital attachment by the late 1920s, a pattern that has continued since then. Hospital affiliations have been necessary for many of the most specialized fields. The relationship between physicians and hospitals in America is sharply distinguished, for example, from the system in Great Britain where only salaried specialists typically have hospital affiliations. Although there has been a rapid increase in the number of salaried hospital physicians in American hospitals in the last decade, the formal separation of doctors and hospitals largely continues, requiring new readjustments as hospitals become part of competing systems.

Past and Present

What emerges out of a review of American hospital history is a set of culture-specific characteristics that mark the hospitals as American institutions. These include the segmentation and diversity of ownership of hospitals, the division between hospitals and the medical profession (a division echoed in the separate development of hospital insurance and medical insurance in the United States), the acceptance of social stratification of the patient population both among hospitals and within different institutions the pervasiveness of the pay or commodity ethos in American medicine, and the general expectation that the role of government is necessary but should be limited to filling in gaps in medical care (through programs such as Medicare or Medicaid) and in providing an atmosphere conducive to the development of services in the private sector.

More generally, the fundamental values attached to the hospital industry and its power structures—its communities of interest—are marked by ambiguity. Strauss and his colleagues observed in Freidson's *The Hospital in Modern Society*, of a single hospital in the 1950s, that because its overall goals were unclear, goals were constantly being negotiated within the established order of the institution. It is useful, in the 1980s, to think of this process of goal negotiation as an intrinsic, continuing element of the national hospital system.

Over and above these general observations, three specific themes mark the continuation of hospital history from past to present. First, American hospitals remain segmented in their interests, communities, and control. Second, decision making continues to be diversified: that is, diffused over communities of interest, ranging from the health professions to individual hospital boards, corporate headquarters, government programs and major purchasers of hospital insurance. Third, American hospitals

are expert at adapting very rapidly to explicit external incentives, usually financial incentives.

Where social needs are made explicit (for example, in civil rights legislation or with the passage of Medicare) American hospitals are socially
responsive institutions. Where there is ambivalence or apathy (for example, in providing medical care to the homeless, uninsured, or indigent)
hospitals look to other institutions—notably to government—to meet such
needs, disclaiming the responsibility of being public institutions. In this
respect, too, hospitals can be seen as socially responsive; that is, as reflecting the messages from the broader culture in which they are based.
Lacking a unified hospital or health system, and lacking consensus about
the appropriate philosophy for an American welfare state, American health
policy is marked by skittishness and change.

In the absence of consensus, decisions about hospital policy have been
left to the jockeying of influence among communities of interest. Part of
the uneasiness about high costs and increased profit making in hospital
care derives from a perceived need to develop a national consensus about
hospital policy without resorting either to a government-dominated health
care system or one dominated by a few massive corporations. A high-
cost system is the trade-off for avoiding either of these two extremes.
The present system allows for organizational experimentation and diversity, for avoidance of draconian management decisions (the specter of
rationing) and overt limitations of care for middle-class Americans, and
for accommodation of conflict among reasonable but opposing points of
view. In this sense the hospital system can be described in terms of con-
structive ambiguity. To those struggling with their implications, rapid
changes cry out for simple theories of explanation and simple solutions.
DRGs became the solution to the rising cost of hospital care in the 1980s,
just as Medicaid was the apparent answer, in the late 1960s, to bringing
the poor into the "mainstream of medicine."

The hospital system can be seen as analogous to the development of
other industries; for example, consolidation of the manufacturing industry at the beginning of the twentieth century, which again followed the
consolidation of the railroads. Under this model, hospitals are small firms
which will inevitably move toward industrial consolidation (and which
may have been held back by the monopoly interests of the medical profession). Such analogies beg the question of whether hospitals are legiti-
mately businesses, and, if so, what does this mean. How far hospital

service may be appropriately compared to manufacturing is another question that demands elucidation; indeed, whether any service industry can be appropriately compared to any manufacturing industry is an important question. The urge for simple explanations remains. Meanwhile, there are those who claim that profit making in health services is ethically wrong and socially dangerous, while others are more concerned that medicine is rapidly being dominated by a "medical-industrial complex" in which the traditional rights of doctors and patients will be swamped by the coming of the monolithic "corporation."

The search for simple theories and the "one best way" of doing things ignores the fact that organizational life in the late twentieth century is messy and complex. Decisions have to be taken in a climate of conflict and negotiation, whether we are speaking of hospitals, factories, government, or schools. Hospitals, like other institutions, carry with them the burdens and potential of their history.

The Business of Childbirth

Jeanne Guillemin and Lynda Lytle Holmstrom

The idea that health care should be left to competitive market forces presumes a good deal about the behavior of ordinary people; it presumes very little about institutional constraints on that behavior. Prospective patients are expected to act like rational consumers, choosing judiciously among a variety of health insurance options, medical professionals, and hospital services. In this way, according to economists such as Alain Entoven, health-minded citizens might think more about early and less costly medical intervention and consequently reduce costly catastrophic medical needs. Yet today the options available for preventing catastrophic medical needs are not readily available and, in the present competitive marketplace phase of hospital care, they show few signs of emerging. In the best of all possible worlds, with 100 percent employment and full insurance coverage for the elderly and disabled, health care could become a buyer's market. Our present situation is characterized by strictly limited alternatives, few of which encourage preventive health care. First, noninsured and underinsured patients have haphazard access to medical care. Many take what they can get: public clinics, public hospitals, or emergency wards. Second, many fully insured patients now confront a health system geared for medical catastrophes rather than their prevention. These restraints apply especially to the area of reproductive medicine, in which many medical problems are exacerbated either by too little health care or too much.

Hospitals, especially major medical centers, have recently discovered that the high technology treatment of mothers and newborns is good business. In part this is because new technologies have been developed and also because invasive acute care has become the accepted American solution to most reproductive problems—from infertility to fetal defects, prolonged labor, and problems of the newborn.

In the United States, the prevention of delivery room disasters—in the form of educational programs, media campaigns, and universal prenatal care—is generally shunned. This is so despite the fact that other industrialized nations and pilot projects within our own country have shown these strategies to be cost effective and beneficial to mothers and infants, especially in the prevention of premature birth, the principle cause of death among newborns. Instead, high technology is now an integral and routine part of giving birth in the United States. Although the home birth movement has been successful in certain communities, nearly all American women give birth in well-equipped hospitals where fetal monitoring, cesarean deliveries, and intensive care for newborns have in recent years become commonplace. In the state of Massachusetts, for example, the cesarean delivery rate is over 20 percent, with no discernible difference between large teaching hospitals and community facilities. This trend is part of a national move toward surgical delivery that has, in the last fifteen years, more than doubled the cesarean rates in the United States, from 8 to 18 percent, with no appreciable improvement in infant health and with some risk to women. Once the decision is made to give birth in a hospital, it is difficult to avoid the complexity of medical technologies routinely used to monitor and solve problems of labor and delivery.

As a further embellishment, large teaching hospitals have developed over the last twenty years an extraordinary capacity to treat critically ill, usually premature, infants. During this time, newborn intensive care has grown from an experimental venture to a complex hospital service for approximately 300,000 infants a year. Its development is in large part a function of institutional capitalization on medical catastrophes, especially prematurity but also birth defects and accidental injuries.

Ideal Patients

From the perspective of hospital economics, any high-use (that is, major surgical or intensive care) patient guarantees good revenues if the patient is fully insured. Short-term, high-use patients are especially attractive when the insurance coverage decreases as the patient's hospital stay lengthens, as can happen with Medicaid and other coverage. Such patients are also desirable when the demand for intensive care beds is consistently high. Once an intensive care unit is developed, the rapid flow of high-cost patients brings a good return on the investment. Even with just standard diagnostic and operating facilities, pregnant women are potentially ideal patients for hospitals to cultivate. Women receiving prenatal care in this country are increasingly prone to batteries of sophisticated tests, particularly ultrasonography. Most women who have cesarean deliveries leave the hospital in a few days, with bills of $2,000 or more. The procedure is major surgery, but obstetricians commonly claim that improvements in surgical techniques and antibiotics allow an early safe discharge of the patient.

Newborns with medical problems represent even greater possibilities. Hospital-born infants begin life as patients and are highly available for referral. In a typical maximum care (Level III) nursery, 30 percent of referred patients are discharged within a week, with anywhere from 15 to 30 percent having died. Even that single week of care can generate large bills. The bed rate for Level 111 nurseries runs from $500 to $800 per day. Many tests are performed daily, and new therapies, adapted from adult medicine, have been perfected for the small premature infants who are the major recipients of intensive care. According to a long range study at the University of California, San Francisco, Hospital, medical care of newborns has shown the most dramatic rise in the decade 1972-82 in hospital expenses of any service, adult or pediatric. In 1982, the average cost for an infant with Respiratory Distress Syndrome, a major symptom of prematurity, was $35,988. Premature infants having surgery had costs averaging $85,368.

If all this medical management were truly necessary, the survival of Homo Sapiens thus far without it would be a mystery—but there is no mystery. What we are seeing today is a change in physician standards of clinical treatment, a movement toward greater involvement in hospital-based technology and, consequently, a dependence on that technology. The national rise in cesarean delivery rates, for example, tells us not that women are reproductively more incompetent than previously (although they might feel that way after the surgery), but that modern specialists have a single radical solution for resolving a diversity of problems. Sometimes the problem is unambiguously medical and serious, as when a fetus is in clear distress and cannot be delivered vaginally. At other times, a cesarean is performed only because the mother has had one previously, not because the procedure is medically indicated. A 1981 National Institutes of Health report cited the mistaken belief "once a cesarean. always a cesarean" as a prime cause of the recent rate increase and advised practitioners to choose natural labor over the automatic repeat cesarean. Between clear indications for surgery and unnecessary surgery lie many and complex reasons obstetricians perform so many of these operations. At the heart of the trend is a fear of injury to the newborn that prompts practitioners to turn to the ultimate solution, surgical invasion. This same overriding sense of concern for the newborn has fueled the expansion of medical intervention for the neonate (the infant in the first month of life).

A heightened sense of risk surrounds pregnancy and childbirth. Among educated working couples who are planning to have a child, hospital birth providing state-of-the-art technological backup is a hedge against potential catastrophes, especially to the vulnerable infant. Since the choice of a single child is currently considered sufficient to experience parenting, the modern, relatively affluent couple is indeed at high risk. Although by socioeconomic criteria, the women from this group should be in good health and not need much medical intervention, they have excellent access to specialized medicine and appear receptive to the benefits it promises. Educated and professional women receive more concerted prenatal care and are more likely to have cesarean surgery than most other women. The elaboration of reproductive medical options, from fetal surgery through newborn intensive care, can be interpreted as insurance against catastrophes for parents worried about damage to their only child.

The same sense of childbirth risks is evident in other Western industrialized countries in which prenatal and postnatal care are covered by comprehensive health insurance. In France, educated professional women have unusually high rates of cesarean birth. In the Netherlands, where home births account for just under a third of all deliveries, educated, relatively affluent women pay extra to have their infants in hospitals and generally leave the day after childbirth.

Protective Sentiments

The protective sentiments of parents are a major dynamic in promoting childbirth technologies. Hospitals provide what parents want, but a main feature of newborn intensive care is that many mothers and fathers are unlikely to know about its enormous capacity and its limits. While most newborns referred to a newborn intensive care unit (NICU) will recover quickly, very premature infants may either have their dying prolonged or survive with severe impairment. As the economist Victor Fuchs has warned, calculating an acceptable margin of error in childbirth—what intervention to accept or reject—is virtually impossible to do rationally at the moment of crisis. To choose against intervention can entail a surrender of the altruism that parents want to express; that sentiment fairly demands exploration of every possibility even in cases of desperation. Crisis decision making can also draw on the spirit of sacrifice that is a mainstay of parenting, but not necessarily in the patient's interest. Given a choice between the risks of major surgery for herself and the remotest chance of asphyxia for her newborn, what woman will hesitate to choose cesarean delivery? Given the choice between not referring a two-pound newborn to intensive care and having a platoon of physicians and nurses labor heroically to save this infant's life, what parents would deny permission to treat? The entire emergency and radical intervention atmosphere commonly attached to the event of childbirth can hinder parents and possibly practitioners as well from reflecting on medical choices in a balanced way. There are some risks, for example, to infants delivered by cesarean and a probable underestimation of mortality and morbidity for women on whom this major surgery is performed. There are also some infants, for instance those born weighing less than 800 grams, for whom the chance of survival is practically zero and the chance of normal development among survivors very poor, no matter what medical care is given.

The real test of parental sentiment is not in the NICU but later, when a premature infant comes home. Studies show that graduates of intensive care, especially those who have been hospital patients for months, take time to adjust to normal parenting. Many are not used to human touch or have learned to associate it with pain because they were frequently subjected to blood tests, tube insertions, and the surgical placement of lines. Much worse than an irritable infant is the newborn whose medical needs—such as oxygen therapy, special feeding, and antibiotics—must be attended to around-the-clock even after hospital discharge. Worst of all is the infant whose problems will never be resolved. These include children with permanent lung damage, deafness, and cerebral palsy. The burdens on parents are financial as well as emotional and physical. The costs of home care, rehabilitation, and institutional care, to say nothing of repeated hospital and medical services, are not by any means fully reimbursed to the parents of children with these needs. Rather than providing certain protection against risks, the new childbirth technologies bring parents another risk, namely the survival of a troubled child.

Other Patients

In addition to the prospective mothers who are calculating the risks of delivery room disasters and hedging their bets with medical intervention, others with few advantages receive a great proportion of emergency and intensive care hospital services. Women in the United States who are nonwhite, have little education, and are in their teens often receive unplanned acute care in the delivery room because they and their infants are at actual rather than feared medical risk. Pregnant women from this group often have their first (and last) prenatal examination in the emergency ward, just prior to a cesarean delivery. A recent report from the Institutes of Medicine tells us that among all women of reproductive age in this country, mothers from this group are most likely to be without medical or hospital coverage. At the same time they are most likely to have newborns who are seriously premature and at highest risk of permanent damage and death. Their choices about delivery room and postnatal medical intervention are especially problematic because almost nothing, including conception, has been planned. Hospital and professional norms are frequently imposed on decisions to operate on this population of women and to refer and to intensify treatment of their infants. Unlike privately insured women, this group may be economically undesirable to the extent that Medicaid and other public assistance fails, as it often does, to cover hospital costs fully and forces the use of charity funds or the acquisition of deficits. When hospitals plan to market perinatal or birthing centers, uninsured and underinsured women are not the intended clients.

These are the two core populations most affected by childbirth technologies: those who actively plan hospitalized childbirth and those who do not. In addition. their children also become patients in the hospital system.

Inventing the Infant Patient

Currently the service of intensive care for newborns is so extensive (about 700 major centers nationally, with hundreds more intermediate care units) that a great diversity of parents have had the experience of watching their infant disappear in an ambulance headed for a central hospital. Or they have been notified that their newborn has been taken from one nursery to another and connected to monitors, an intravenous line, and a respirator. Medical investment in childbirth technologies has resulted in the remarkable invention of a new patient, the neonate. Thirty years ago, the body of a newborn infant was a mystery. As William Silverman describes the early years of neonatal medicine, the field was full of experimental pitfalls and dead-ends. Infants born very prematurely or with major defects were often set aside to die or categorized as stillbirths. The identity of the newborn was, as far as institutional records were concerned, barely distinguishable from that of the mother. Today, there is hardly a therapy, from mechanical respiration to kidney dialysis to brain surgery that has not been adapted to newborn physiology, including the needs of very small premature infants. These innovations mean that a newborn can be perceived by physicians and by parents as an insolable patient with the same right to medical care as an adult. The total dependence of the infant on parents becomes, in the hospital context, a secondary issue when choices about medical treatment must be made, just as family matters are presumed essentially irrelevant in the treatment of adults. An adult patient with no loving spouse at home to continue postoperative care is not denied surgery in favor of a patient with a caring spouse. Similarly, the newborn infant is now perceived as a person with potential autonomy and actual civil rights, regardless of parental attitudes. This idea of autonomy extends as well to the fetus and parallels investigations in fetal medicine. While anti-abortionists lobby for a constitutional amendment to protect the fetus from the moment of conception, physicians are perfecting the sequence of removing a defective fetus from the uterus, surgically correcting the defect (for example, hydrocephalous), and replacing the fetus in the mother's body.

As is often the presumption in adult medical care, the denial of medical treatment has been repeatedly put forth as the greatest danger to the newborn. The current federal Baby Doe regulation, for instance, threatens to cut off funding for those hospitals whose physicians withhold or withdraw treatment from any newborn and especially those with birth defects (referred to as disabilities). The regulation allows nontreatment only for infants clearly "born dying" or in a state of irreversible coma, in short, for hopeless cases.

Ironically, this focus on medical neglect comes at a time when neonatology has expanded the kinds and numbers of treatable newborn cases. Especially important is the clinical drive to treat smaller and smaller premature infants. There would have been little expansion of newborn intensive care over the last ten years without the publication of several reports about improved prognosis for infants born weighing less than 1500 grams. Until around 1973, there was little enthusiasm among obstetricians for referring these infants to a special care nursery because their prognosis for survival was not good. At about this time, experimental use of oxygen therapy for newborns in this birth weight range, 1200 to 1500 grams, proved successful insofar as most infants survived. Generated by several teaching hospitals, the studies reporting these successes were based on small samples, as few as a dozen cases. Yet they gave license to other pediatricians in major medical centers to treat very premature infants with respirator therapy and intravenous feeding. The survival rates, as far as we know, did improve and gave obstetricians greater confidence in referring newborns to intensive care. As these more fragile infants have become routine referrals, the NICU technology has become geared to their needs and to the needs of even smaller and more experimental cases. In the same way, progress in the surgical treatment of spina bifida, brain hemorrhages, heart defects, and other more unusual infant problems are widely heralded in professional journals and in the media.

Structuring the System

The recognition that mothers and newborns are potential consumers of advanced hospital technology is best evidenced in the growth of regional centers that coordinate childbirth technologies. The newest version of these service packages is the perinatal center that combines childbirth in a community hospital with access to a Level III NICU in a central hospital. The idea is to persuade local obstetricians and their patients that quality care means quality emergency services. The community hospital promises a choice of delivery rooms. One is designed to look like a standard American bedroom, softly lit and pleasantly decorated. The other is stark and technical and signals the readiness of medical intervention. Even the bedroom-type birthing room is only minutes away from the operating room. The custom in many hospitals seeking to attract prospective parents is that a free champagne celebration comes with the service. In addition, rapid access to a Level III nursery is assured if the newborn should have an emergency medical problem. In this way, maternity beds in the smaller hospital are filled while a certain volume of infant patients is directed to the high-level nursery.

The success of any perinatal center is directly determined by, first, good relations between obstetricians and neonatologists and, second, the belief of parents and practitioners in the efficiency of centralizing hospital resources in large regional centers. Obstetricians, who now handle more than 80 percent of births in this country, are more frequently sued and pay higher malpractice insurance rates than any other specialists. They are bound to be concerned with liabilities and, especially with the new Baby Doe regulation in effect, are under great pressure to insure the best treatment for all newborns, regardless of condition. The state-of-the-art technology and resources available in a Level III nursery is good protection against anyone—parents, state child abuse officials, federal agents. or special interest groups—who might want to take legal action against a private practitioner.

Neonatologists, in turn, depend on obstetricians for referrals and in general have no vested interest in imposing admission standards that would restrict case volume. To the contrary, many maximum care nurseries represent themselves as moving progressively toward even greater success than the survival of the 1200-gram newborn. Newborns of 600 and 700 grams are not unusual patients in the Level III nursery. Neonatologists with a sense of mission envision the 500-gram infant as a frontier case which, with improved techniques, might be made to survive outside the uterus. While no NICU staff wants to admit hopeless cases—that is, infants born dying—the spirit of progress extends to every newborn.

Not only technology but expertise defines the value of a newborn intensive care service. The physician/patient ratio is often one to five because NICUs are usually located in teaching hospitals and rely heavily on residents to provide around-the-clock bedside care. The nurse/ patient ratio is often one to three. The regional NICU will also have a retinue of consulting physicians, perhaps the most prestigious being the pediatric surgeon who is willing to operate on very small patients.

Along with professional interdependence, newborn intensive care has developed because of a widespread belief in centralization or regionalization in hospital services. If one model of the perinatal center is a constellation of community hospitals that refer newborns to a regional NICU, another is the equally regionalized major medical center which provides both high technology maternity care and the Level III nursery. Fifteen years ago there was nothing less profitable than a maternity bed in a community hospital; most women giving birth needed little medical attention or only minor intervention. A declining birth rate seemed to depress the market. At this time, many community hospitals began closing down maternity wards and the argument for centralized childbirth facilities began to be heard and acted upon on a national level. The reasoning was that it was more efficient for prospective mothers to come to a central source of medical care than for small hospitals to bear the burden of unprofitable beds. High volume would offset the drawback of supporting maternity beds in central hospitals. Few people foresaw that childbirth itself—possibly because of the shift to more central, high technology hospitals—would become medicalized and be seen in a new economic light.

The argument for the efficiency of regional newborn intensive care centers was even easier to make. Why should community hospitals duplicate costly technology and skilled personnel that could be centrally located? Newborns with acute medical needs could be more efficiently transported to the central hospital.

Diminishing Role of Parents

In retrospect, the regionalization of childbirth technologies has had important unpredicted costs. The ballooning of surgical costs was not predicted. Also unpredicted were the experimental forays to save extremely premature infants, who when they survive can cost in the six figures for just the first months of life. The long-range costs of handicapped survivors have yet to be rationally calculated.

Some costs have been more than financial. One is the problem of separating parents and newborns. The critically ill infant can become so well integrated into the hospital system that parents are virtually denied their proper role as guardians of the newborn's interests. Geographic separation is one part of the problem. The Level III nursery itself can exclude parents on the basis of its intimidating atmosphere. Under pressure to provide emergency care to a constant flow of small patients, the NICU is ordinarily not communicative with parents. Even with long-term patients, the typical staff is oriented to the infant as a patient, not as anyone's child. Important medical decisions tend to be made first by physicians and then presented to parents as ultimatums.

There are other signs that parents have diminished control over the new childbirth technologies and consequently over their children and family life. For the pregnant woman, the issue can be control over her own body. The increasing number of court-ordered cesareans is one indication of this trend. There is also debate over whether a pregnant women defined by a physician as abusive to the fetus should be legally restrained. In a recent Hastings Center Report, the case was presented of an insulin-dependent woman in her third pregnancy who refused special treatment and, hospitalized after a threatened miscarriage at twenty-one weeks, wants to return home. Is her physician justified in seeking a court order? From one point of view, the risks of birth defects to infants of diabetic women mandate careful medical management and enforced hospital treatment. But, as Barbara Katz Rothman pointed out, two presumptions supporting this position are not warranted. One is that the history of success in obstetrics is so good that all statements about the well-being of the fetus can be taken as authoritative. Twenty-five years ago the woman who refused her DES treatment, disdained diuretics, and gained more than thirteen pounds might, by current ethical standards, be liable for criminal action for endangering her unborn child. By current medical standards, she probably saved the child's life by defying her physician's orders. The other presumption is that a pregnant woman is just a vessel for the precious infant, the means to the end of reproduction. In present medical parlance, women are referred to as "the maternal environment" rather than as human beings.

The history of medical care for women is unfortunately full of episodes of unnecessary and even barbaric therapies. Today the emphasis is not on clitoral excision, hysterectomies or even radical breast surgery, but directly on childbirth, on human reproduction. This means, as childbirth is medicalized, that fathers as well have reduced control over what will happen to their children. If parents have only a rudimentary idea of the causes of their newborn's illness and only a rudimentary notion of the benefits and drawbacks of therapy, they cannot exercise their responsibility as guardians of the child's interests. This is all too frequently the situation that obtains in newborn intensive care.

The loss of parental advocacy at the infant's bedside would be little cause for concern if medicine could offer miracles. Then neonatologists would succeed in what they try to do, give parents back healthy, normal infants. In many cases, the infants discharged from the NICU are just that, if their birth weight was not too low or if their defects were minor. For infants in the more experimental birth weight categories, the uncertainties about outcome are serious. Even more to the point, physicians and other nursery staff members have few incentives to tell parents about these uncertainties. This part of the perinatal package is based on referrals, not on the personal cultivation of parents as clients. Most parents and their treated infants are not seen again by the nursery staff. If the children have medical needs, they will probably be addressed in some other hospital, by some other physician. The personal experience of knowing the parents and seeing how the families fare is a less serious deficiency than clinicians' present ignorance of the medical condition of previous patients. The regional system is so complex that even finding former NICU infants for follow-up studies is a dilemma. Instead, neonatologists are forced to rely on immediate diagnostic feedback to gauge the efficacy of treatment. To counteract the most subjective interpretations, some published studies inform neonatologists of the general odds that govern treatment. For example, a Rhode Island report on 247 infants weighing between 500 and 999 grams at birth states that the overall mortality rate was 68 percent, with 26 percent of the survivors showing, between the first and fifth years, moderate to serious impairment. By the standards in adult medicine, these cases would be experimental. Yet knowing the odds, most practitioners would continue to treat with maximum care because they are willing to take the chance. The chance they think of is the death of the newborn, a clinical failure, rather than the infant's long-term survival with injuries.

If parents are summarily excluded from crucial decisions affecting the newborn patient, the risk to the infant is that impersonal and routine hospital norms will govern that treatment—and not always in the patient's interest. This pitfall is exactly the problem that the Baby Doe regulation, for better or worse, is intended to remedy. Among its strongest advocates are representatives of the disabled who are conscious of the peril to Down's syndrome infants with surgically correctable defects and to spina bifida newborns whose parents tell physicians not to treat these physically imperfect patients. If these infants potentially are in jeopardy, it is also possible that very premature infants can be subject to abuse by overtreatment, not particularly because parents seek aggressive medical care but because professionals and institutions proceed automatically without reference to the family. Parents. since they are legally responsible for their child, should be informed of the experimental nature of the treatment. Even better, since Level III units are not likely to lose their impersonal aura, routine treatment of such small infants should be governed by scientific protocols that make physicians responsible for defining and reporting on the goals of their work.

Redefining Perinatal Care

The increased use of childbirth technologies relies on their emergency care emphasis. Maximum medical intervention is justified because certain awful things might happen to the infant. This heightened sense of childbirth risks has defined United States perinatal care as addressing only what happens just before and just after delivery. In other industrialized countries, the term has a different meaning, one that covers prenatal visits as well as postnatal, at-home medical attention for the mother and infant.

Expanding the connotation of time in perinatal programs would help redefine the curative approach now taken to important problems such as premature birth. In the last thirty years there has been only a slight decrease in the proportion of low birth weight infants born in this country, from 7.5 to 7.0 percent. Instead of attacking this problem only after it occurs, a recent Institutes of Medicine (IOM) report reviews the literature and strongly advises universal prenatal care as a way of combating premature births, which is the same as combating infant mortality.

If this advice, which is not new, is unpopular, it is not simply because Americans apply to their infants the same belief in miracle technologies that motivates adult medicine. Poverty and racism are intrinsic parts of the prematurity/infant mortality problem. For the years 1977 through 1979, for example, there was a dramatic difference between the health and survival chances of white and black newborns. The national infant mortality rate was 13.6 per 1000 live births. For white infants, the rate was 11.9, and for black infants, 22.8. Black infants accounted for 16.5 percent of all live births in these years, but for 30 percent of all low birth weight deliveries and 34 percent of very low birth weight infants (1500 grams or less). As the IOM report made clear, economically disadvantaged and nonwhite women, the same women liable to be uninsured or underinsured for childbirth, are most likely to have premature infants.

If the heavy investment in costly childbirth technologies continues, the two-tiered system emerging will not decrease rates of premature births. Its effect may be to turn perinatal centers into luxury services which refuse Medicaid and indigent patients and thereby selectively increase neonatal and infant mortality rates. Unwanted patients, mothers and infants, would get standard public hospital care which might become a synonym for minimal medical intervention. This change could also mean that if severely damaged infants from lower-class and black families are not turned into inmates of chronic care institutions, neither are the only moderately premature newborns given the benefit of intensive care. While more affluent, privately insured parents can afford prenatal care, utilize the maximum hospital technology, and enjoy options eventually to become powerful advocates for their infants, other parents at higher medical risk will be even less able to help themselves or their children.

The mixed blessings associated with childbirth technologies and newborn intensive care in particular affect the entire discussion of access to hospital care for women and infants. Are the more extreme experiments being conducted in the name of clinical problem solving an actual benefit for those patients? Are invasive therapies an unmitigated good for large proportions of pregnant women and infants? It is access to prenatal care that distinguishes privileged women from disadvantaged women. That kind of medical attention seldom demands specialists' services or hospital resources, nor does it require that women's bodies be envisioned as passive vehicles for the fetus. Prevention in this area offers none of the incentives—professional, institutional. or cultural—that insure the current success of the hospital high technology approach to human reproduction.

Silent Knife:
Cesarean Section in the United States

Nancy Wainer Cohen and Lois J. Estner

The cesarean delivery rate in the United States has reached epidemic proportions. We know that statistics do not make exciting reading, but the facts and figures speak for themselves, and what they have to say is appalling.

The fact is that America has fallen in love with machines, computers, tools, and gadgets. We have not yet entered an era of computerized childbirth, but it is surely not far off. In the meantime, the birthing stage is set with mechanized props that turn a warm, human, natural event into a cold, impersonal performance. We see the cesarean knife as the ultimate symbol of technocratic interference in the process of childbirth.

The "silent knife" is carving a new image of childbirth in our country. Having long ago defined birth as a medical event, America is now on the threshold of accepting it also as a surgical event. As we tolerate one invasive procedure after another in the birthing rooms of our land, we lose our horror of the knife; indeed, we sometimes welcome surgical delivery as the end to a poorly managed labor. Many cesarean mothers describe an initial feeling of relief when the "need" for a cesarean is discovered; surgery provides an escape from the tortures of the hospital labor room.

According to Robbi Pfeuffer's "The Hazards of Hospital Childbirth," the number of invasive procedures used in hospital deliveries "increases every year." They now include placing the woman flat on her back, restricting her food intake, artificially inducing or stimulating her labor,

---

Reprinted from *Silent Knife: Cesarean Prevention and Vaginal Birth after Cesarean* by permission of Bergin & Garvey Publishers.

rupturing her amniotic membranes, routinely using intravenous fluids, analgesia, anesthesia, electronic fetal monitors, episiotomies and forceps, and routinely separating mothers from their babies. "Routine cesarean section might also be added," Pfeuffer notes, "for in one Boston teaching hospital, one out of every four babies is born by cesarean section."

That figure is outrageous, but, regrettably, it is not atypical. One out of every four babies is born by cesarean section in New York City, too; and the 1979 Massachusetts Health Department statistics listed seven Boston area hospitals with cesarean rates over 25 per cent, one with a rate of over 30 percent! We have heard rumors of physicians with 80-100 percent cesarean rates. It becomes hard to remember that as recently as 1968, the overall cesarean-section rate in the United States was 5 percent, a rate deemed normal by generations of obstetric and nursing textbooks, although a bit high by us. If we (reluctantly) accept a 4 to 5 percent cesarean section rate as "normal," then it is clear that over 80 percent of today's cesareans are an unnecessary surgical intervention! Perhaps we need to take a look at who is doing the intervening.

In "Unnecessary Cesareans: Doctor's Choice, Parent's Dilemma," Susan G. Doering reminds us that until quite recently, "one could judge a physician by his section rate: the lower it was, the better obstetrician he must be." She recalls Kroener's statement:

> One of the long held principles of obstetrics has been that the cesarean section rate was inversely proportional to the quality of obstetrics practiced. Any physician with a high section rate was evaluated for the quality of his obstetric care and accused of trying to pad his financial remuneration.

As an example of that bygone philosophy, Doering describes the "stress and concern" of a group of Los Angeles physicians who, in 1956, were placed on probationary status by the Joint Committee on Accreditation because their hospital section rate was almost 10 percent. Doering's remark that "things have changed a lot since 1956" is an understatement. Now it almost seems that physicians and hospitals pride themselves on their high cesarean rates, and that high rates are considered synonymous with good obstetric care.

Let us contrast those distressed, concerned Los Angeles physicians with Dr. John Sutherst and Dr. Barbara Case, writing in the April 1975 issue of a British journal, and quoted by Gena Corea: "It may well be that during the next 40 years *the allowing* of a vaginal delivery or attempted vaginal delivery may need to be justified in each particular instance" (our emphasis). When a physician is able even to contemplate such a trend, it becomes apparent that the medical profession is no longer holding itself accountable for its excesses; that, as *Williams Obstetrics* notes, "in modern obstetric practice, there are virtually no contraindictions for cesarean section. "

This complacent attitude is reflected in the skyrocketing cesarean rate. Between 1970 and 1978, the cesarean birth rate in the United States increased about threefold, from 5.5 percent to 15.2 percent, an almost 200 percent increase. In 1979, officials at the National Institute of Child Health and Human Development (NIH) became concerned about the rising cesarean delivery rate in the nation and decided to hold a consensus development conference on cesarean childbirth. A nineteen-member task force was appointed to gather and analyze data for a preliminary draft report. By the time the conference convened in September 1980, the cesarean-section rate in the United States had reached 18 percent, with northeastern states such as New York and Massachusetts running consistently ahead of the national norm. This translates into approximately 14,850 cesareans in Massachusetts and 647,640 cesareans in the country, in 1980 alone.

The regional variation in cesarean rates can be seen on a smaller scale in the rate differences among doctors and hospitals. Diony Young and Charles Mahan, authors of *Unnecessary Cesareans: Ways to Avoid Them*, remark that factors such as age, medical training, personal attitudes, habit, location, style of practice, availability of facilities and personnel, financial incentives, and convenience affect the differences among individual physicians. Among individual hospitals, factors such as hospital size and number of beds influence the rate, with more cesareans occurring in the larger hospitals. Additionally, the rate of cesareans is higher in teaching than in nonteaching hospitals. Young and Mahan caution that "an unusually high physician or hospital rate may indicate that the physician or hospital is receiving referrals for complicated pregnancies that require cesarean section." Then again, it may not.

The trend toward rising cesarean rates is "pervasive," according to the NIH conference report, "affecting hospitals and patients in all parts of the country [and] is also evident internationally." But at twice the British rate and approximately four times the West European average, the United States has by far the highest rates. With 98 percent of cesarean mothers in the United States opting for repeat surgical deliveries in subsequent pregnancies, it is likely that things will get much worse before they get better—unless we, as consumers, begin to exercise our rights and make demands for change. Now.

What has happened to childbirth in America? How have we allowed cesarean section to become an acceptable alternative to vaginal birth? Why did we relinquish our rights as healthy, normal birthing women and join the johnnied ranks of ailing hospital patients? When did we start believing that surgical delivery is safer and better for our babies? These questions and more must be answered before we can even hope to bring the cesarean epidemic under control. Let's start at the beginning.

Legend has it that Julius Caesar was born by cesarean section and that the procedure was named after him. It is more likely that the name of the operation comes from the *lex caesaria* of Roman law, which required that abdominal surgery be performed on a dead or dying woman in a late stage of pregnancy to save her baby for the state. It may also come from the Latin *caedere,* to cut.

In any case, we know from early mythological references and ancient folklore that surgical delivery has been practiced for centuries. It was first performed to provide a separate burial for the fetus of a dead mother, then to extract a living baby from a dead mother in an effort to save it. Not until the sixteenth century was the surgery performed with the intent to save both mother and baby.

The first cesarean sections in America probably occurred in the late 1700s or early 1800s. The death rate for both cesarean mother and baby was quite high, as uterine suture was not yet practiced, and the importance of sterile techniques had not yet been recognized. In 1882, when Adolf Kehrer and Max Sanger closed the wound of the uterus with silk sutures, the most important advance in cesarean surgery was made.

It was not until the late nineteenth century that reports of cesareans became common, and the early 1900s brought the first hospital records of cesarean deliveries. In 1916, when Dr. Craigin originated the phrase "Once a cesarean, always a cesarean," surgical delivery was still a very conservative procedure done for an absolute contracted pelvis, a recurring condition. By the 1930s, hospital was replacing home as the place to give birth, making surgical delivery a more convenient option and allowing it to become an alternative to high- and mid-forceps on the impacted fetus. With the advent of sterile technique, improved operating methods and anesthesia, and the availability of blood and antibiotics, the risks of cesarean surgery were greatly reduced. Still, the cesarean rate remained fairly stable.

Until the 1960s, hospital birth usually meant delivery under general anesthesia and a lengthy hospital stay, whether delivery was vaginal or abdominal. Then the "back to nature" movement of the sixties made women realize how far from nature hospital childbirth practices had strayed, and the resurgence of the women's movement gave them a strong voice with which to be heard. Maternity care, responding to consumer demand, began to undergo remarkable changes. Childbirth preparation and regional anesthesia allowed women to experience consciously the births of their children, and they insisted that their husbands be made partners in the experience. Maternity care in many of the larger hospitals became family-centered, with baby rooming in and siblings coming to visit. By the early 1970s, childbirth environments and practices had begun to be humanized in response to the demands of childbearing families. Each forward step for natural childbirth, however, took the cesarean experience, by contrast, a leap behind. Ironically, it was just at this very time that cesarean birthrate began to soar.

So Many Reasons Why

While consumer groups worked to humanize and naturalize the childbirth experience, medical groups were working to eliminate the risks of childbirth to mother and baby. On the surface, it would seem that the two groups would be united in a joint effort, with the potential for phenomenal results. At closer look, however, we see that the new drugs, machines, and procedures espoused by the physicians are often counterproductive and result in more complications than they are intended to prevent. Moreover, the benefits and safety of this "new obstetrics" have yet to be proved.

In *An Evaluation of Cesarean Section in the United States,* her 1979 report to the Department of Health, Education, and Welfare, Dr. Helen Marieskind identifies in order of significance twelve factors that contribute to the burgeoning rate of operative deliveries. We would like to present them here in some detail.

Threat of malpractice suits is the most frequent reason given for the increase. Doctors are concerned about the threat of malpractice suits if a cesarean is not performed and the outcome is a "less than perfect baby." Many physicians feel pressured to practice "defensive medicine" in order to be "covered" if they "produce" a defective infant. They feel that if they have performed a cesarean, they have done everything they can. When questioned, physicians freely agreed off the record that fear of a suit prompted cesareans and that this is commonly discussed among colleagues. Few, however, know of a colleague who has been sued. One obstetrician said that fear of malpractice suits rather than medical criteria is the reason for the rise. Upon examination of data from insurance claims, it is not clear that the threat of malpractice suits for failure to perform a cesarean justifies the rapid increase in cesarean deliveries. However, obstetricians feel "at risk."

The policy of "Once a cesarean, always a cesarean" has become standard obstetrical practice in the United States. In a 1974 professional activities study, only 0.9 percent of 358 women who had previously had cesareans delivered vaginally. The subjects were a random sampling from all over the country, with eight cases the most at any one hospital. The cesarean repeat rate in our country is almost 100 percent, and the policy accounts for approximately one-third of the indications for cesarean deliveries in the United States and Canada. Marieskind reports, "In 1976 alone, we could potentially have saved about 95 million dollars had a policy of individual evaluation and subsequent...[vaginal birth after cesarean] been followed. From all reports, the mothers and babies would have had at least equally as favorable an outcome as from routine repeat cesareans."

Lack of training makes physicians ill-prepared to manage labor. We believe that the idea that labor has to be "managed" is responsible for many problems. Many physicians stated that they are not familiar with normal labor but have received extensive training in the use of highly technical equipment. Others commented that the art of obstetrics is no longer being taught, and that residents have little or no experience with vaginal-breech deliveries or such obstetrical maneuvers as external version. In most medical centers, anesthesiologists train residents in general, not local, anesthesia. Many physicians complained that regular reviews of deliveries were rarely offered; when they were, only difficult cases were discussed. Patients with similar cases who were successful at vaginal delivery were not discussed. It was also stated that delivery-room nurses' estimates of cesarean sections in particular hospitals were more accurate than the estimates by the chiefs of staff. If that is true, then it is unfortunate that the nurses are not the ones responsible for keeping the records.

Most physicians believe that a cesarean section results in a superior outcome. "Superior outcome," however, has not been proved. Other factors, such as the availability of neonatal intensive-care units, improved nutrition and prenatal care, and the availability of abortions may be more influential in regard to improvements than acknowledged. In fact, fetal mortality and morbidity rates have shown little change in the decade since the cesarean rate took wings and flew. The United States, with the highest cesarean rate in the world, ranks fifteenth and sixteenth in infant mortality.

In "The Cesarean Epidemic," Gena Corea states: "there is no evidence whatever that liberal use of the c/ section has done *anything to raise the mental performance of children*" (emphasis in original) or to "reduce the incidence of neurological disorders in our population." The belief that birth is a dangerous process for babies is simply unfounded and unsubstantiated. In fact, it is a tried and proven means of entering this world.

Have increased cesarean delivery rates resulted in lower neonatal mortality rates? Dr. Diana Pettiti, a member of the NIH task force, used New York City birth certificates from 1968–69 and 1976–77 to study the relationship between neonatal mortality and method of delivery. She found that for term deliveries complicated by dystocia or by fetal distress, there were *no significant* differences in neonatal mortality between vaginally delivered and surgically delivered infants. Her conclusion:

This analysis raises serious questions about the extent to which the rising cesarean delivery rate has had a beneficial effect on pregnancy outcome...[and] provides strong evidence for the need to inquire more closely about the risks and benefits of the present high cesarean delivery rate.

"Superior outcome"? Hardly.

Dr. M.G. Kerr says that it might be "both misleading and dangerous" to attribute improvements in pregnancy outcome to the efforts of physicians. "We may have assumed too lightly that more sophisticated management necessarily brings benefits to women." He concludes, "There is virtually no reliable information to determine the benefits of obstetrical innovations in terms of fetal well being," and points out that even if benefits can be measured, they have to be balanced against the costs— not just hospital costs and doctors' fees, but also "the unwanted side effects of interference in terms of physical trauma, discomfort, emotional and social distress and the detrimental effects this technology may have on the aspects of maternity care." We agree.

The changing indications for cesareans contribute to the rising rate. There is increased use of cesarean delivery for cephalopelvic disproportion (CPD), failure to progress, and breech presentation. Many doctors commented that a section may be safer than a vaginal breech birth because few doctors had sufficient experience with the latter. Marieskind has questioned whether the seemingly superior outcome of cesareans-for-breech is because of the surgical intervention per se or because of the fact that cesarean-breech data are being compared with data of vaginal-breech deliveries managed by people increasingly unskilled at such deliveries—an extremely important issue. Several physicians stated that no one knows how to do breech vaginals anymore. Why don't they learn? Dr. Marieskind quoted one physician as follows:

> Section is remarkably safe, but we did have two deaths two years ago, in both of which the operation itself played a role. We have seriously infected patients from time to time. By and large, I think American obstetrics has become so preoccupied with apparatus and with possible fetal injury that the mothers are increasingly being considered solely as vehicles. In many instances, small and uncertain gain for the infant is purchased at the price of a small but grave risk to the mother. I don't think I have to spell out the politics of this for you.

Age, parity, and fertility characteristics have been cited as contributors to the rise. Older women and women bearing their first babies have increased in the childbearing population. The declining fertility rate and decrease in average family size have led to the concept of "premium babies." Marieskind states that an analysis of national data does show changing ages, but they are not of significance to justify the increase in cesarean sections. She says that demonstration of shifts in parity and ages by itself contributes little toward an understanding of cesarean incidence.

Economic incentives are involved: increased earnings for obstetricians—more money for less time, a predictable expenditure of physician time, added length of hospital stay with increased hospital earnings, and greater reimbursement by third-party payment for a cesarean— provide little incentive to support vaginal birth or adopt a "wait and see" attitude that could culminate in a vaginal delivery. Several physicians stated that they simply "couldn't afford not to do cesareans" because of fear of malpractice suits or because of time constraints involved in attending deliveries and keeping office hours. Marieskind suggests that a policy of accommodating deliveries to the "working day" also contributed to the cesarean increase.

Technological interventions appear to contribute to the rise in the cesarean rate. Interventionist procedures have permeated obstetrics. Marieskind reports that while these developments may help some people, they have "side-effects," one of which is increased cesarean sections. She adds:

> There are many who argue that the woman is protected from technology—and therefore the potential of its promoting a cesarean—by the concept of informed consent. Unfortunately, this point of view ignores the practice of many hospitals to *insist* on interventions. It also ignores a very human dilemma; when a woman is pregnant or in labor and is told that "what we'll do will save your baby," she is most unlikely to refuse.

Birth weight is cited as a reason for the rising cesarean birth rate. Bigger babies would contribute to CPD. Marieskind points out that this reason is unsubstantiated because the average birth weight has increased only two ounces during the years in which the section rate has doubled. Cesarean section, however, is used as part of an "aggressive approach" to save low-birth weight infants.

Management of women with *chronic diseases* like diabetes and heart disease has improved to the extent that these women can now carry a pregnancy to term, and often their medical management includes delivery by cesarean section.

Herpes II is on the increase in the United States. Infants infected by vaginal herpes as they pass through the cervix can suffer from brain, kidney, or lung damage or can die. To avoid this possibility, the baby is delivered by cesarean. It is generally agreed that if cultures are negative late in pregnancy, if cervical smear shows no shedding, and if there are no lesions present in the vagina during labor, a vaginal delivery is appropriate.

Miscellaneous other factors contributing to the cesarean epidemic have been identified. Multiple pregnancy was listed, although opinions differ greatly as to appropriate management in multiple gestations. Some physicians advocate cesarean section because the second twin is frequently in a breech or transverse position. Others advocate cesarean only for the second twin.

Several physicians commented that the increase in natural-childbirth patients showed *no differences in obstetric outcome* between those women who had taken classes and those who had not. Included in miscellaneous factors is the statement by a few physicians that women are really afraid of labor and want a cesarean (rather like a man fearing intercourse and preferring to be castrated!).

Lastly, Marieskind mentions physician attitude to cesarean section. Cesareans are now regarded as commonplace, she says. This is evidenced by many physicians who predicted that the section rate would climb because they are "just so easy." For whom, we ask? Several physicians asked: "What's so great about delivering from below, anyway?" This, about the miracle of birth, from obstetricians.

Cesareans are done for many reasons. In addition to the legitimate ones, these include power, control, money, fear, and prestige. However, we believe that the most important reason is that most physicians totally lack understanding and respect either for women or for birth. Repeat cesareans are done for the same reasons, with risk of uterine rupture the *excuse* for this deplorable crime. The word obstetrician means "to stand before," to stand before a birthing woman in awe and reverence, not before an operating table, knife in hand.

Medical Indications

When is cesarean delivery really necessary? Marieskind divides the indications for cesarean section into two categories: *absolute indications,* those which determine that there is no other method by which a healthy, living child can be delivered, and *relative indications,* those where the physician determines that a cesarean delivery will offer a better outcome for mother and baby.

The absolute indications for a cesarean section are life threatening and extremely rare. Maternal pelvic contraction is one example. Here the pelvis is clearly incapable of accommodating a mature fetus. Pelvic contraction may have been caused by injury to the pelvis, as in a car accident, or by extreme malnutrition, such as that suffered by American slaves in the early nineteenth century. A normal, reasonably healthy woman rarely has maternal pelvic contraction.

Prolapse of the umbilical cord, where the cord precedes the baby in the birth passage, is another absolute indication for a cesarean, as the pressure of the descending head on the cord can cut off the baby's blood and oxygen supplies. Hemorrhagic conditions also indicate the need for a surgical delivery. These include complete placenta previa, where the entire placenta has implanted over the opening of the cervix, and placenta abruptio, where the placenta separates from the uterine wall before the birth of the baby. Finally, a baby that stubbornly refuses to budge from a transverse presentation must be delivered by cesarean.

Between "absolute" and "relative" reasons is a "gray area" of cesarean indications that depend on individual circumstances. In the past, diabetic mothers were almost all delivered by cesarean section to avoid the intrauterine fetal death that frequently occurred if pregnancy went beyond 38 weeks. However, medical advances in the care of the pregnant diabetic are now allowing some diabetic women to carry to term and deliver vaginally. The same is true for women with heart disease. In some cases of placenta previa, if the placenta is only partially covering the cervix, a vaginal delivery is possible. Women with active vaginal herpes have also until recently been delivered by cesarean section, as exposure to the virus during vaginal birth could be lethal to the baby. Now it is known that vaginal birth can be safely achieved, depending on the location of the open herpes lesion. Another fetal indication for cesarean delivery is RH hemolytic disease, where the mother's RH-negative blood and the baby's RH-positive blood are incompatible. This indication is becoming virtually nonexistent, because of new methods of preventing maternal sensitization. If the fetus is endangered by anemia as a result of RH disease, and the delivery cannot be induced safely and successfully, a cesarean delivery is required. A failed induction to end toxemia of pregnancy may also lead to a cesarean.

It is the relative indications for cesarean section, however, that are responsible for the increasing rates. These are the ones that are doctor-determined and, we believe, often doctor-caused, or iatrogenic.

According to the NIH Conference summary report, a diagnosis of dystocia is responsible for 30 percent of the increased cesarean rates. "Dystocia" is a catch-all term that encompasses two groups of currently accepted indications for cesarean section. The first group includes problems such as cephalopelvic disproportion and feto-pelvic disproportion, where the baby's head or the whole baby is deemed too large to be accommodated by the mother's pelvis. The second group has to do with problems of labor dysfunction, with such names as "failure to progress," "prolonged labor," and "uterine inertia." Of the 130,000 abdominally delivered pregnancies reviewed by the NIH for its study, dystocia was the indication for approximately 43 percent. Additionally, many reports list CPD as the primary cause of cesarean section and the primary indication for one-third to one-half of the operative procedures.

CPD differs from maternal pelvic contraction in that it places the blame for the problem on both the baby and the mother. Because it is common for each successive baby to be a bit larger than its predecessor, many physicians tell a CPD cesarean mother that she will never give birth vaginally. We are happy to report that they are full of beans.

What we want you to remember is that CPD is fast becoming a grab-bag phrase, that it is an easy diagnosis for a physician to make when your baby refuses simply to fall out of you, and that it *never* contraindicates an attempt at labor or vaginal birth after cesarean (VBAC). Louis R. Saldana states that "previous fetopelvic disproportion does not rule out the possibility of vaginal delivery"; R.A. Bartholomew has recommended that patients who were sectioned previously for disproportion should not be denied consideration for vaginal delivery; and G.A. Morewood agrees that "a previous cesarean for CPD does not rule out subsequent vaginal delivery."

Ina May Gaskin, author of *Spiritual Midwifery*, tells us that because of natural selection over millions of years most ladies' pelvises are completely adequate in size to give birth to a normal-sized child. It is important to remember, she says, that neither the pelvis nor the baby's head is a fixed size. Even if the pelvis is small, a fine natural delivery is still possible, provided the mother is strong and patient, "the rushes strong, and the vibrations good."

In 1946, O.S. Heyns reported on the Bantu women in South Africa. He said that these women deliver babies spontaneously, although they have pelvises so small that Western women would most assuredly need cesareans to deliver the same size babies. Heyns believes that psychological differences account for stronger uterine contractions, which help the baby be born:

> It is submitted that in the European world there is an unfavorable emotional background which has an inhibitory effect on efficient uterine activity. [When] there is emotional stability supported by unwavering resolution to push through with the task of spontaneous delivery, [any woman can equal] the achievement of the Bantu. Simple dystocia due to contracted bony passages can almost be eliminated by fostering the will in the parturient [that's you!] to deliver herself.

We need to learn from our sisters in South Africa. They have much to teach us. Another culture, reported on by L. Marchand in 1932, believes women are better off dead than unable to bring forth their children by themselves. They either birth or die, and they prefer birthing.

A diagnosis of CPD made prior to the onset of labor is particularly suspect. During labor, the muscle fibers stretch, the central portion of the perineum thins, and the connective tissue ligaments of the pelvis soften and relax to give more room; in addition, the flexible bones of the baby's head mold to decrease its circumference. If a squatting position is assumed during pushing, the size of the pelvis may be increased more than a centimeter. A preliminary X ray in the late stages of pregnancy cannot possibly account for the changes that will occur during labor. What it can do is begin a chain of events that will ultimately lead to a cesarean, for even the slightest mention of CPD is enough to undermine the first-time mother's confidence in her ability to birth. A labor and delivery-room nurse notes:

> The doctor examines the laboring woman and mentions on his way out that he's a bit worried about the pelvic margin. You can see the woman's approach change after that. Her heart goes out of it. Naturally, t a few hours later, she' s off to surgery.

A woman who has once delivered a baby vaginally is almost never diagnosed as CPD in subsequent deliveries. Marieskind says, "It is possibly significant that while cephalopelvic disproportion can be determined by clinical or x-ray pelvimetry prior to delivery, neither it nor failure to progress can be determined by any quantifiable measure after the birth."

"Failure to progress" is the other category of dystocia that by contemporary obstetrical standards necessitates a cesarean. Even as you read these words, thousands of laboring women in hospitals across the land are failing to progress. One of the roots of the problem is Friedman's curve, a graphic definition of "normal" labor patterns based on a study of the labors of a "large number" of women. *Williams Obstetrics* calls the limits set by the Friedman chart "admittedly arbitrary." The NIH draft report states:

> Functional definitions of abnormal labor progress, pioneered by Emanuel Friedman, are typically based upon a concept that the slowest progress experienced by a population of laboring gravidas is abnormal...the concept that slow progress constitutes abnormal progress permeates current obstetrical thinking, and although less easily documented, may also conceptualize the patient's expectations. Thus, delivery for all patients in *less than 24 hours* has been advocated, as has intervention after *two to four hours* of poor progress in active labor. [Emphasis added.]

"Although less easily documented" than the physician's expectations, the laboring woman's preconceived notions of normal labor do undermine her confidence when progress is slow. "I was found wanting at five centimeters," says the woman in Chase Collins' story "Random Voodoo." Soon after that, she is on her way to a cesarean.

We have so many questions to ask about functional definitions of labor progress. How does one define the "beginning" of labor? (We know women who have experienced mild contractions for days and even weeks!) What is "normal" labor? How does one allow for the notorious slowing down of contractions under epidural anesthesia? What is "poor progress"? Does it generally indicate too-early arrival at the hospital? How is the labor being managed? Is the slowly progressing woman walking and taking nourishment and squatting when she pushes? Is she offered kind words and gentle encouragement when she becomes disheartened? Or is she lying flat on her back, I.V. in place, fetal monitor clattering away, food and drink denied, and all manner of analgesia and anesthesia offered when she shows signs of frustration? Has anyone put a time limit on her labor? We hope not. The idea of an optimum length of labor with its accompanying time constraints horrifies us. We have an image of a blustery physician charging into the labor room, shouting, "Time's up!" (That would be enough to make any uterus stop contracting!) We know that failure to progress is seldom an issue with home births or with midwife-attended births, and we contend that the mere idea of a time limit for delivery can be enough to cause labor dysfunction.

In *The Cultural Warping of Childbirth*, Doris Haire cites the belief of Dutch obstetricians that "when the labor of a normal woman is unhurried and allowed to progress normally, unexpected emergencies rarely occur." Their belief is shared by the midwives of The Farm in Tennessee, a self-sufficient spiritual and farming community that delivers its own babies. Ina May Gaskin, the farm's first midwife, cautions:

> The mother's rushes may or may not cause her cervix to dilate at a steady rate. You don't have to have any preconceived notions about what is too long for the first stage. If the mother is replenishing her energy by eating and sleeping, rushes are light, the baby's head is not being tightly squeezed and the membranes are still intact, the first stage can stretch over three or four days and still be perfectly normal.

Few physicians are willing to take such a laissez-faire attitude toward a long labor, and the methods used to speed things along often lead to surgical delivery.

When we consider that the maternal mortality ratio for dystocia is 41.9 deaths per 100,000 cesarean births, compared with 11.1 deaths per 100,000 vaginal births, the need to evaluate dystocia as an indication for surgical delivery becomes even more compelling. In the meantime, it is important to remember that failure to progress, like CPD, never contraindicates VBAC for future deliveries. C. Pauerstein found in his VBAC study that "success in giving birth vaginally was not…related to the degree of cervical dilation attained in the previous labor or to whether the woman had labored at all."

In fact, success in giving birth vaginally after a cesarean section is not related to much that occurred in the prior labor. Yet, prior cesarean delivery is second only to dystocia as an indication for cesarean section, accounting for almost 30 percent of the increase in the cesarean rate and for over 30 percent of the surgical deliveries performed. In the United States, more than 98 percent of the women who have cesarean sections go on to deliver their next children surgically; in other words, less than 2 percent of cesarean mothers have subsequent children vaginally. The amount of unnecessary surgery performed via elective repeat-cesareans is staggering. Ours is the only country where routine repeat-cesarean is a matter of national policy.

When Edwin Craigin made his "Once a cesarean, always a cesarean" presentation to the New York Medical Society in 1916, the cesarean birth rate was less than I percent, and the classical incision was in use. This incision extends vertically into the upper segment of the uterus and has a slightly higher potential for instability (1–3 percent) then the lower-segment incision (0.S–1.5 percent). The lower-segment incision is a low, horizontal "smile," or "bikini," cut that came into use in the 1930s for the purpose of allowing subsequent vaginal delivery. The lower-segment incision is used in over 90 percent of current cesarean surgery, yet the idea of VBAC has yet to gain general acceptance with the American medical community. Says W.I. O'Connell:

> Vaginal delivery following cesarean section is neither unique nor experimental. There are several reports in the literature that attest to the feasibility of such a procedure, but the medical profession as a whole seems to exhibit a profound reluctance to accept the fact.

As R.G. Douglas and associates remark, while "most dogmatic medical concepts are noted for their impermanence, Craigin's dogma is self-perpetuating because of fear of legal reprisal." Fear of malpractice suits, fear of rupture, and fear of the relatively unknown combine to make many physicians reluctant to accept the realities of VBAC.

Other physicians, however, are learning to judge each labor on its own merit and not by the records of past deliveries. "The medical literature should encourage medical practitioners to seriously consider allowing a trial of labor," says S. McKay, editor of *ICEA Review*; and, indeed, the medical literature is starting to do just that. R. Gordon Douglas reports:

> With all facts entered on the ledger sheet, we have concluded after observing over 3,000 patients who have had a previous cesarean section that vaginal delivery is better for both mother and infant when there is no recurring or new indication for cesarean section. If progress is unsatisfactory or some complication develops during the course of labor, flexibility is maintained and *cesarean section can be resorted to at any time.* I feel that the results so obtained are superior to those obtained by routinely performing an elective repeat cesarean section. [Emphasis added.]

Those who favor routine repeat cesarean because of its "ease" and "safety" need to be reminded that "all the factors that make cesareans so safe nowadays also serve to make VBAC safe, and more rewarding." We agree with F.P. Meehan when he says that "elective repeat cesarean section is meddlesome obstetrics unless there is a recurring indication."

One indication for cesarean that is not a recurring indication is breech presentation, which occurs in 3–4 percent of all pregnancies. Ina May Gaskin describes three major types of breech presentation. In the *complete breech,* the thighs and knees are flexed, with the buttocks and feet presenting, and the baby is in a sort of upside down fetal position. In the *incomplete, or frank, breech,* the baby is in a jackknifed position, with the buttocks presenting and both feet touching the head. This is the most common breech position and the easiest presentation for a vaginal-breech delivery. The *footling breech* presents one or both feet first and is the least common breech position. Breech presentation is associated with greater risk factors than the vertex (head down) position, yet cesarean delivery for breech babies is a fairly recent trend in American obstetrics. Some blame the increasing use of cesareans for breech on the failure of medical schools to train physicians to perform vaginal-breech deliveries. One obstetrician reported:

> Recently I had two breeches close together, assisted at each delivery by a first- or second-year resident. I discovered that these fellows knew practically nothing about

breech delivery. They assumed that every breech was going to be delivered by cesarean section, and when it came to the delivery, they knew nothing about getting the arms out, about delivering the after-coming head, the use of Piper forceps, or any such things. Their first thought was—a breech; we do a cesarean. It seemed to me that there was too much science and not enough art. They knew all about ultrasonic monitoring, scalp sampling, all the ultrasonic things, but nothing about the actual technique and art of delivering a breech.

Others cite superior infant outcome as the reason for resorting to surgical breech delivery, although this contention is largely unsubstantiated.

In any case, the proportion of breech presentations delivered by cesarean rose from 11.6 percent in 1970 to 60.1 percent in 1978, accounting for another 10–15 percent of the increase in the cesarean rate during those years. Approximately 12 percent of the cesareans performed are done because of breech presentation, and many institutions report that 60–90 percent of their breech presentations are delivered surgically. Some physicians choose to deliver all multiple births by cesarean because often one of the babies is in a breech position. It is important to note here that the dramatic rise in the use of cesarean section for the delivery of breech babies has not been, accompanied by measurable improvement in infant outcome. In fact, "there has been no overall decrease in mortality over a 10-year period for the total group of breech presentation." A review of 457 breech deliveries at the Medical Center Hospital in Burlington, Vermont, showed "no significant improvement in death and morbidity rates for breech babies delivered by c/section over those born vaginally."

So-called fetal distress is responsible for another 10–15 percent of the increase and for 5 percent of the cesareans performed. There is no evidence that the actual incidence of fetal distress has changed; however, the diagnosis of fetal distress has become much more common over the past ten years. Many critics point an accusing finger at the electronic fetal monitor.

By NIH definition, "fetal distress during labor is a condition resulting from inadequate fetal oxygen supply and carbon dioxide removal." Signs of possible fetal distress are meconium in the amniotic fluid or irregularities of the fetal heart rate. The NIH draft report notes, "In some instances infants predicted to be normal may have in fact experienced fetal distress and are depressed at birth. On the other hand, some infants predicted to be distressed appear normal at birth." When fetal distress does in fact occur, it is tragically often the result of interventions in the normal course of labor and birth. Labor stimulants such as pitocin (which is generally accompanied by analgesia to make the exaggerated contractions bearable or used to speed up labor once analgesia has slowed it down) put a great deal of stress on the fetus, as does artificial rupture of the membranes cushioning the baby's head. The common use of the flat on-the-back position during labor allows the pressure of the uterus to rest on the inferior vena cava (the main blood vessel bringing blood back to the heart from the lower body) and to cut down the blood supply to the uterus. Lester Hazell warns that there is no way of knowing how many cases of fetal distress are caused by the mother's remaining immobilized on her back because of a fetal monitor or I.V. Any interference in the rhythm and pattern of a woman's labor has the potential for distressing her baby.

More than any other indication for cesarean, fetal distress shows that the emphasis of the medical profession is on the fetus rather than the mother. The view of the baby as a delicate creature endangered by the turbulent forces of birth, a view held by the mother as well as by the physician, paves the way for many labor interventions and problems. In *Birthing Normally,* Gayle Peterson says that when we can see the baby as resilient and ready for the transition to outside the womb, and when we can see labor as a healthy process that stimulates the baby for breathing, then we have achieved the attitude for a healthy delivery. In the meantime, we have to wonder why so many "fetal distress" babies are cut from their mothers' stomachs with Apgar scores of 9 and 10. Fetal distress as an indication for cesarean section is clearly in need of more accurate definition.

Induction of labor is of two types: *medical* (use of drugs like pitocin) and *surgical* (artificial rupture of the membranes). Both types put a great deal of stress on the baby and on the mother, both of whom are unprepared for a violent surge in active labor. The United States Food and Drug Administration has banned the use of oxytocin for elective induction of labor (induction for the convenience of the woman or her physician) because of the potential hazards of prematurity, fetal distress, newborn jaundice, rupture of the uterus, and higher cesarean rate. It is now used primarily as a follow-up to artificial rupture of the membranes, which has a high failure rate and leaves the woman, in the eyes of her physician, highly susceptible to infection. When both surgical and medical induction have failed, a cesarean is performed to protect the woman from infections, which used to threaten within seventy-two hours but which recently for some reason have reduced their delay to only twelve hours. The NIH summary report points out the need for a safe and effective method of labor stimulation for those women who should not carry to term because of medical problems such as diabetes and toxemia. For all healthy, normal women, labor induction should be seen as the first step on the road to surgical delivery and, as such, should be heartily avoided.

Finally, low-birth weight and premature babies are often delivered by cesarean because it is believed that they are unable to tolerate labor. Improved survival rates for these infants may be the result of recent innovations in newborn care rather than of surgical delivery. Which women are the most likely candidates for cesareans? Statistics show that by today's obstetrical standards, any pregnant woman is likely to fall prey to the knife. But Marieskind suggests that women who have the highest incidence of cesarean section are as follows:

- Women with the least and most education. The 1972 National Natality Survey showed the highest cesarean rate among women who were college graduates.
- Women with the lowest and highest incomes; that is, women who don't have to pay and women who can afford to.
- Women of the youngest and oldest ages. Women in the under-15 age group are particularly high-risk, and there has been a substantial increase in births among this age group. In women over 30, dysfunctional labor and/or malpresentation have been reported to be almost double. One study found that a higher incidence of sedation occurred in older women, that dysfunctional labor could generally be associated with sedation use, and that women 35 years and over were five times more likely to experience cesarean section. "In general, women outside the prime childbearing years of 20–29 are potentially at higher risk and may have more complications with their pregnancies, thereby making a cesarean delivery more likely."
- Women with the lowest and highest parity. Women who are *primiparous* (first delivery) or *multiparous* (six or more deliveries) are likely to have cesareans. Primiparas generally have a higher rate of CPD, of hemorrhage, of dysfunctional labor, and of preeclampsia. According to Marieskind, it seems quite reasonable to expect that the number of complications reported in primiparous women may be in part attributable to the physician's unfamiliarity with the patient herself and both the physician's and the patient's unfamiliarity with her ability to manage labor and delivery. Older women who are multiparas are more likely to have placental accidents and more likely to have multiple births, which increase the chances of toxemia and hemorrhage.

- Women with public insurance and women with the most comprehensive private insurance.
- Women who have no prenatal care and women who have the most prenatal care (perhaps because they are "high risk" to begin with).
- Women who use general municipal hospitals and women who use exclusive private hospitals.
- Women with low- or high-birth weight babies.
- Women with low- or high-gestational-age babies.
- Women who have lost a baby (and come to this birth with tension and fear).
- Women with multiple births.
- Women who are private as opposed to nonprivate patients.
- Women who have taken childbirth-education classes and expect to be in complete control.
- White women (a slight difference).
- Metropolitan women (including high-risk women who have come to the city for better prenatal care).

Still, the most likely candidate for cesarean section is the woman who has already had one, and the uterine scar remains the single greatest indication for cesarean delivery.

For most of this century, the integrity of that scar has been the subject of debate and controversy. When women consider VBAC, the scar is what makes us hesitate. Our doctors point at it knowingly and sadly shake their heads. It is as if we had been branded "high risk" down at the O.R. Corral, so that in every obstetric territory they will know we come from c/section. If we think about straying from the herd, they threaten us with "rupture"— a terrifying idea. "Rupture" is the risk they talk about when they warn us against VBAC. And what are the risks of cesarean section? "Oh, none," they tell us, "it's so safe that there's really no reason not to do it!"

Niles Newton remarks that physicians in the nineteenth century did a very successful advertising campaign to convince women that birth was dangerous. We would add that physicians in the twentieth century have done a very successful advertising campaign to convince women that cesarean section is safe. Right now we will take "equal time" to give you some very frightening information about cesarean section.

Risks to the Mother

This quotation from N.J. Eastman appeared in an issue of the *ICEA Review* that focused specifically on vaginal birth following cesarean section:

I gather the impression that, except in our own clinic, nothing ever goes wrong with a patient who has a cesarean section. Anesthetic mishaps are never mentioned, nor does appreciable blood loss or need for transfusion seem to occur (although everyone knows that the average blood loss at section is at least 700 cc.). These sectioned patients in the literature, however, appear to be immune to pulmonary embolism, and the ubiquitous staphylococcus passes them by; as for postoperative distention, one gets the impression that this complication is now of historic interest only. But in our own experience, the course of cesarean section is not always so tranquil, and once or twice a year we are scared to death by some section patient who acts up with one or another of these complications. True, we have not lost a section case for a good many years, but I wonder sometimes if our luck has not about run out. In any event, on the basis of my own experience, I find it difficult to believe that cesarean section, even today, is quite as safe as having a haircut, statistics to the contrary notwithstanding!

Eastman's skepticism, or at least his admission of it, is unusual. Most physicians would have us believe that a cesarean is a simple little operation, that it is, indeed, "quite as safe as having a haircut." Not true! "The statement that cesareans have never been safer for the mother," notes Susan Doering, "simply means that the surgery is safer now than it was twenty or fifty years ago." Despite all the wonderful advances in recent medical history that serve to minimize the risks of cesarean delivery, a cesarean is still major abdominal surgery, with all the risks inherent in any surgical procedure.

In order to prevent any further comparisons between a cesarean section and a haircut, we would like to share with you Michelle Harrison's description of the cesarean delivery of a baby. We thank Dr. Hamson and her publishers at Random House for allowing us to quote so extensively from her new book, *Woman in Residence:*

In the morning the woman is wheeled on a stretcher to the L&D (Labor and Delivery) suite, and then to the delivery room, which doubles as a section room. For epidural anesthesia, the woman is placed on the operating table on her left side. She is told to curl into a fetal-like position to allow a needle to be inserted between the vertebrae of her curved spine. When the needle is withdrawn, leaving a tube in the spine, the woman is placed flat on her back and the table temporarily tilted slightly to lower her head in order to establish a level of anesthesia that is high enough to make the woman's abdomen numb, but won't affect her ability to breathe. There is only a fine margin of both safety and comfort: if the level is too low, she will have pain during the surgery; if it is too high, she will have difficulty breathing and will require mechanical assistance.

The woman's bladder is next catheterized and the tube left in the bladder to keep urine draining. During the surgery the bladder is cut away from the surface of the uterus as there is a greater risk of perforating or cutting into it if it is full.

Preparation of the surgical site consists of scrubbing and draping the abdomen, with only that portion to be cut left exposed. It is similar to any other surgical preparation except for the inhibited discussion if the woman is awake.

I had been wondering why I always got so covered with blood and amniotic fluid during a Caesarean section, while the surgeon would come out so much cleaner. I would be soaked through my gown, my greens and my underwear. It was finally explained to me: "The table is tilted slightly so the blood and fluid run onto the assistant and not onto the surgeon."

As soon as the woman is draped, the anesthesiologist tilts the table to one side and signals for the surgeon to begin. The surgeon takes a scalpel from the nurse and with one strong and definite motion creates a crescent-shaped incision along the woman's pubic hairline. As the skin is cut, the subcutaneous tissue bulges upward as though it had been straining to get through all the time. Within moments this fatty tissue, interconnected by thin transparent fibers, becomes dotted and then covered with blood that oozes out of tiny vessels. With scalpel and forceps—delicate tweezers—the surgeon cuts deeper beneath the subcutaneous tissue, to a thick layer of fibrous tissue that holds the abdominal organs and muscles of the abdominal wall in place. Once reached, this fibrous layer is incised and cut along the lines of the original surface incision while the muscles adhering to this tissue are scraped off and pushed out of the way. The uterus is now visible under the peritoneum, a layer of thin tissue, looking like Saran Wrap, which covers most of the internal organs and which, when inflamed, produces peritonitis. The peritoneum is lifted away from the uterus and an incision is made in it, leaving the uterus and bladder easily accessible. The bladder is peeled away from the uterus, for the baby will be taken out through an incision in the uterus underneath where the bladder usually lies. When a Caesarean is done as an emergency procedure and speed is essential, the bladder is not removed and instead the incision is made much higher in the uterus. This produces weaker scar tissue and greater chance of rupture during a subsequent pregnancy and labor.

The uterus of the pregnant woman is large, smooth and glistening. Shaped like a huge pear, the top and sides are thick and muscular, the lower end thin and flexible. With short careful strokes of a knife, a small incision is made through the thinner segment. Special care is taken not to cut the baby or the membranes surrounding the baby which, if still intact, now bulge through the tiny hole in the uterus. The room becomes silent: the quiet presence of the baby about to be born causes time suddenly to stop.

The obstetrician extends the initial cut either by putting two index fingers into the small incision and ripping the uterus open or by using blunt-ended scissors and cutting in two directions away from the initial incision. If the membranes are still intact, they are now punctured with toothed forceps, and the fluid spills out onto the table. In the normal position, the baby's head is down and under the incision, so the obstetrican places one hand inside the uterus, under the baby's head, and with the other hand exerts pressure on the upper end of the uterus to push the baby through the abdominal incision. The assistant also uses force now to help push the baby out. Once the baby's head is out, the throat is immediately suctioned with a small ear syringe, and then the shoulders and rest of the body are eased out. Held in the air, the baby usually begins to cry. The cord is clamped and the baby handed over to a nurse holding a warmed towel. Sometimes, en route to the nurse, the infant is momentarily held over the woman's head with its genitals facing down into the mother's face, as she is told, "Look, it's a boy/ girl!" The assumption is always made that the woman wants most to know and see the sex of her child. For many women, including those delivering vaginally, this is all they see of their babies at the time of delivery.

The rest of the surgery is more difficult for the woman. There is more pain and women often vomit and complain of difficult breathing as we handle their organs and repair the damage. This period may also be more difficult because there is no longer the anticipation of waiting to see the baby born. Sometimes the woman is given sedation for the rest of the surgery.

The placenta separates from or is peeled off the inside of the uterus. Then, since the uterine attachments are all at the lower end, near the cervix, the body of the uterus can be brought out of the abdominal cavity and rested on the outside of the woman's abdomen, thus adding both visibility and room in which to work.

With large circular needles and thick thread a combination of running and individual stitches is used to sew closed the hole in the uterus. A drug called pitocin is added to the woman's IV to help the uterus contract and to decrease the bleeding. Small sutures are used to tie and retie bleeding blood vessels. The "gutters," spaces in the abdominal cavity, are cleared of blood and fluid. The uterus is then placed back in the abdominal cavity. The bladder is sewn back onto the surface of the uterus, and then finally the peritoneum is closed. Now sponges are counted to be sure none have been left inside the abdominal cavity, and then the closure of the abdominal wall begins.

Muscles overlying the peritoneum are pushed back in place, and are sometimes sewn with loose stitches. Fascia, the thick fibrous layer, is the most important one, since it holds all the abdominal organs inside and keeps them from coming through the incision, especially if the woman coughs or sneezes. Therefore this layer is closed with heavy thread and many individual stitches so that, even if a thread breaks. the stitches won't all come out. The subcutaneous tissue, most of which is fat, is closed in loose stitches that mainly close any air spaces which might become sites for infection. Skin, the final layer, is closed with silk or nylon thread or metal staples. The appearance of the final scar is generally considered important, since many people judge whether a surgeon is good or not by the scar's appearance.

A dry bandage is placed over the woman's incision and then taped to her skin. The drapes are removed. A baby has been born.

However, for far too many women and their infants, the trauma is not over.

In "Complications of Cesarean to Mother and Infant," Madeleine Shearer summarizes the physiologic costs of cesarean section to the mother. Some of these are pain and depression, gas, infection, hemorrhage, adhesions, injury to adjacent structures, blood transfusion complications, aspiration pneumonia, anesthesia accidents, cardiac arrest, and death.

Death. Although we tend to think of cesarean section as a life-saving rather than a life-threatening procedure, the maternal mortality rate for cesarean patients is not insignificant. John Evrard and Edwin Gold, in their eleven-year study of maternal death associated with cesarean section in Rhode Island, found that "the risk of death from cesarean section was 26 *times greater* than with vaginal delivery" (emphasis added). A recently completed analysis of maternal deaths in Georgia showed a mortality ratio of 59.3/100,000 births by cesarean section as compared with 9.7/100,000 vaginal births. A California study showed the risk of maternal death associated with cesarean section to be two to three times greater than that for vaginal delivery. All of these studies took into account the conditions that necessitated the cesarean and only included deaths that were caused by the surgery itself.

Maternal mortality statistics are difficult to assess because maternal death is notoriously underreported (or covered up!). The *Ob./Gyn. News* for July 1980 describes a study of cesarean sections performed in Georgia in 1975, where eleven deaths were determined by routine surveillance of death certificates. Upon further investigation, five more cesarean-associated deaths were identified. By obtaining additional information from the medical examiner's reports, the hospital records, the police reports, and the women's physicians and families, researchers attributed nine of the total sixteen deaths to the surgery itself. The reported cause of death in those nine cases was pulmonary embolism, in six women, and complications of anesthesia, in three. In this article, Dr. George L. Rubin stated that earlier studies had underestimated the risks of cesarean section and that physicians should carefully assess the risks whenever they are considering performing a section.

Maternal death is defined as one related to pregnancy and/or the process of childbirth. An article in the Winter 1981 issue of *NAPSAC News* warns that "the time span of consideration" for maternal death often extends only to the sixth week following a live birth, so that the death of a mother after this time span is not attributed to pregnancy-related causes even when it should be. Additionally, many maternal deaths that occur closer to the time of birth are not recorded as maternal mortalities because the woman with severe complications has been moved from maternity to another wing of the hospital and is no longer considered a maternity patient.

The *NAPSAC* article cites a study of childbirth-related deaths that found a significant number of maternal deaths to be caused by complications of cesarean delivery. Yet the death certificates of many of these women made no mention whatever of the cesarean surgery or even of the fact that they had been recently pregnant. This article suggests that maternal deaths in the United States may be double the rates reported. "Theoretically," it says, "the period of time during which a maternal death could occur would begin with conception and extend through the year following birth."

The NIH draft report cites the fact that maternal deaths are underreported in vital records—probably seriously underreported—as one of the major problems in data evaluation. Most of the NIH data on maternal mortality comes from the Professional Activities Study (PAS), an organization that collects data from a large number of hospitals throughout the United States and provides the largest single tabulation of information on cesareans in the country. Of interest to us is the PAS finding that the relative risk of maternal death in a repeat cesarean delivery increased during the eight-year period 1970-78 (you might like to have that bit of information to offer your doctor when you are discussing VBAC with him!). The NIH task force determined that "cesarean delivery carries about four times the risk of maternal mortality of a vaginal delivery" and that "cesarean delivery for previous cesarean carries two times the risk of maternal mortality of all vaginal deliveries." We believe these figures to be conservative.

The NIH task force also determined that maternal morbidity (disease) rates are generally five to ten times higher after cesarean delivery than after vaginal delivery:

> A cesarean delivery is a major operative procedure and as such is associated with many complications leading to maternal morbidity that are never encountered in a vaginal delivery. Examples of these complications include operative injuries to the urinary tract and bowel, wound abscess, wound dehiscence, evisceration, operative and postoperative hemorrhage, and paralytic ileus. In addition, complications such as pulmonary emboli, venous thrombosis, and anesthesia related morbidity are more common following a major operative procedure. Consequently, maternal morbidity associated with cesarean delivery is substantially higher than the morbidity associated with a vaginal delivery.

"Infections constitute the greatest portion of this morbidity," the NIH summary report concluded, and "the most common infections are endometritis, urinary tract infections, and wound infections." But hemorrhage is also not uncommon, with the average blood loss following cesarean section estimated to be about 1,000 cc, double the usual blood loss following vaginal birth.

Most of the studies we have read report a 50 percent morbidity rate associated with cesarean section. What this means is that 50 percent of all new mothers delivered by cesarean section have some serious illness such as infection or hemorrhage! "Almost half of all cesarean patients had one or more operative complications," Madeleine Shearer found in her study, "including a respectable number of severe complications which compromised future child-bearing or were potentially lethal. "

McGaughey and associates add that "maternal morbidity in repeat sections is high." Their study of pregnancy and labor following cesarean section showed that the complications of repeat cesarean section "were of sufficient magnitude in many cases to cause severe, even if limited, disability," and that "the incidence of wound infection and disruption, pneumonia, bladder injury, septicemia, and pelvic thrombophlebitis indicates that the procedure is not benign."

Like maternal mortality, maternal morbidity associated with cesarean section is seriously underreported. Few follow-up studies are done once women leave the hospitals, and physicians do not talk about the postoperative complications they treat—especially not with their pregnant clients. Few women are even remotely aware of the risks to which they subject themselves when they submit to surgical delivery. No one tells them about the risks of infection and hemorrhage. No one tells them about the risk of adhesions that result in intestinal obstruction, or the risk of postoperative urinary-tract symptoms resulting from the adherence of the bladder flap to the uterus. No one talks about possible injuries to the bladder during abdominal delivery. The only risk that is discussed with the cesarean patient, if she is lucky and there is time, is the risk of anesthesia; and while she is made to feel that she has a voice in the decision about which one to use, she generally does not have the option to refuse it altogether. The role of anesthesia is an important consideration when assessing the risks and benefits of cesarean section, for anesthesia is a necessary component in the operative procedure.

Exposure to anesthesia always carries a risk that, Marieskind notes, increases with each successive episode; and, given the current policy of repeat cesarean section, most cesarean mothers will undergo additional surgery for subsequent pregnancies. The possibility of an anesthesia accident is a risk inherent in any surgical procedure, but it has the potential for being doubly tragic in cesarean surgery because there are (at least) two patients involved. Maternal deaths related to anesthesia continue to occur, and most of these are avoidable. But in every case, use of anesthesia can cause serious problems. Appropriate selection and better technique can reduce these risks. Both the physician and the mother have responsibilities in this regard.

> The best that obstetricians can do is to be aware of the knowledge about drug effects on the mother, the labor, and the fetus, and when they are truly indicated, use the minimum amount of the apparently safest medication to achieve the necessary result. Similarly, the mother must also make herself aware of the results which may ensue from medications used during labor, and temper both her demands and her acceptance of such medications with that knowledge.

A knowledge of the types of anesthesia used for cesarean section, and their inherent dangers, is necessary for every pregnant woman.

General anesthesia works quickly and requires less skill to administer than other anesthesia. Its well-known disadvantages are an unconscious mother, the hazard of aspiration of gastric contents into the lungs (a common cause of anesthetic death), and a depressed newborn. In addition, women are generally groggy and depressed themselves for days following the use of general anesthesia. Having missed not only the birth but also the critical bonding period, they often feel alienated from the baby and from the birth experience itself. Mothers who have had general anesthesia have much more difficulty integrating and accepting their cesarean sections.

Because of those disadvantages, most women today who are allowed a choice select regional anesthesia instead. Regional anesthesia is of two types: *spinal* and *epidural.* Spinal anesthesia involves the injection of a local anesthetic into the lumbar subarachnoid space. Its disadvantages are its effects on the baby and its possible complications: hypotension (reduced blood flow), total spinal blockage with respiratory paralysis, anxiety and discomfort, spinal headaches, and bladder dysfunction. The incidence of maternal hypotension after spinal anesthesia, estimated to be as high as 80 percent, is a contributory factor to maternal anesthesia-related morbidity .

Lumbar epidural anesthesia also involves the injection of a local anesthetic into an area of the spine, but this time into the epidural space. Often a catheter is inserted so that reinforcement of pain relief may be provided, as larger doses of local anesthetic are required than with the spinal. The disadvantages are the greater amounts of anesthetic required, the effects on the baby, and the possibility of inadvertent spinal anesthesia when the dura is accidentally punctured. As with spinal anesthesia, epidurals also carry the risks of hypotension and convulsions, or even cardiac arrest resulting from central nervous system stimulation.

An additional concern with epidural anesthesia is the likelihood of "spottiness" in pain relief. Areas called "windows" may be unaffected by the anesthesia, with the result that the woman can feel everything that is going on in that particular spot—cutting, pulling, stitching, everything! As you can see, choosing your anesthesia is really deciding which is the least of the evils.

Seldom mentioned in connection with cesareans and drugs is the cesarean mother's increased need for *post*partum drugs. It is as if no one wants to talk about how much she is going to hurt. The fact that the surgery is so painful is often a surprise and a difficulty. There is a Catch 22: you can take medication and be too groggy and weak to hold the baby, or you can not take it and be in too much pain to care about holding the baby. "My baby and I, we just lay there and cried together," one woman wrote, "he in his bed and I in mine—I couldn't even lean over to pick him up." In "Unnecessary Cesareans: Doctor's Choice, Parent's Dilemma," Susan Doering says:

> Not only are 50 percent of surgically delivered women actually sick postpartum, but virtually 100 percent experience a great deal more pain, weakness, problems moving around, and difficulties caring for their newborns. In my own research, I observed that women who had been delivered by cesarean were significantly more negative about their birth experience, were much more miserable physically, required far more drugs postpartum, experienced more serious and longer-lasting depression, and did not "feel like a mother"…till much later than the vaginally delivered women. Many other researchers have reported on the shock, deep disappointment, feelings of failure, and other negative emotions experienced by cesarean mothers postpartum. Surgery is never a pleasant experience, but becoming a mother through major abdominal surgery is particularly difficult. Helpless, dependent newborns cannot wait until their mothers "recover"—they need mothering at once.

When we look upon the cesarean section as major abdominal surgery, we are able to see the risks of a whole range of physiologic complications. When we look upon it as the birth of a baby, we need to examine its potential for psychological trauma and consequent mothering difficulties. The psychological complications can be as debilitating as the physiological ones.

Gayle Peterson says, "How a woman gives birth has been found to influence her confidence and ability to mother." The cesarean mother is at a decided disadvantage; she is a mother, yes, but she has not given birth. Having lost control over her childbirth experience, she is likely to feel cheated, disappointed, angry, frustrated, guilty, regretful, helpless, and depressed. In addition, she may experience a sense of failure, distaste for her scar, and envy of those who have given birth vaginally. These are not healthy feelings with which to welcome a newborn, and others will soon grow impatient with her.

Often there is little sympathy for a cesarean mother the first few days after surgery. "C'mon, Sally, let's get going here. You've only had a baby. Let's not pamper ourselves. Hop out of bed!" (Hop? Hop? How about a shuffle?) No one would expect someone who had just had an appendectomy to begin caring for another person within hours after the operation; yet the cesarean mother, having undergone the same kind of major abdominal surgery, is expected to do just that. Or, at the other extreme, she is separated from her baby immediately after delivery and only allowed to see him for a few moments every four hours. ("You must get your rest, dear. We're taking lovely care of him in the nursery!") There is a balance, and it's up to the hospital staff to find it. Those who tend to the cesarean mother postpartum need to remember that the psychological assimilation of the birth process is generally longer for her than it is for the mother who delivers vaginally.

In "The Cesarean Section Patient Is a New Mother, Too," Betsy Bampton and Joan Mancini advise nurses to pay special attention to the cesarean mother's needs as a maternity patient. They emphasize the importance of communicating with her—before the surgery, to prepare her; during the surgery, to reassure her; and after the surgery, to comfort her. They also point out the importance of making sure that the new cesarean mother has access to her baby immediately after the delivery and often thereafter. Providing her with emotional and physical comforts and the opportunity to get to know her baby in a nonthreatening way will give her the time and energy to try to integrate all that she has just gone through:

> The cesarean section patient needs to relive her labor and delivery experience so she can finalize her pregnancy, face the separation from her fetus, and integrate this experience into her life pattern. The experience may be traumatic. She may misunderstand events, forget moments of the experience or her response to it because of fear and apprehension.

On the other hand, the new cesarean mother may feel fine, be delighted with her baby, and take her departure from the hospital without any extraneous emotional baggage. The woman who readily accepts her cesarean experience is not necessarily healthier, just different.

Risks to the Baby

When we talk about the risks of cesarean section, it is sometimes easy to forget the smaller, less verbal, and more helpless patient involved. But the risks of surgical delivery to the infant must not be overlooked; they are every real, quite dangerous, and too common. Among those listed by Madeleine Shearer are jaundice, fewer quiet and alert periods after birth, iatrogenic respiratory distress, neonatal drug effects, abnormal or suspect neurological exams, low birth weight, neonatal acidosis resulting from maternal hypotension, inadvertent infant-to-placenta transfusion, and neonatal death.

We have long known about the danger of anesthesia to the unborn child, and this is the most obvious fetal risk of all surgical deliveries, in first and repeat c/sections combined. Doris Haire warned years ago about the role that medication plays in our "staggering incidence of neurological impairment." She cautioned that an infant who showed no signs of respiratory distress and scored well on the Apgar scale could, upon closer investigation, show lingering signs of oxygen deprivation resulting from obstetrical medication administered to the mother. She noted that "we can no longer assume that the apparent recovery of an asphyxiated infant after successful resuscitation is a guarantee that the infant has come through unharmed." Haire went on to say that a baby with a heartbeat after cardiac massage may appear to have recovered but, in fact, may be "irreversibly brain-damaged. "

Our confidence in drug-testing programs should have been weakened by what happened with thalidomide and diethylstilbestrol. Yet many of us continue to assume that science and government protect us and our infants from drug-related tragedies. All pregnant women should be warned that the Food and Drug Administration has no regulations whatever regarding drugs and the childbearing woman. It does not require that obstetrical drugs be proved safe for the fetus.

It takes only seconds or minutes for anesthesia (or in fact any medication) to cross the placenta and enter the circulatory system of the unborn infant; it takes days and even weeks for the newborn's immature excretory system to rid his body of the effects of these medications. The sluggishness and depression exhibited by the medicated newborn may mask other problems that require immediate attention. At the least, they serve to interfere with the infant's sucking reflexes, thus preventing him from getting the full immunologic advantage of his mother's colostrum and inhibiting the start of the breast-feeding relationship.

In addition to lower Apgar scores and an "alarmingly high incidence of asphyxia" (December 1979 *ICEA Review)*, cesarean newborns exhibit problems such as a greater intracellular water content, wet lung, lower blood volumes, and lower plasma levels. Dr. Mary Ellen Avery, in a study of the effects of cesarean delivery on the fetus, concluded that "morbidity and mortality are greater among infants delivered by cesarean section."

Fetal mortality rates. Some figures show greater mortality rates among vaginally delivered babies, which would tend to support those cesarean advocates who claim better results from surgical delivery. However, R. Gordon Douglas gives three reasons why their claims are unjustified:

- When a fetus is known to be dead, a physician will not perform a cesarean. Therefore, intrauterine death becomes part of the vaginal-birth mortality statistics.
- When a fetus is very small for date, it may be delivered vaginally. Thus many premature or low-birth weight babies, who are known to be high risk, may be part of the vaginal birth statistics.
- A baby known to have severe congenital abnormalities will not be delivered by cesarean and so is likely to join the vaginal-birth mortality statistics.

Douglas concluded that there is "no evidence that vaginal delivery per se is responsible for a higher perinatal mortality than cesarean section. In fact, our data indicated that a number of infants delivered by elective cesarean section were premature and died as a result of pulmonary complications."

For elective repeat-cesareans, fetal mortality statistics are available, and they are high. Studies have shown death rates varying from three to seven times higher in babies delivered by scheduled cesarean than in those whose mothers were allowed to start labor. A 1969 study showed that 1 out of 100 mature infants died after elective primary- or repeat-cesarean with no trial of labor. R.C. Benson determined that neonatal mortality was twice as high in infants delivered by repeat-cesarean without labor when compared to a vaginally delivered control group. He also found that four times as many cesarean babies had dangerously low five-minute Apgar scores (0.3 range) and that reasons for favoring vaginal delivery were evident at both the four-month and one-year pediatric neurologic exams. Diana Petitti reports that a comparison of neonatal mortality rates for 1976–77 for vaginally delivered infants with those delivered by repeat cesarean showed a higher rate of neonatal mortality in the repeat-cesarean group for all birth weights. These studies support Douglas's contention that "cesarean section should not be done until there is definite evidence of labor."

The villain in elective cesarean delivery (whether it be primary or repeat) is iatrogenic prematurity, or the doctor's miscalculation of the baby's readiness to be born. (This also occurs commonly in inductions.) In addition to low birth weight, the danger of prematurity is an immature respiratory system, which can cause respiratory distress syndrome or hyaline membrane disease. Prematurity is estimated to exist for 5–22 percent of c/section babies as compared with 6–7 percent of babies born vaginally.

Respiratory problems in the premature newborn are caused by a deficiency in alveolar surfactant. Surfactant develops in the lungs at about thirty-six weeks and helps get oxygen to the body tissues. There is a test to measure its presence and thus the lung maturity of the baby: the pulmonary phospholipids in surfactant are synthesized by the lung and secreted into the amniotic fluid. A sample of fluid can be removed by a procedure called amniocentesis, which itself carries many associated risks. The fluid is analyzed, and the ratio of two of the phospholipids, lecithin and sphingomyelin, is used as the internal standard. This is called the L/S test. Like all the other tests, it measures only one aspect of fetal maturity and has the potential for being inaccurate; but it is better than most educated guesses when a woman must be sectioned without benefit of labor.

Much of the perinatal mortality and morbidity from iatrogenic prematurity is preventable. First of all, the physician should encourage his patients to work toward vaginal birth after cesarean rather than elective repeat-section. If VBAC is impossible, he can wait until the woman goes into labor before he delivers her by cesarean. This has the advantage of establishing fetal maturity and stimulating lung action in the fetus (the "thoracic squeeze") by the contracting uterus. It also thins out the uterus and minimizes blood loss.

Second, the physician must be convinced that a simple clinical estimate of fetal age and maturity is not an adequate means of determining optimal birth date. He must learn to perform routinely the available tests for maturity on any woman for whom labor is contraindicated. While the L/S test has the potential for greatly reducing the risk of iatrogenic prematurity, the trial-of-labor test has the potential for pretty much eliminating it altogether. Louis Saldana found that infants delivered following a trial of labor had reached optimal fetal growth and maximum lung capacity.

We have shown how cesarean section endangers mothers and how it endangers infants. Cesarean delivery also threatens the mother/infant relationship.

In *Bonding: How Parents Become Attached to Their Babies,* Diony Young states that "a positive childbirth experience appears to create in the mother an increased self-esteem and self-confidence." This, in turn, may foster maternal bonding. On the other hand, Young tells us, "A negative birth experience, where fear and pain predominate, may adversely affect a mother's feelings toward her child." Because a cesarean delivery is so often a negative experience, colored by fear and pain, the cesarean mother and child are at a decided disadvantage as they begin their life together. Often the mother is medicated, sluggish, depressed, angry, disappointed, and all those other feelings we have mentioned. The baby is groggy or fussy because of the effects of the anesthesia and other complications. And these two are supposed to be gazing into each other's eyes with everlasting love?! Add to this hospital procedures that routinely separate cesarean mothers from their newborns, and this couple is off to a very difficult start.

Recently, because of studies by Marshall Klaus and others, there has been a great surge of interest in the issue of bonding—the early development of the unique attachment between mother (and father) and baby. Research by Marshall Klaus and by Lee Salk demonstrated that the first twenty-four hours postpartum are a crucial period for the development of the normal mother/infant bond. Moreover, it was pointed out that hospital routines, which generally separated babies from their mothers during that postpartum period, served to inhibit rather than encourage the mother's nurturing instincts.

It was not long before parent groups, studies in hand, began to bang on the doors of hospital administrators demanding change. And it was not long before the hospitals responded to consumer demand and began to institute rooming-in, whereby mother and baby became roommates and touched, stared at each other, got to know each other, smiled at each other, and bonded. Although rooming-in has become pretty much standard fare in hospitals across the country, it is still routinely denied many cesarean mothers. The cesarean newborn is still required by too many hospitals to spend the first twenty-four hours—bonding time!—in a special-care nursery, in an artificial warmer, alone and apart from the one person who knows his needs best, away from what Doris Haire calls "the most logical of warming devices," his mother's arms.

The immediate results of all this are that the mother is more a hospital patient than a mother, and the baby is lying alone, at the peak of his sucking reflex, not learning how to nurse. Both Klaus and Salk demonstrated that maternal response and nurturing are adversely affected for a full month after birth when the mother and her baby have been thus separated. (It is significant that of all the risks associated with cesarean section, this risk to the mother/infant bond is the one that makes consumer groups the most irate. Forget morbidity and mortality: bonding is the issue around which they rally. "You can take my health, and you can take my life, but you can't take my relationship with my child!" they seem to say.)

What are the long-range effects of early mother/baby separation? Klaus and his associates feel that the "battered child syndrome" may be one. M. Lynch reported, in a study of child abuse, that bonding failure is related to the mother's pregnancy, her labor, her delivery, and the amount of neonatal separation she endured. Also mentioned in this study was the high incidence of prematurity among abused children. Others question whether the mothers of abused children have a higher cesarean rate than the general population. Given the greater likelihood that the cesarean baby will be premature and will be separated from his mother immediately postpartum, the implications for his future warrant further examination.

Despite all of these physiological and psychological maternal and fetal risks, the force that ultimately turns the cesarean tide may well be the economic cost of cesarean section to the consumer.

The costs of a cesarean vary widely throughout the United States, but they are always greater than the costs of a vaginal delivery. In general, physicians charge about a third more for a surgical delivery, and the hospital stay for both mother and baby is about double. Marieskind warns that sometimes there are additional charges for the use of the operating room, the use of the recovery room, additional supplies, anesthesia, lab work, pharmacy items, I.V. equipment, blood transfusions, oxygen, and X rays.

All of these expenses also hold true for the cost of a repeat-cesarean as compared with a trial of labor and a vaginal delivery. In a study by Shy and associates, the cost difference between an elective repeat-cesarean and a VBAC averaged $500 per patient. As we have already mentioned, the Marieskind report estimated that " in 1976 alone, we could potentially have saved about 95 million dollars had a policy of individual evaluation and subsequent vaginal deliveries been followed." Many are starting to look at midwives and home birth as a way to cut costs and avoid the interventions that lead to cesareans. Charles Mahan, as reported in the *ICEA Review* in 1979, predicts that when the insurance companies and the professional-service review organizations start to realize the tremendous cost savings of VBAC, they will exert economic pressure to end the practice of routine repeat-cesareans. But until that happens, American babies will continue to be "from their mothers' wombs untimely ripp'd."

In its summary statement, the NIH task force concluded that the rising cesarean-section rate is a "matter of concern." Its members agreed that the cesarean trend could be stopped and indeed reversed "while continuing to make improvements in maternal and fetal outcomes."

We also conclude that the rising cesarean-section rate is a matter of concern. It is a matter of grave concern. The cesarean epidemic must be brought under control. Too many mothers and their babies are being needlessly exposed to avoidable risks, and too many physicians are refusing to admit it. As it becomes increasingly apparent that the medical profession is not going to put constraints upon itself, it becomes more and more obvious that we, the consumers, are going to have to take control.

In the meantime, the silent knife continues to slash its way across the stomach of America, maiming our confidence in our bodies and murdering our hopes and dreams for our children's births. Its quick, stealthy flash cuts through to the core of our being, stripping us of our illusions of control and leaving us wounded and vulnerable.

Hospital Care for Profit

Geraldine Dallek

In 1961, four men set out for a game of golf. Two were real estate agents; two, young lawyers from a prestigious Louisville, Kentucky, law firm. That golf game was the beginning of what was to become an international corporation with $2.6 billion in annual revenue—Humana, Incorporated. Only a few years later, in 1968, two Nashville doctors met with Jack Massey, a founder of Kentucky Fried Chicken, and Hospital Corporation of America (HCA), the nation's largest for-profit hospital chain, was born. By 1984, HCA owned or managed 260 hospitals in 41 states and grossed more than $3.9 billion from its hospitals and nursing homes. By the mid-1980s, proprietary hospitals controlled 12 percent of the acute care hospital market in the United States, 21 percent in the South.

It is possible to understand the rapid growth and impact of these proprietary chains only by examining the environment that nurtured them. In many ways, the medical care industry is like the defense industry. First, the goals of each—protecting our nation and protecting our health—are intrinsically valued by our society. Second, medical care and national defense are extremely costly. We spend $300 billion on defense each year, three-fourths as much as the $400 billion spent on health care. Third, both industries, in what is clearly aberrant free-market behavior, have been permitted to set the price of the goods and services they produce. In defense, it is the weapons contractors who have been virtually given a blank check: in the medical industry, hospitals, nursing homes, drug manufacturers, and physicians have, until very recently, also had carte blanche to determine how much their product is worth. Given these factors, is it any wonder that both industries are highly profitable?

The ability to make money from the delivery of medical care is not new. In the late nineteenth century, as hospitals became safe and attractive places in which to care for the ill, small for-profit hospitals sprung up in the United States and Western Europe. In Europe, individual for-profit hospitals faded from the scene as government assumed more responsibility for ensuring the provision of health care. By contrast, the for-profit hospital industry in the United States flourished.

In the early 1980s, for-profit chains were the darling of Wall Street with a 20 percent growth rate. During 1982, a recession year for most businesses, stocks of the top four hospital chains rose 30 percent. Profits of the twenty largest chains went up 38 percent in 1983 and 28.5 percent the following year. In 1984, HCA's chief executive officer was the second highest paid executive in the nation, and the head of National Medical Enterprises (NME) beat out the movie moguls as the highest paid executive in Southern California.

What accounts for the rapid expansion and huge profits of these new hospital organizations? Traditional reimbursement policies go far to explain the attractiveness of the hospital industry to entrepreneurs. Hospitals, until adoption of the new Medicare diagnosis related group (DRG) payment system in 1983, were generally paid by a retrospective cost-based reimbursement system. This open-ended system for paying hospitals, begun by Blue Cross plans (acting almost as agents for the hospitals) after World War II, was adopted by the federal government as the quid pro quo for the hospital industry's support of Medicare and Medicaid legislation in 1965. The potential for profits in this reimbursement system cannot be overstated. "It was hard not to be successful," commented the chief executive officer of National Medical Enterprises in a 1985 *Wall Street Journal* article. Profits could be made by simply buying existing hospitals and making sure that bills to both private and public insurers contained an add-on profit.

Hospitals could be bought easily in the seventies and early eighties. For-profit chains' access to capital through the sale of stock gave them an advantage over their nonprofit brethren for purposes of both building and buying hospitals. Because of their large revenue, assets, and equity base, they were viewed as sound financial risks.

The major growth of for-profit chains came from the purchase of financially troubled hospitals. Between 1980 and 1982, 43 percent of the growth of the six largest for-profit chains came from the purchase of other for-profit hospitals, mostly independent facilities. A third of the growth came from the construction of new hospitals and a fourth from the purchase of public and voluntary nonprofit hospitals. Following a for-profit purchase, ailing hospitals were brought back to health by building new facilities to attract physicians, substantially increasing charges, and reducing services to those who could not pay. Public hospitals owned and run by local governments were often receptive to being bailed out by for-profit chains. Faced with aging facilities, unable to attract privately insured patients, and confronted with increased numbers of the poor seeking care, public hospitals awash with red ink were all too happy to sell to for-profit chains.

In assessing the impact of the for-profit hospital industry, we must go well beyond the counting of beds. The industry has had a far-reaching impact on the cost of hospital care, the delivery of services to the poor, and the behavior of other health care providers.

Costly Care

For-profit chains have often been viewed favorably because of their promise to bring managerial efficiency to the "wasteful" nonprofit sector. It does not appear that they possess superior managerial talents. After reviewing a number of studies on multihospital systems, Ermann and Gabel concluded in a May 1985 article in *Medical Care* that "There is little empirical evidence that [multihospital] systems have realized economies of scale of mass purchasing or use capital facilities more efficiently." Nor have chains served as a competitive catalyst to an industry grown fat by its insulation from free-market forces. Theoretically, competition and efficiency would lead to reduced costs. Judged by this standard, for-profit hospital chains also failed, as they increased, not lowered, the cost of hospital care.

For-profit chain costs have been higher than nonprofit hospital costs for three reasons: they mark up charges well above expenses; they use more expensive ancillary services than nonprofit facilities; and charges must cover their higher capital costs. According to several studies, the difference in costs between for-profit and not-for-profit hospitals is substantial. A comparison of charges at 280 California for-profit and nonprofit hospitals showed that for-profit hospital charges per admission were 24 percent higher than those of the voluntary hospitals and 47 percent higher than public hospital charges. According to this study—by Robert Pattison and Hallie Katz, reported in the August 1983 *New England Journal of Medicine*—huge profits were made in ancillary services such as pharmacy and laboratory services. The study also showed that despite the claims of administrative savings, costs for "fiscal services" and "administrative services" (which include costs to maintain corporate headquarters elsewhere) were 32 percent higher in for-profit chain hospitals than in voluntary hospitals. The authors concluded that the data "do not support the claim that investor-owned chains enjoy overall operating efficiencies or economies of scale in administrative fiscal services."

Results of a more recent study, by Lewin and Associates and health policy analysts at Johns Hopkins University, of eighty matched pairs of investor-owned chain and not-for-profit hospitals in eight states were remarkably similar to the Pattison and Katz study: prices charged by for-profit chain hospitals were 22 percent more per admission than those charged by matched not-for-profit hospitals.

For-profit hospitals also charge more for several procedures, according to a 1983 Blue Cross/Blue Shield of North Carolina study. Comparing charges for three commonly performed hospital procedures—gall bladder removals, hysterectomies, and normal deliveries of babies—at six for-profit hospitals and six matched nonprofit hospitals, the study found that in all but one case the average total charge was from 6 percent to 58 percent higher in the for-profit hospitals.

Patients have generally been insulated from higher for-profit charges by their third party coverage. Nevertheless, at least one Las Vegas man found the cost of care at his local for-profit hospital upsetting. In a June 1985 letter to the *Las Vegas Review Journal,* the gentleman recounted how he had:

> recently had the misfortune of requiring emergency room treatment at Humana Sunrise Hospital for kidney stone problems. This was my second encounter with this problem. The first encounter occurred last July, and I was treated at Southern Nevada Memorial Hospital.
>
> As the treatment was almost identical, I have had the opportunity to compare the costs of the two facilities. I was not surprised to find that Humana hospitals were more expensive; however, I was shocked to discover that the cost was fully 50% above that of Southern Nevada.
>
> As I was curtly informed by administrative personnel at Humana, the costs were higher because Humana is a "private" hospital, and Southern Nevada is a county hospital. Now this is a point well taken and probably could account for a 15 or 20% difference, but 50%—Come on, who does Humana think they are fooling?

For-profit hospitals have also increased health care costs indirectly by building unneeded hospitals. For example, primarily because of the growth of for-profit hospitals, twelve Florida counties, underbedded in 1972, had 6,600 excess beds three years later. The for-profit chains that had controlled 16.7 percent of beds in 1972 had built 60 percent of the new beds.

If efficiency is measured by maximum use of the physical plant, for-profit chains are once again found wanting. In 1985, average hospital occupancy rates for the four largest proprietary chains ranged from 46 percent to 56 percent. Empty beds were not as important under the old cost-based reimbursement system, as charges to insurers for patients in the occupied beds could be increased to cover the cost of unoccupied beds. This changed with Medicare's new reimbursement system which pays a flat rate based on a patient's diagnosis and vigorous cost containment programs begun by Medicaid and private health insurers in 1983 and 1984.

The old cost-based reimbursement systems not only rewarded hospitals for providing extra services and hiking up prices but failed to penalize them for empty beds. Medicare's new flat rate reimbursement scheme provides opposite incentives: it rewards hospitals for reducing services (the fewer services provided, the more money made) and penalizes them for their empty beds. This dramatic change in the way hospitals are paid would, it could be supposed, hurt most those hospitals that had taken greatest advantage of the old system. This seems to have happened. In October of 1985, announcements by the leading chains of flat or reduced earnings stunned Wall Street and resulted in a steep decline in their stocks.

In response to changes in hospital reimbursement and declining hospital revenues, chains began to diversify—investing in more lucrative areas of medical care, including nursing homes, insurance companies, health maintenance organizations (HMOs), neighborhood emergi-centers (often called doc-in-the-box), and home health agencies. Their proven ability to maximize profits from the provision of medical services will thus be tested in new arenas. Called a "managed system" approach, this vertical integration of the health industry gives proprietary chains added power to shape the future of health care delivery in this country.

Analysts may argue over the exact impact of the growth of the proprietary chains, but most agree that in subtle and not-so-subtle ways chains have irrevocably changed the milieu in which hospitals operate. Nowhere has the change been more profound than in the provision of hospital care to the poor.

Turning Away the Poor

Chains make no secret of their view that health care is nothing more than an economic commodity to be sold in the marketplace for a profit. One Humana senior vice president put it this way: "health care is a necessity, but so is food. Do you know of any neighborhood grocery store where you can walk out with $3,000 worth of food that you haven't paid for?" Chain spokesmen are also commonly heard to claim that their hospitals' commitment to the poor is taken care of by the payment of taxes. Given this view, it is not surprising that several state studies have found large disparities in the amount of care for the indigent provided by for-profit hospitals and voluntary and public hospitals. Typically, public hospitals provide the lion's share of uncompensated care; voluntary hospitals come in a poor second, with for-profit facilities running a dismal third.

Although for-profit hospitals constituted 32 percent of Florida's hospitals in 1983, they provided only 4 percent of the net charity care provided within the state. Florida's Hospital Cost Containment Board openly criticized for-profit hospitals in its 1983–84 annual report for their failure to share the burden of serving the uninsured poor. According to a report by the Texas Task Force on Indigent Health Care, for-profit hospitals made up 19.1 percent of the hospitals in that state in 1983, but provided less than I percent of the charity care and only 2.7 percent of the bad debt. Nonprofit hospitals, while making up 36.1 percent of the hospital facilities in Texas, provided 13.1 percent of charity care and 42.8 percent of the bad debt. Texas's public facilities provided most of the care of the poor: public hospitals, constituting 44.7 percent of the hospitals in the state, provide 86.9 percent of the charity care and 54.6 percent of the bad debt.

Some national data on provision of care for the indigent are available from the January 1981 Office of Civil Rights (OCR) survey of all general, short-term hospitals in the United States. An analysis of OCR data on inpatient admitting practices showed that 9.5 percent of all hospital patients were uninsured in 1981; yet only 6 percent of patients treated at for-profit hospitals were uninsured while 16.8 percent of those treated at hospitals owned by state and local governments were uninsured. Alan Sager also used OCR data in his study of hospital closures and relocation in 52 cities. He found that of the 4,038 patients categorized on admission as charity care patients (not to be charged) during the OCR survey, only I received care at a for-profit facility.

To some extent, the amount of charity care provided by for-profit hospitals is limited by their locations—in suburban white communities where few of the poor reside. When those hospitals are matched with similarly located nonprofit facilities, the amount of care to the poor differs little by ownership. However, geography does not explain why chain hospitals located in areas with significant numbers of uninsured populations provide so little in the way of charity.

The plight of one fifty-six-year-old uninsured laborer described in a recent *Washington Post* article is a case in point. Mr. G.R. Lafon sought care for third-degree grease burns on his side and back at the hospital nearest his home, a for-profit facility. The hospital and two other for-profit hospitals refused him emergency care because he did not have a deposit ranging from $500 to $1,500. One of the hospitals did take the precaution of inserting an intravenous tube and a catheter to stabilize his liquids before sending him on his way. After seven hours and a seventy-mile trek, Lafon arrived at Parkland Memorial Hospital in Dallas, the city's public hospital, where he was immediately admitted. Lafon required nineteen days of hospitalization and a skin graft for a cost of $22,000. Soon after discharge, he began receiving notices for an overdue hospital bill—not for the $22,000 owed to Parkland (that will be written off because Lafon is poor and uninsured) but for $373.75 from the for-profit facility to cover the cost of the catheter and intravenous tube.

Similar horror stories can be heard all over the South. In Memphis, for example, the city's largest HCA hospital threatened early in 1985 that it would stop chemotherapy treatments for a farmer with lung cancer when his family ran out of cash to continue the treatments. It was not until the day a suit was to be filed against the hospital claiming abandonment, denial of emergency medical care, intentional infliction of mental distress and extortion, that the HCA relented and agreed to continue treatment.

Voluntary hospitals and even some public hospitals also turn away the poor. What distinguishes the actions of for-profit chain hospitals from those of individual voluntary or public facilities is that the for-profit hospitals' policy denying access is established at corporate headquarters and affects all their facilities throughout the nation. Although many voluntary hospitals are reducing their uncompensated care load in order to survive, others continue to view care for the poor as part of their mission.

The impact of care to the uninsured goes beyond the number of poor that proprietary chains do and do not serve. In the past five years, 180 public hospitals have been bought or managed by for-profit companies. This has resulted in an inexorable diminution of care to the poor: public officials do not sell hospitals in order to continue providing indigent care; they do so in order to relieve themselves from what they perceive as an onerous burden. These sales, in turn, add to the financial troubles of the public and voluntary hospitals which continue to serve the indigent population. Chains also have had one other far-reaching effect on the provision of care to the poor: they have caused what Louanne Kennedy of the City University of New York describes as "the proprietarization of voluntary hospitals."

Beat 'Em or Join 'Em

Nonprofit hospitals have long had a split personality, torn by the need to make money (their business side) and the need to succor the poor and sick (their humanitarian or social side). The rapid growth of for-profit chains forced nonprofit facilities to come to terms with this dichotomy. In the process, hospitals became more businesslike and less concerned with humanitarian goals.

Interestingly, for-profit chains did promote competition in the delivery of hospital services but not, as the supply/demand curve predicts, on the basis of price. In the middle and late seventies, as the number of empty beds increased, hospital survival became increasingly predicated on attracting physicians who would admit their privately insured patients. In the competition for doctors, a hospital belonging to a large chain with easy access to capital had distinct advantages over the local voluntary and especially the public facility. A choice between a thirty-year-old public hospital with its leaky roof, overcrowded emergency room (filled with poor people), and frequent equipment breakdowns and the spanking new Humana or HCA hospital with the latest in diagnostic equipment and nary a poor person in sight, was no choice at all.

Chains also had the money to recruit doctors to their hospitals. For example, an April 5, 1982, Humana's recruiting letter to pediatricians offered the following inducements to join a five-physician multispecialty group in Springhill, Louisiana:

guaranteed income—$5,500 per month for the first six months; the lowest projected first-year income is $150.000;

rent-free office—absolutely no business or other overhead expenses the first year; this includes a paid nurse, secretarial and office equipment and furniture, free utilities, and more;

paid health/dental/life/malpractice insurance;

company car; paid moving expenses; paid country club membership; paid on-site visit.

The most famous for-profit hospital recruit. Dr. William DeVries, was brought to the Humana Heart Institute in Louisville, Kentucky, with the promise of 100 artificial heart transplants.

In the competition over physicians, chains did not ignore the patient. Although price was not a consideration, well-heeled patients were lured to specialized chain facilities which touted the latest in sports medicine, treatment of diet disorders, wine and candlelight dinners for new parents, and a free hairstyle with a "tummy tuck." If patients were to be appealed to directly, then chain products had to be merchandised, and so advertising budgets became part and parcel of the cost of providing medical care.

At the same time as voluntary hospitals were losing private, paying patients to the new hospital on the block, they were also getting less money for the private, paying patients still filling their beds. Generally, under the blank-check reimbursement system, hospitals simply passed on the costs of their nonpaying patients to their privately insured patients whose care was paid for through employer-subsidized insurance. Thus, employers were subsidizing care for the poor through higher insurance premiums. While hospital access for the poor has been far from universal, a great deal of service was paid for by this cost shift. The health insurance industry estimated that it was charged an extra $8 billion in 1983 to subsidize the provision of care to those who could not pay and were uninsured.

As hospital costs kept spiraling (in some years by 20 percent) and as the number of uninsured poor increased, commercial insurers and business interests became less willing to pay this cost shift or what they called a "sick tax." Arguing that they should only have to pay premium costs to cover care for their work force, not the nation's poor, employers demanded and got reductions in their premium costs and the beginnings of competition based on price.

Voluntary and public hospitals subsidizing the poor are at a distinct disadvantage in any game based on price competition because they are, according to policy analysts, playing on an "uneven playing field." To even stay in the game, they are forced to act like their opponents, which means toughening up their billing and collection practices and managing their indigent patient load. Unfortunately, "managing" is often synonymous with "excluding." An American Hospital Association study found that in 1981 and 1982 about 15 percent of nonprofit hospitals adopted limits on the amount of charity care they provided, and 84 percent increased billing and collection efforts.

There is no question that many tax exempt charitable institutions provided little or no care to the poor well before the proprietary chains came on the scene. For these hospitals, for-profit chains made barring the poor an acceptable way of doing business. For nonprofit hospitals that took their charitable status seriously the chains made it difficult and in some instances impossible for them to continue fulfilling their mission. The traditional behavior of tax exempt hospitals that provide little or no charity care is being challenged in state courts. A June 1985 decision by the Utah Supreme Court denied tax exempt status to two nonprofit hospitals owned by Intermountain Health Care, a nonprofit hospital chain, because the hospitals did not meet their obligation to provide charity care.

"If you can't beat 'em, join 'em," was a slogan adopted by a large number of voluntary and public hospitals in the early eighties. In addition to conscious efforts to reduce services to the poor, nonprofit hospitals embarked on a mad scramble to buy nursing homes, establish home health agencies, "unbundle" hospital services (remove services such as pharmacy, laboratory, and X-ray from the hospital to get the higher reimbursement rates), specialize in highly profitable ventures such as sports medicine and wellness centers, structure patients care to achieve optimal reimbursement, consider terminating unprofitable services, and advertise.

While most hospitals argue these changes are necessary for survival, others maintain their efforts are directed toward continuing to subsidize charity care. This latter justification is commonly used by public hospitals which began in 1984 and 1985 to undertake corporate restructuring as an alternative to outright sale or transfer of management to a for-profit firm. While the exact configurations vary, the basic idea is to create several new nonprofit and for-profit subsidies. One of the nonprofits will lease the existing hospital for a nominal amount and operate it for the actual public owners, blurring what had once been a clear-cut distinction between for-profit and public hospitals.

Nonprofit hospitals copied the for-profit giants in one other way. Finding strength in numbers, voluntary hospitals began to form their own nonprofit chains. Although some chains of voluntary facilities (such as religious hospitals) predated the rise of for-profit chains, the impetus for increased horizontal integration among nonprofit hospitals in the early 1980s was competition from the proprietary chains.

Good Business or Basic Care?

In 1979, one health analyst commented that "We could wake up in a few years with a few Exxons controlling half the hospitals." It did not take long for this prediction to come true. By 1990, it is likely that ten or so for-profit and nonprofit managed systems will compete with one another to serve the paying customer, while the few public hospitals left (primarily large inner-city facilities which cannot be closed for fear of adverse political repercussions) will continue their struggle to serve the impoverished of the nation. Is this the legacy of the proprietarization of American hospitals? The answer is no. The growth of for-profit chains was simply the natural development of a society that never viewed health care as a right, guaranteed to every citizen, and a government adverse to bucking the prevailing notion that medical providers should be left to their own devices to shape the nation's health care delivery system. If, in the shaping, no space was available for millions of Americans, so be it.

Uwe Reinhardt, a Princeton economist, argues that America's political ideology—its fear of big government—helped to create a medical system that tolerates "visible social pathos in our streets." This system accepts the existence of 35 million uninsured, most of whom are poor and near-poor; denial of prenatal and sometimes delivery care to poor women; the transferring or "dumping" of 500 patients a month from private Chicago hospitals to Cook County General, a public facility; excessive markups on drugs needed to control hypertension and other chronic illnesses; inhuman conditions in many of our nursing homes; and, lately, the premature discharge of elderly patients from hospitals when Medicare payments prove inadequate to cover the costs of care.

Our response to this social pathos depends in large degree on how we view the delivery of medical care. If, as for-profit hospitals maintain, health care is a business, if HCA and Humana are no different than a McDonald's or a Macy's, then our response is obvious: protect against the grossest anticompetitive behavior, but generally adopt a laissez-faire attitude and let market forces dictate the supply and price of goods. If, however, we believe that health care is more than a business, but a societal good, then our response is different indeed. Laws will be needed to assure that prices are controlled, profits limited, and people guaranteed the provision of basic health care.

Which is it? To date, we have either ignored the question or, when forced to confront it, tried to have it both ways. This has led to ambiguous policies at best and huge holes in the nation's health care safety net. The "let's have it both ways" mentality is evident in the government's Medicare policies. Although the provision of medical care to the elderly and disabled is clearly seen as a societal good, the federal government's Medicare reimbursement policy with its substantial return on investment and unlimited passing through of capital costs resulted in huge profits for investor-owned hospital chains and more money going for fewer services. It is only recently, with the advent of DRGs and 1986 legislation to eliminate return on equity (over three years) and proposals to cap federal reimbursements for capital costs, that we have begun to realize that unlimited profits may be at odds with the nation's commitment to providing health care for the elderly.

States have not been any more certain of how to reconcile the needs of the ill and the needs of the medical care marketplace. A few northeastern states have controlled the growth of for-profit hospitals through hospital rate regulation; by limiting rates hospitals can charge, states limit the profits hospitals can make. These states also include payment for care of the indigent in their controlled rates. Other states have sought to require good citizenship of all their hospitals, for-profit and voluntary alike. Florida, South Carolina, and Virginia tax hospitals in order to pay for increased care of the indigent. Tougher emergency room laws in a few states, most notably Texas, have made it more difficult for hospitals to refuse emergency care to the poor or inappropriately transfer them to the nearest public hospital. Efforts have also been made, primarily through the health planning program, to require hospitals wanting to build or modernize to provide a small amount of charity care. North Carolina now requires for-profit hospitals that buy public hospitals to continue to provide care to the poor of the community.

Unfortunately, these efforts are too little too late; the poor and, increasingly, the middle class with inadequate insurance are not guaranteed access to even basic hospital care when ill. Neither the federal government nor the states have been willing to limit profits made from providing hospital care, to require all hospitals to serve a minimum of uninsured and Medicaid recipients, or to provide health care coverage for all in need.

Unlike other Western industrialized nations, we treat medical care as a commodity to be bought and sold in the marketplace. This marketplace mentality is allowing corporate medicine to distort our medical care system into one that costs us a great deal even while it serves a diminishing share of our people.

Public Prospects

Robert G. Hughes and Philip R. Lee

Public hospitals are as old as the republic, and many of these institutions are facing a crisis in financing that will affect their future. Crisis, particularly financial crisis, is not a new experience for public hospitals, but the current crisis may prove more damaging than many in the past. To cope with the crisis and deal with it effectively, the roots of the current problems must be understood and appropriate policy and management responses initiated.

Approximately one-third of the 5,500 general acute care hospitals in the United States are public hospitals (owned or controlled by a state or local government). These hospitals collectively represent a vital part of our health care delivery system, yet many of them, especially the larger urban public hospitals, are being adversely affected by a number of factors—including the residues of the recession of 1981–82, federal and state health policy changes affecting the organization and financing of health care, and other federal policies (for example, the increased allocation of funds for military purposes) that have limited resources available for domestic social programs. Changes at the state level and in the private sector that have given rise to the wave of enthusiasm for competition in the health care industry are adding to the problems facing public hospitals.

Some public hospitals have closed. Many of the largest remaining public hospitals have reduced their number of beds, cut staffs, postponed capital improvements, and gone back to their local government sponsors for additional financing to maintain their level of service to the poor. In the face of fiscal distress, aging physical facilities, civil service constraints on personnel, and the emerging acceptance of competition and the growth of proprietary enterprises as a rationale for cost containment, public institutions face an uncertain future. The choices available for

211

these hospitals range from closure, sale to proprietary organizations, or creative restructuring, to relying on institutional inertia to see them through the next decade. What is the future role of public hospitals in our health care system?

Hospital ownership falls into three broad types: public, voluntary (private, not-for-profit) and proprietary (private, for-profit). Public hospitals differ from voluntary and proprietary hospitals in important ways. On average, public hospitals are more likely to offer primary medical care services than other hospitals, and they serve people who are poor, less educated, and have less access to physicians than people served by voluntary or proprietary hospitals. These differences are consistent with the historic community role of public hospitals: they are the providers of last resort that care for people who, because of the political and socioeconomic structure of our society, are unable to obtain care elsewhere. Rural public hospitals fill geographic gaps and make services accessible in many sparsely populated areas that would otherwise be acutely underserved. Public hospitals located in cities care for a disproportionately large share of the poor and the uninsured in their communities while other voluntary and proprietary hospitals serve primarily the insured and the nonpoor. Overall, public hospitals fill gaps in our health care system by providing over 17 percent of all hospital care, primarily to the poor and uninsured who would otherwise go without care, be sicker, and die sooner.

Despite their common role as provider of last resort, public hospitals are not homogeneous. The diversity of public hospitals and the roles they played in their communities was an issue addressed by the Commission on Public General Hospitals, established in 1976 by the Hospital Research and Educational Trust (an affiliate of the American Hospital Association). The commission's purpose was "to examine the present health care delivery roles of public general hospitals and to identify future roles, if any, for these hospitals." Recognizing the variation among public hospitals and the need to take account of these differences in assessing their future, the commission divided public hospitals into four groups: (1) urban public general hospitals, or those located in the nation's 100 largest cities; (2) public general hospitals in metropolitan areas outside the 100 largest cities; (3) rural public general hospitals; and (4) university public hospitals.

By far the largest group was the rural public general hospitals, which made up almost three-fourths of all public hospitals. These hospitals, as might be expected, are small (with an average of seventy beds) and provide only 40 percent of the patient days provided in public institutions. They have fewer specialized facilities than other hospitals, fewer physician specialists on staff, and are often the only hospital serving the community in which the hospital is located. The large number of small rural hospitals makes them an important part of our health care system, but they are sufficiently different from large urban public hospitals that it is appropriate to consider their futures separately. These rural public institutions are more likely to be influenced by their monopoly status— that is, by being the sole source of inpatient primary and secondary care in a geographical area with their diverse clientele (not just the poor)—than by the factors that are adversely affecting large, urban public institutions, which, in part, stem from their location in communities with many other hospitals and from their role as major providers of inpatient and outpatient care for the indigent.

The other three groups of hospitals identified by the commission were the large urban public general hospitals (90), the medium-sized metropolitan public general hospitals (357), and the hospitals owned by public universities (45). The commission's report argued that the future of these three groups was likely to be different from each other. The medium-sized metropolitan public hospitals, many of them district hospitals, were found to be similar in many respects to private hospitals in the same settings—in size, financial health, and proportion of paying patients— and thus were not expected to encounter obstacles different from those encountered by such hospitals generally. University owned hospitals were distinguished by the extent to which their future depended on societal decisions about financing graduate medical education and the future role of complex, higher cost tertiary care technology in health care. Their educational and research roles, as well as their specialized tertiary care role, are likely to be the overriding determinants of their future.

The remaining hospitals, the large urban public hospitals. have attracted the most attention from policymakers and others, including the commission. These hospitals are large (with an average of 503 beds) and have traditionally served as provider of last resort in their communities. The report of the commission summarized their situation:

> By tradition, these hospitals serve many patients who have no other source of financing for their health care. The also serve many neighborhood residents for whom they are the hospital of choice, and they frequently provide the community

as a whole with certain highly specialized and emergency services. As a group, the urban public-general hospitals are extremely susceptible to financial problems because they serve large numbers of unsponsored patients and provide many services, including ambulatory care services, that are not adequately reimbursed by third-party payers. Many of these hospitals today are in serious financial difficulty because of inadequate local government appropriations and a growing caseload of unsponsored patients. Further, a number of them are encumbered with outdated and outmoded plant and equipment. Because of their weak financial position, they have difficulty in raising capital, even for renovations to bring them into compliance with fire and life safety codes. Many of these urban public hospitals are engaged in training large numbers of physicians and other health professionals, and their medical staffs often are composed of full-time attending physicians who, with medical residents, provide physician services.

Among all hospitals, the urban public-general hospitals, as a group, have the most serious and persistent problems.

Why did these hospitals emerge as a major focus of the commission's work and why do they continue to attract a disproportionate share of policy attention today? In large part it is because their role, which has its roots in their historical mission of providing care to patients regardless of their ability to pay, has resulted in these hospitals absorbing the costs generated by the structural defects of our health care system and of our fragmental system of health care financing. The stresses on these institutions are accentuated by the changes in financing affecting all hospitals.

Urban Crisis

The most fundamental force in the current transformation of our health care system is the effort to control costs. Historically hospitals and physicians have been paid by methods that provided no incentive for efficiency and, indeed, often provided incentives for delivering ever more specialized and expensive services. Increasingly sophisticated technology, potential malpractice suits, rising public expectations, hospital market structure, and the nature of hospital-physician relationships, in combination with perverse economic incentives, contributed to health care expenditures absorbing an increased share of the gross national product, particularly during the past twenty years. During this period, the organization of health care was relatively unconstrained by lack of external resources. Physician supply increased rapidly. Physicians continued to practice in relatively the same way and in the same settings as in the past; hospitals, although perhaps inconvenienced by regulatory efforts such as Certificate of Need and health planning programs, for the most part did not significantly alter their organization or financing, and many were able to modernize, expand, and add new services. Financing mechanisms adopted during this period often were designed to accommodate the professional interest groups of physicians and hospitals.

Recently, vigorous efforts to control costs have forced hospitals and (to a lesser extent) physicians to examine their organization and financing with an eye toward responding to externally imposed constraints. These constraints have emanated primarily from government. other third party payers. and employers who have paid for their employees health insurance. The federal government's implementation of the prospective payment system for Medicare, based on diagnosis related groups, has been important not only for its actual financial consequences, but because it symbolized the extent to which organizations external to hospitals have taken action to explicitly influence hospital behavior. Such actions include selective contracting, utilization review, preadmission screening. prospective pricing. and monitoring lengths of stay; collectively these have been aimed primarily at the costs of inpatient hospital care.

One consequence of these cost-control actions has been a reappraisal of the ways hospitals have allocated the costs of providing care to patients who cannot pay. Approximately 17 to 25 percent of the United States population under sixty-five years of age are uninsured or underinsured, and these people have more need of health care than the general population. In the past they often received care, and the costs were covered internally within hospitals through cost shifting. By increasing charges to paying patients, hospitals can offset the costs of caring for nonpaying patients, as long as they have a relatively large number of paying patients and a small number of nonpaying patients.

In theory, costs for nonpaying patients could be distributed across other citizens through insurance if all participated in the same group insurance, or across the entire population via national health insurance. In fact, these costs have been covered intra-institutionally via cost shifting, with the hospitals performing the social function of redistributing costs. As third party payers became more active in cost-control efforts, they began to negotiate with hospitals on price and to limit cost shifting, thus forcing hospitals to critically reexamine their traditional ways of financing care for the poor. Hospitals began to pay much more attention to the proportion of their budget devoted to charity care or covering bad debts. Patients who require charity care or who appear likely to incur debts that they cannot repay become a severe institutional liability in such a climate. Increasingly these patients are referred to public hospitals for care.

These organizational and financial changes have adversely affected the large urban public hospitals in two ways. First, the hospitals serve a disproportionate share of nonpaying patients so they are the most affected by restrictions on internal cross-subsidization and the increased "dumping" of nonpaying patients by private hospitals. Second, their historic role as "provider of last resort" has put them at risk of attracting even more nonpaying patients as other hospitals take actions to control their own costs by reducing their numbers of nonpaying patients. These adverse effects are magnified as the federal government seeks to reduce its Medicaid responsibility for financing health care for the poor. Cost shifting has moved from intra-institutional to inter-institutional, with the costs of providing care to nonpaying patients exported to large urban public hospitals. They are the safety valve for nonpaying patients and other hospitals in their communities, and they are increasingly taking on the burdens generated by the systemic changes in health care financing.

Many public hospitals are financially subsidized to some extent by the government that controls them. A county hospital, for example, might operate at a deficit for the year, with a county board making up the difference through an annual appropriation. Revenue from sources such as Medicaid, Medicare, other third party payers, and patients often falls short of expenses. The changes described have increased such deficits, putting even more pressure on public hospitals to seek additional funds via appropriation, yet at a time when many of their government sponsors are unable to afford increased subsidies. This has caused many governments to seek alternate means of operating their hospitals or, more drastically to find ways of getting hospitals out of their budgets altogether. Some governments have contracted with private firms to take over management of their hospitals; other public hospitals have been sold outright to private organizations; and still other hospitals have undergone a corporate reorganization that established a new governance mechanism (and budgetary responsibility) independent of the former governmental sponsor.

The current difficulty of the large urban hospitals that have remained public are a result of their role in the overall system of health care, a role that has been advantageous to other hospitals, medical schools, and many third party payers. Systemic costs for indigent care have been exported to these hospitals—the last resort not only for patients, but for other local institutions that, by dint of the existence of a public hospital, are not faced with the unavoidable demands of providing for the poor.

Efforts to control health care costs are inextricably linked to access in our decentralized, pluralistic health care system. As individual hospitals and multihospital systems take steps to ensure their own long-term financial viability, they make strategic decisions that determine the types of patients that will have access to their institutions. For example, a decision to locate a new hospital in an affluent suburban area, to offer services more likely to attract insured patients, or to institute a rigid credit and collection policy—these decisions foster paying patients and discourage nonpaying patients. More subtle, but not necessarily less powerful, forces also affect the payment status of patients likely to use that hospital, such as the extent to which patients who appear indigent are treated with respect and a hospital's reputation for serving anyone in the community.

Actions by individual private hospitals or hospital systems that respond to cost controls in a reasonable way to assure their fiscal viability have the consequence of eroding the fiscal viability of public institutions and reducing access to the system as a whole. The dilemmas facing large urban public hospitals are a consequence of their role relative to other hospitals in the communities and changes in the environment of hospitals generally. Their problems do not stem primarily from internal hospital characteristics such as mismanagement, civil service constraints. demands of unionized workers, or the inefficiencies of bureaucratic medicine; they are overwhelmingly the consequence of factors external to hospital operation—changes in the financial and organizational structure of our health care industry and in the ideas our society has apparently accepted as a rationale for behavior among health care institutions.

The Reagan administration has lead the ideological shift affecting health care through two main themes: New Federalism and competition. New Federalism has emphasized the responsibility of state and local governments for many functions that had increasingly been performed by the federal government over the past forty years. The administration's policies and legislative initiatives have been, in theory, designed to reverse this shift of responsibility. Competition has been adopted as the most appropriate means of distributing goods and services, including health care, within a classic market model. This model encourages discussion of health care primarily in economic terms, using economic concepts such as market share, price competition, and marketing. Health care is viewed increasingly as a commodity purchased from profit-maximizing firms that are part of an industry, and less as a service expected to be available to all citizens. We do not share the Reagan administration's confidence in competition as the most appropriate means to assure access and control costs. The combination of New Federalism and pro-competition policies in health care have had the predictable effects of putting strain on the local institutions that provide care for citizens unable to enter into the competitive market because they lack the means: urban public hospitals serving the poor. Medicaid policies, although not the same in all states, often add to the problems facing local public hospitals.

Medicaid is a federal-state assistance program that finances care for low-income blind, aged, disabled, or welfare family members. The Omnibus Budget Reconciliation Act of 1981, legislation whose content was predominantly dictated by the Reagan administration, resulted in federal Medicaid payment reductions of 3 percent in 1982, 4 percent in 1983, and 4.5 percent in 1984. More than one million citizens, primarily the working poor and their children, lost Medicaid eligibility between 1981 and 1985. Of the 20 million people covered by Medicaid, most still have less coverage than citizens with conventional third party insurance; indeed, the extent of that coverage varies markedly from state to state, and it does not begin to address the problem of poor or uninsured citizens uhose incomes put them above governmental definitions of poverty or who are excluded through other restrictive criteria. Medicaid now covers only about 40 percent of Americans living in poverty.

Federal policy since 1981 has simultaneously increased the number of citizens without means to pay for care, transferred responsibility for these citizens to state and local governments, and encouraged private sector competition for paying patients. Paying patients are primarily those insured through their place of employment, with the employer paying most of the premium. Urban public hospitals care for a disproportionate share of Medicaid patients, and these patients do not change institutional providers when their benefits are cut or when the state reduces the level of payment to hospitals as it has in California and other states. Medicaid patients that become ineligible may seek care at the public hospital because they know they will receive care regardless of their ability to pay.

Urban public hospitals are facing a crisis generated by reduction in federal programs, limits on local revenues, increased demands for services to people who cannot pay, and the transformation of all facets of health care delivery into an industry dominated by corporate actors. Underlying these changes is an apparent shift in societal values. This is toward acceptance of a federal government overwhelmingly preoccupied with controlling its own spending on health care and away from expectations that governmental policies will be directed at alleviating this country's major inequities in access—inequities unsurpassed in any developed country. Given the current situation, how can large urban public hospitals survive and prosper in the coming decade?

Urban Strategies

Discussions about the fate of large urban public hospitals are not new. Their current situation, fueled by increases in uncompensated care, is even more precarious than in the past. One result of the dramatic increase in the number of uninsured or underinsured patients requiring care, with the increased burden on public hospitals, has been a growing national and state focus on the issue of financing health care for the poor. This has moved to the top of many state and local policy agendas. The survival of the large urban public hospital is tied directly to state and national responses to this issue. Without adequate levels of payment for those who are uninsured or underinsured, large public hospitals cannot survive except as second-rate institutions providing less and less adequate care for the poor.

Health care funding for low-income citizens is essential for these hospitals. The preferable source of this money and the mechanisms of collection and distribution will vary by state and locality, and urban public hospitals will need to adopt approaches tailored to their particular situation. Regardless of the mechanisms, increased funding to pay for these services should be the primary objective of those trying to save these institutions. At both federal and state levels, large urban public hospitals should work collectively and use their firsthand knowledge of the inequities caused by inadequate funding and their access to the political process to press for a resolution. They should rely on the value of equity in our society and demonstrate the inequities that do exist with strategically selected concrete examples. The current crisis of uncompensated care should be used to educate the public about the hospitals' unique community role.

Previous analyses of the problems facing urban public hospitals have concentrated on characteristics of internal management and corporate structure. Such analyses can be considered as a form of institutional victim-blaming. By directing attention to internal difficulties inside the hospitals, these analyses ignore the external factors that are the primary causes of urban public hospital problems. Nevertheless, internal management changes should be considered, but only as part of an overall strategy aimed at increasing the hospital's negotiating power within its local health care system and with state and local government agencies that provide much of their funding. The success that does come from internal management changes and corporate reorganization will depend on how much they help the institution respond to and influence its environment.

Strategies for large urban public hospitals must begin with the recognition that, for many of the institutions, continuing to function in established ways while the environment and other hospitals change will result in additional decline and leave them moribund. Hospital environments are changing drastically. Physician supply is increasing rapidly in many areas of the country. Large employers are forming local and regional health care coalitions to take advantage of their large market shares and control their costs. These coalitions, as well as insurance companies and governments, are negotiating over price and contracting with hospitals and physicians. Health maintenance organizations, preferred provider organizations, and a potpourri of physician-hospital arrangements are proliferating. This realignment and formalization within the health care system will establish its structure for the next several decades. Public hospitals need the ability to operate on an equal basis with their competitors in the organizational, economic, and political processes that will determine their futures.

Within this changing arena, urban public hospitals have the advantage of their traditional mission, which is congruent with deeply held values of equity in our society. But these institutions cannot rely solely on the intrinsic value of their mission. They must also recognize that all health care institutions, even those that clearly provide important services that otherwise would simply not be available, will be subject to economic as well as social criteria of performance.

Governmental agencies and insurers will apply the same economic criteria used to evaluate the performance of private hospitals to public hospitals. The traditional mission of "provider of last resort" will not exempt urban public hospitals from a comparative analysis of performance. They must demonstrate that they have confronted economic issues directly. For example. they should invest effort in strengthening their credit and collections policy by increasing collections from patients who can pay (often via insurance) and developing institutional accounting for those who cannot pay. This will provide the hospital with information about its own operations, which is an essential component of any strategy for change. For example, a large urban public hospital needs a client profile to document its role to politicians, accurate cost data to negotiate with payers, and an accurate description of the amount of charity care and bad debt to get local political credit for the charity care and to demonstrate responsible control of bad debt.

A successful hospital must have management and leadership skills that are directed at influencing governmental policy and negotiating favorable agreements with other organizations. Such leadership and management skills are essential for hospitals to negotiate agreements with physicians, a medical school, other hospitals, insurers, state Medicaid programs, or patient groups. At a national level, this approach has been adopted through the formation of the National Association of Public Hospitals. This organization monitors national legislation that will affect its constituents, testifies at hearings, and works with Congress and its staff to bring the perspective of the large urban public hospitals to bear in the policy process. A similar organization, the California Association of Public Hospitals, has operated on a state level in California.

Despite the bleak current status of large urban public hospitals, they have strengths and characteristics that can be strategically used, in establishing their future roles. Many offer services not available at any other hospital. These monopolized services can be the basis of favorable negotiations with other hospitals and payers. The hospitals often have high levels of occupancy (80 to 90 percent) in contrast to declining occupancy in many community hospitals; and it seems unlikely that politicians will close the doors on a hospital that is full of the sick and injured. A hospital full of patients can be an effective bargaining tool in an era of excess hospital-bed capacity.

Bargaining implies an entrepreneurial orientation, and this may seem to contradict the role of these institutions; but an entrepreneurial orientation is not necessarily inconsistent with the traditional values of large urban public hospitals. Such an orientation simply recognizes that effective management and leadership of these institutions will require skills that fit a competitive environment. It does not mean that individual leaders or the hospitals must adopt profit as a primary purpose. Women and men who both possess these skills and are committed to the traditional role of these institutions could, if given the opportunity, have a major impact on the future of these hospitals. Important as such strategic actions by the hospitals themselves may be, the future of public hospitals as a valuable health resource for our country does not rest ultimately on their actions: it rests on the historical resolution of our society's ambivalence toward health care.

Two views of health care have been at the heart of this country's unprecedented expansion and operation of health care delivery during the past several decades, and these views contain opposing answers to the basic questions concerning the government's role in health care delivery. In one view, health care is placed squarely in the context of this country's political economy. The economic characteristics of delivering health care are given primacy, and the dominant criterion by which health care is judged is efficiency. This view of health care underlies most of the cost control efforts initiated in the public sector in the last decade; it also underlies corporate decision making in the vast private proprietary component of health care delivery. In the other view, health care is placed squarely in the moral sphere; it is a right. The obligation of a society toward its members is given primacy in this view, and the dominant criterion for our health care system is equality of access.

Each view emphasizes different aspects of health care, either economic or moral, and each has logical implications when extended into the other's sphere. The economic view, which is this country's ideological heritage means competition, implies that health care should be provided on the basis of ability to pay. Conversely, the logical extension of the view that health care is a right allows for no legitimate principle by which to allocate limited resources. Each view, when logically extended into the opposite sphere, implies a perspective unacceptable to most Americans—that no limits should be put on costs for health care or that health care should be rationed by ability to pay.

Both views are based on values at the heart of American culture: on the one hand, equity; on the other hand competition and merit. Neither view of health care has gained sway over the other, and as a result they both have contributed to, and been strengthened by, an expanding health care market. They grew side by side, opposite in principle, but seldom forced to reconcile. By the late 1970s, the disproportionate expansion of the health care sector within the United States economy generated a demand for fundamental shifts in health care delivery. Reconciling the two views of health care—as a right and as a business—is a need most acutely felt in urban public hospitals. They are the institutional representation of a fundamental value conflict in our societal views of health care, and their future can be watched as a symbol of our country's attempt to resolve the contradictions in economic and moral perspectives of health care.

Opiate of the Managers

Alan Sager

Despite the visible growth of for-profit chains in recent years, most Americans receive their inpatient care in voluntary, nonprofit hospitals. About 60 percent of our hospitals are nonprofit; they contain 70 percent of all acute care beds. These institutions are beleaguered and fearful. They are attacked by free-market advocates as flabby, poorly managed, and unimaginative in comparison with the for-profit sector. Advocates of more equitable access complain that they fail to provide enough free care to uninsured citizens. Public and private groups that pay for most hospital care decry high costs.

Powerful opinion has fastened on increased competition as the preferred method of controlling spending on health and building a more desirable system of care. Competition has many aspects. Some, such as more efficient internal management, are socially desirable on balance. Others—such as marketing more profitable services, serving fewer uninsured citizens, and possibly reducing levels of care below medically appropriate levels—are less desirable. The mixture of good and bad depends in part on the degree to which the assumptions for pure and perfect competition can be met in health care.

Nonprofit hospitals' most visible response to competition has been to accept and embrace it, with little public criticism. To understand the societal pressure for increased competition, and its attractiveness to so many hospital managers, it is helpful to examine a few recent trends in health care finance and delivery. Such an examination reveals the drive toward competition as the most recent manifestation of policy by spasm in United States health care. It suggests that if we worship competition instead of using it as a tool when appropriate, we will achieve health services that provide more care for fewer people at greater cost.

Policy by Spasm

In 1950, we spent $3.9 billion on hospitals, equal to 1.4 percent of the gross national product. By 1984, this had reached $157.9 billion—4.3 percent of a much larger GNP. Much of this is attributable to a method of paying hospitals by reimbursing their costs. If hospitals incurred certain allowable costs in treating patients insured by Blue Cross, for example, Blue Cross reimbursed these costs. If hospital costs rose during the following year, Blue Cross raised its premiums and paid the hospitals more money. Medicare did the same thing until recently. By giving hospitals something close to the power to tax, this method spurred and supported spending increases.

Although cost reimbursement did not restrain hospitals financially, it was not designed with evil or profligate intent. Rather, when patched together during the 1930s and 1940s, it was intended to help meet hospitals' pressing needs for cash and patients' equally pressing needs for financial security. Few of the nation's voluntary hospitals, which became established as visible social institutions only between 1880 and 1920, had ever had much money. Depression and war strained most of them badly. Cost reimbursement was designed for financially starved nonprofit entities that had never spent extravagantly. Few expected that reimbursing their costs would markedly change their behavior. How then did this happen? Nonprofit hospitals' responses to cost reimbursement were modulated in important ways by simultaneous changes in economic conditions, physician-hospital power relations, patients' expectations, and medicine's capacities. In a sense, cost reimbursement arrived on the scene at exactly the wrong time.

Having little money historically, hospitals had even less in the way of management structure. Before World War II, their administrators typically supervised housekeeping functions and kept rudimentary accounts. They had little authority and seldom were asked to perform the operating or financial tasks demanded of managers in the economy at large. Trustees made the major financial and physical plant decisions; physicians allocated available medical resources. Endemically low budgets, punctuated by financial crises during recurring recessions, obliged all parties to keep costs as low as possible.

Cost reimbursement worked on this penurious environment like a rainstorm on dried seeds in a desert. Hospital trustees and managers accustomed to counting syringes and bedpans suddenly and unexpectedly had access to vast resources. Taking hospital frugality for granted, and unable to imagine the level of postwar prosperity. Blue Cross's creators had not seen a need to design it to encourage careful hospital financial management. The overall growth in the insured population during the 1950s and 1960s, rising real incomes, an economy apparently protected against serious recession, and favorable public attitudes toward medical advances and health care meant that there was no force working to restrain hospital spending.

There was also a powerful internal force for higher spending. Before the war, a relatively tight hospital bed supply and a relatively loose physician supply prevailed. This meant that hospitals could exact from physicians seeking admitting privileges such concessions as unpaid service in clinics. After the war, large numbers of beds were built, encouraged in part by federal Hill-Burton grants. Physician/population ratios declined, as older physicians began to retire in large numbers and as medical school enrollments were kept low. Hospitals seeking to fill their beds increasingly depended on the physicians who decided whether and where to hospitalize. Physicians were able to oblige hospitals to hire residents and support staff and to buy equipment. As a result of these changes, which depended on the confluence of cost reimbursement with several other forces, more patients were served in more costly ways.

In 1965, a Congress anxious to assure older citizens' access to health services moved to protect them against these rising costs by legislating Medicare. Worried that hospitals might refuse to participate, the federal government initially paid them even more generously than did Blue Cross. Passing Medicare without simultaneously instituting financial controls or incentives to spend money carefully, accelerated the rate of increase in hospital spending. There was little recognition in 1965 of the need for financial controls, and no constituency for imposing them on a hospital industry anxious for federal money without strings attached. The inevitable tensions among cost control, access enhancement, and improved effectiveness were either ignored or shrugged off for a time. This manifests the making of health policy by spasm.

Many in Congress quickly saw this error. The unexpectedly high costs of Medicare's hospital and physician benefits blocked both the addition of meaningful long-term care (nursing home and home care) services under Medicare and the passage of national health insurance. Almost two decades of halfhearted efforts to control Medicare's spending on hospitals followed. While the desire of many in Congress and in HCFA (the federal Health Care Financing Administration, responsible for Medicare and Medicaid) to control costs was strong, there was little constituency pressure to offset vigorous hospital lobbying to retain steady access to public funds.

Several types of steps were taken to limit costs. Without strong political will, these resembled efforts by right-thinking Lilliputians to restrain a Gulliver. Among the first of these steps was Medicare's refusal to pay some costs of individual hospitals that exceeded a certain proportion of the average for their type and region. These reimbursement caps were largely evaded by shifting costs to uncapped services and by time-consuming administrative appeals.

In the absence of a clear and effective national policy to control health costs, HCFA and various state officials irritatingly skirmished with hospitals about relatively small sums. Under cost reimbursement, payers could save money mainly by identifying certain costs for which they would no longer compensate. In response, hospitals could either eliminate the expenditures for which they were no longer reimbursed or suffer financial losses. They could not improve their financial positions by initiating cost reductions, because these would engender reimbursement cuts. The major strategy of the hospitals was to make a game of the reimbursement system. For example, older patients could be placed in the newest building, obliging Medicare to pay more than its proportionate share of capital costs. HCFA sought to reduce opportunities for gaming by requiring uniform financial reporting. This would have allowed HCFA to compare costs across hospitals and then to disallow costs that seemed to be associated with inefficiency.

Hospitals successfully combated implementation of this reporting requirement by claiming that their compliance costs would be burdensome. They did not wish to allow federal regulators access to information that might label some hospitals as inefficient and that might reduce the benefits of fairly unrestricted cost reimbursement. In part because cost reimbursement did not allow hospitals to improve their bottom lines by becoming more efficient, and in part because some legitimate costs (such as those of uncompensated care of the uninsured) were often disallowed, hospitals' financial officers typically focused on wringing as much money as possible out of the cost reimbursement formulas. HCFA and the hospitals found it impossible to shape a cost reimbursement system both could live with.

Realizing that cost reimbursement was an invitation to add capacity and—once extra beds were built—to provide more care, Congress attempted to control spending by requiring the states to review hospital requests for additional beds or equipment through certificate of need (CON) programs. Because states paid little for hospital care, they lacked reasons of their own to disapprove more than a few hospital requests. But the administrative procedures were time-consuming, and many hospitals resented the obligation to explain their intentions and to demonstrate their reasonableness. In these areas—reimbursement caps, uniform financial reporting, and CON—and others as well, regulators and hospitals skirmished ineffectually and irritatingly. Prior to the early 1980s, almost all federal efforts to regulate hospital spending were largely ritualistic. We should not conclude that strong regulation failed; it was never really attempted.

By 1983, a number of forces combined to end the sparring. Some were economic; others political. In the private economy, sharper foreign and domestic competition was combining with soaring health insurance premiums to sensitize many employers and unions to the need for change. These groups could look sympathetically at parallel and mutually reinforcing public efforts. Politically, budget deficits were compelling attempts to control costs. Since the passage of Medicare, limiting hospital spending had been largely an aim internal to Congress and HCFA. High federal deficits vastly strengthened this internal pressure. A combination of ideology, policy analysis, and political strategy dictated that cost control be accomplished—or appear to be accomplished—by competition-enhancing mechanisms.

Congress decided that Medicare would pay hospitals very differently. The prospective payment system (PPS) would apply formulas to determine hospitals' payments independent of current costs. If hospitals could treat Medicare patients for less than the sums they received, they would make money; if not, they would not. PPS is the most recent example of policy by spasm in the United States health care system. It relies on only a few years of testing, in one state. For its size, PPS is the second least-studied law in modern history. The first is the Omnibus Budget Reconciliation Act of 1981, which failed to balance the budget by cutting taxes and increasing defense spending.

After a phase-in period ends, PPS will pay hospitals by their case mix, adjusted only for area wage rates and certain other costs, such as medical education. Each of the some 470 diagnosis related groups (DRGs) used to capture case mix is supposed to be fairly homogeneous, and is assigned a weight that is supposed to reflect the resources required to treat the average patient with that DRG. The average DRG would have a weight of 1.00; a DRG with a weight of 2.00 is thought to be twice as costly to treat. There are several problems with this. DRGs are probably not very homogeneous, and the weightings do not always reflect actual costs of treatment. Each problem provides hospitals with opportunities for guiding their total revenues. These opportunities, along with the new incentives to control costs, give hospital managers and physicians new powers to shape their bottom lines.

Federal powers are far greater. PPS is prospective in that it starts with certain actual base-year costs of treating patients in each DRG and inflates these to reflect those increased costs (such as price increases in the economy at large) over which hospitals could not be expected to exercise control. The formulas for inflating DRG payments are in federal hands, permitting annual decisions about how generously to pay hospitals. Thus, while PPS provides hospitals with some incentives for behaving efficiently, it for the first time gives the federal government the tools needed to control Medicare spending. As such, it constitutes the most sharply regulatory federal intervention in the United States health care system. Why, then, does it masquerade as one competitive solution to the health cost explosion?

The rate of increase in spending on hospitals in the United States is being slowed because the major payers—governments and employers— have resolved to pay less. Realizing that cost reimbursement had meant surrendering fiscal power to the hospitals, payers have taken back that power. This has not been easy to accomplish. A variety of interests and arguments have converged on a pro-competition package of reforms in health finance and delivery. Payers might see in competition a way to make lower total payments palatable. Some care givers might embrace competition because they fear they have no choice; others, because they have been trained for it.

Advocates of competition in health care draw on a growing belief in the free market in society at large. (Regulation, by contrast, was perceived as a burdensome failure in society generally and in health care specifically.) This is partly ideological. The seductions of the invisible hand are powerful; so little serious thought and effort promise so much. It is partly founded on such perceived competitive victories as the lower prices that seem to accompany airline or telephone deregulation. In health care, greater competition has won genuine victories by cutting the cost of a few standardized products, such as eyeglasses and drugs, without apparent harm to their quality. It has been embraced by many in the business community who hope to force hospitals to bid lower prices for the right to serve their workers.

The apparent successes of three competitive elements in health care seemed to argue for increased competition even while threatening many nonprofit hospitals with loss of patients. Chains of for-profit hospitals grew rapidly between 1975 and 1985, especially in burgeoning Sunbelt states. Much of this was due to the historic for-profit hospital advantage in responding quickly to rapid population growth. For-profit hospitals also grew because a traditional nonprofit strength, access to philanthropic fundraising, was eroded by the declining purchasing power of the philanthropic dollar in health care. Despite the importance of these environmental factors, the successes of the for-profit hospital chains were sometimes facilely ascribed to inner efficiency, productivity, superior management. and the ability to control costs.

For-profit ambulatory surgery centers also thrived, competing with the hospital's traditional core services of operating room and inpatient recuperation. Ambulatory surgery offers lower prices by avoiding both the hospital's overhead and the real costs of inpatient recovery. Overhead and sicker patients remain with the hospital, increasing its average costs. The appearance of higher costs sharpens critics' attacks. Hospital ability to cross-subsidize care of more costly patients by earning surpluses on less costly ones is weakened. Most important may be the total societal cost increase due to the building of more operating rooms in ambulatory surgery centers, often owned by physicians. This allows excessive numbers of surgeons to perform equally excessive amounts of surgery, free from the control of hospital utilization review committees.

Memberships of Health Maintenance Organizations (HMOs) have been increasing rapidly, reflecting successful competition with the traditional fee-for-service cost reimbursement system of finance and delivery of care. Because enrollees prepay a monthly fee, HMOs have no incentive to overprovide care. Members use substantially less hospital care; this helps drive down hospital costs and occupancy rates. Some reductions can be accomplished without sacrificing effectiveness of care; but by presenting financial incentives to provide less care, HMOs can become vehicles for inappropriate underprovision. This did not loom as a problem to the reformers who promoted HMOs as alternatives to fee-for-service and cost reimbursement in a lush financial environment. They envisaged idealistic salaried physicians largely insulated from financial considerations—made neutral to money. As with cost reimbursement itself a financial system designed for one institutional and social context grew explosively and dangerously in another. Today, growing numbers of HMOs are operated for profit, and physician compensation is increasingly calibrated inversely to amounts of care delivered. Far from financial neutrality, this is an incentive to underserve that must be resisted.

Growth of HMOs, for-profit hospitals, and ambulatory surgical centers strengthened the political appeal of competitive solutions to exploding costs. Coupled with this was the delegitimization of traditional authorities—physicians and those who ran hospitals. Physician resistance to Medicare and to expansion of medical school enrollments undermined respect for the profession in some quarters. An even greater threat may be posed today by the research into physicians' patterns of practice by Wennberg and others. Wide variations in surgical rates and inpatient admissions seem to suggest unscientific allocation of health care resources. Also disheartening have been the studies of professional decision making that reveal considerable interphysician variations in treatment decisions. Unhappily, organized medicine has vehemently rejected public evaluation of the efficacy of various therapies. Advocates of competition might conclude that financial pressures on physicians to do less might not undermine outcomes. Although cost reimbursement and fee-for-service engendered overcare, it does not follow that undercare is preferable—only that it is cheaper.

Hospitals are blamed for several things; among them the irresponsible overprovision of beds. It is not clear that we have more beds than other nations, but we now think we have more beds than we need. For decades, public policy declared the nation to be underbedded in reference to a standard of 4.5 beds per 1000 citizens. In the mid-1970s, as we approached this level, 4.0 was thought the proper number. There may never have been a day when we had the right number of hospital beds. This is disheartening; it resembles the physician shortage that turned into a glut, and it leads some to despair about the prospects for rationality. The bed surplus has become both an argument for competition and means of using competition to drive down hospital spending.

Most nonprofit hospitals have embraced competition. Some find it attractive; others fear that they have no choice. Competition appears to be an anodyne against cost containment. We may have less money, but spending it will be more exciting. If others are already competing, a response in kind is obligatory. Similarly, when California's Medicaid program won the right to force hospitals to bid for its patients, Blue Cross demanded the same right because it feared that hospitals would seek to overcharge Blue Cross patients to make up losses on Medicaid.

Competition seemed more attractive than the irritating regulation under which hospitals had been suffering. Many nonprofit hospitals had been recruiting larger administrative staffs composed of well-trained managers. These individuals, many with business degrees, sought opportunities to use their training to enhance their organizations' interests. They believed that cost reimbursement left them unable to respond to competitive attacks from several directions. Hospitals sought freedom of action.

Many nonprofit hospitals have concluded that their numbers will be reduced by lower spending on health care: competitive pressures from for-profits, HMOs, and ambulatory surgery; and increased price sensitivity of patients to health costs (engendered by steadily rising out-of-pocket costs to patients). Each hospital wishes to survive. The alternative of eliminating a few beds from most hospitals is thought not to save enough money, but this choice probably deserves closer attention. Most hospitals that believe themselves vulnerable, and many that do not, are working to strengthen their market position.

The strategies being employed can be distinguished by their aims: lowering costs or enhancing market position by other means. Costs are lowered internally in part through tighter management. This signals a turn, although with modern techniques, toward the style of tight internal cost control that preceded cost reimbursement. Efficiency—reducing costs of testing, providing meals, heating the building, nursing the patient, or cleaning the carpet—is the aim. This is the main proper scope of improved pure management in the hospital. Unhappily, most hospitals' relations with their workers remain primitively (and, for a service industry masochistically) confrontational, inviting trouble when they pursue efficiency.

As complexities of prospective payments and the strategic planning demands of a more competitive environment strengthen the power of managers, they seek to influence not only cost per unit of care but also the amounts of care—the number of days a patient stays in the hospital, and the number of tests and other ancillary resources employed in treatment. Substantial savings can be won through more miserly or careful clinical practice. Most administrators walk carefully in these areas; they compare costs engendered by physicians treating similar patients and urge reductions that do not endanger effectiveness of care. Other managers, under fiercer competitive attack, are pressuring physicians to cut care that may be needed. "Quicker and sicker" discharges of Medicare patients are said to be more common under DRGs. Still others hope to avoid the appearance of high costs by creaming, serving less needful patients.

Pressures toward lower costs, when clinically appropriate, are what competition advocates have had in mind. They can be desirable. Other means of competing do not clearly control costs or achieve other goals worthwhile to society. Hospitals have sought to strengthen their market positions through vertical integration, corporate diversification, and selective bidding and price discrimination.

Through vertically integrated contracts with physicians and nursing homes, hospitals hope to assure themselves of both a steady flow of patients to admit and sites for prompt discharge. Integration is proceeding to include hospital-controlled HMOs and even insurance companies. Nonprofit hospitals are forming holding companies that will conduct allied for-profit activities. These arrangements also help hospitals shelter revenues from regulators. Some hospitals are offering low prices to attract volume business. such as that from HMOs. These hospitals seek to keep enough of their beds filled with paying patients to weather the harsher competitive storms. They hope that, when some of their competitors are forced to close, they will be able to restore some of the price cuts they have been forced to endure. The more financially stable hospitals can best afford this strategy.

From payers' standpoints, competition does double duty. It is a device to induce hospitals to bid for patients—either formally as under California's Medicaid program or informally, as when individual hospitals cut deals with HMOs or the new preferred provider organizations (PPOs). It is clearly in payers' interests to promote competition at a time when slack physician and hospital bed supplies inevitably mean that the payers will enjoy market power. By allowing hospitals to retain any surpluses they manage to earn, it eases hospital acceptance of the lower payments inherent in Medicare's DRG system.

An Affordable Society

This nation seems to be moving simultaneously toward less equal income distributions and more costly necessities—among them housing, transport, defense, education, and health care. This is inherently undesirable and productive of greater social tensions. We should be working toward a society we can afford to maintain for all. This should be easy to do in health care since, by international standards, we are already spending the right amount of money in total.

Competition will help payers save money, but it will not move us directly toward a health care system of which we can be proud. On balance, competition seems likely to harm access and effectiveness of care; to the extent that it controls cost, it will probably do so in ways that create still more serious financing problems in the future. By refusing to build a health finance and delivery system that pays deliberate attention to balancing equitable access, cost control, and effectiveness of care, we will achieve through competition what we did through cost reimbursement—tougher choices among less attractive alternatives.

An invisible hand may point pure and perfect markets toward efficient disposition of consumers' purchasing power, but each of the requirements for such competition is largely absent in health care. These include many small buyers and sellers of care, free entry and exit of sellers, absence of artificial influences on behavior, and good information about the costs and values of what is exchanged. We have a few large purchasers of care. Entry of unlicensed care givers is not allowed. Health insurance is an artificial influence on care-seeking behavior, and most sick people would not have it any other way. Information about which care works, who needs it, and how to provide it is both unequally distributed and in short supply. There is no reason to believe that the bottom lines of impure and imperfect markets register a public interest. Those who do well do not necessarily do good.

Access is harmed. As bad money drives out good, so competition drives out cross-subsidies borne of altruism toward uninsured citizens or those with illnesses costly to treat. As panic-stricken hospitals stampede for the chance to compete by price, they become much less willing to overcharge paying customers in order to cross-subsidize care of the uninsured or the severely ill. Very needful patients may have trouble finding care—just as sick people have trouble buying health insurance or poor people securing bank loans. As payers seek to force insured patients to pay more out-of-pocket, to mimic market conditions, patients seek less care.

Effectiveness is diminished as well. Converting health care into a commodity erodes the trust of patients in their physicians. Many physicians exposed to increasingly powerful financial and administrative pressures to give or authorize less care are likely to bend. Others will risk loss of patients or income. The institutional contexts in which health financing operates from day to day are centrally important. Cost reimbursement might have worked well in the penny-pinching hospitals for which it was designed. Similarly, prospective payment was designed for nonprofit HMOs and successfully pioneered by them. We cannot sanguinely transfer prepayment into intensely competitive environments.

We cannot even expect competition to do a good job of cutting total costs. We would like it to reduce the two kinds of waste prominent in American hospitals—administrative and clinical. Himmelstein and Woolhandler assert in a recent *New England Journal of Medicine* article that marketing, billing, recording, paying, and other administrative overheads generate some $78 billion in waste in the United States health care system. They argue that up to half of this could be saved if we employed methods of managing money that have been in use in other nations for decades. Much of this cost is systemic, associated with our financing methods, and cannot be controlled by individual hospitals. The rest is intimately associated with competitive behaviors per se. More competition will mean more such waste. Only competing care givers require strategic planning, marketing, and pricing overheads. Enduring mistrust between payers and care givers multiplies record keeping for each.

Competition is not a good vehicle for reducing the clinical waste associated with care that is ineffective or unnecessary. It pushes for less care, but is not able to distinguish whether fat or lean is cut. The variations in physician practice patterns and hospital use rates that have helped to delegitimize professional influence in health care do not inspire confidence in the abilities of managers to reduce spending wisely. If the combination of these efforts does reduce total cost, total administrative and clinical waste may still increase as a proportion of hospital spending.

Equally important, it will cause serious long-term harm to health care financing. As a share of GNP or as real dollars per capita the United States spends about as much on health care as most Western European nations. Unlike them, we do not assure equal financial access to care; we deprive between one-tenth and one-third of our citizens of this access. Davis and Rowland have found that the uninsured use only about half as much physician and hospital care as those who are insured. Abandoning spasmodic policymaking would mean cutting costs in ways that mobilize saved funds on behalf of the underserved. Competition does not do this. Instead, it returns savings to payers. Once gone, this money will be very difficult to recapture.

We should consider four steps toward a system of care affordable for all. These will be socially desirable and also, before long, professionally and financially attractive to many hospitals and physicians. First, we should financially entitle all Americans to health care. This will preclude controlling costs through rationing by ability to pay. A related symbolic measure will be to rename HCFA, the federal Medicare-Medicaid agency, Health Care for All. Second, we should cut clinical costs by identifying what care works and what does not. This is proper. What is needed is a series of large-scale clinical trials and other studies aiming to validate medical knowledge. This is a huge task, one requiring cooperation and resources simply unavailable under competition, but we should make a beginning. Our $400 billion health care system, in a sense, has the nervous system of a dinosaur, with a small brain and enormous sets of neurons governing the body. We could make rapid progress in identifying clinical waste if we devote a fraction of the money now wasted in processing health insurance claims to studying what works.

Physicians who continue to claim that medicine should remain an art, and not become a science, should be asked to seek payment not from Medicare but from the National Endowment for the Arts. Physician resistance to learning what type of care works is an international scandal. Organized medicine's destruction of the National Center for Health Care Technology during the first year of the Reagan administration testifies to medicine's dislike of science. Bernard Fisher's struggle to evaluate radical breast cancer surgery was described in a *Technology Review* article titled "Science Comes to Medicine—Slowly."

Physicians have fought for both medical and financial autonomy. In part because the costs of the latter have undermined respect for the former, they are in the process of losing both—to managers. Their only prospects for regaining professional autonomy are to surrender financial autonomy. Validated standards of care will prove sensible rationing devices, bulwarks against managerial meddling in physician-patient relations, and indispensable defenses against malpractice litigation. In the latter area, a lack of standards once protected all but the most glaringly incompetent physicians against suit; today, they expose all.

A third step toward a system of affordable health care is that we save needed hospitals from closing and needed physicians from driving cabs. Today, empty hospital beds may only in part reflect overbuilding. Just as fields were plowed under while citizens hungered during the depression, so may we close needed hospitals owing to maldistributed purchasing power. Witness the closing of very large numbers of urban hospitals during the past three decades—40 percent of those opened before World War II—located disproportionately in minority neighborhoods. Physicians and hospitals should abandon their lemming-like love of competition, designed and promoted by their adversaries. They should embrace a secure system that covers all who need care, including those who are today uninsured or in danger of being underserved. This natural congruence of interests—care for all in exchange for employment for all—should overcome at least some care givers' traditional failure to advocate visibly on behalf of the underserved. Care givers have nothing to lose. The fear of government involvement that helped explain care giver silence has already been realized.

A fourth step is to slice administrative fat. Several dozen billion dollars would be saved if we moved toward the simpler methods of paying hospitals and physicians. Budgets and salaries, when combined with responsibility for defined populations, are powerful inducements to spend money carefully.

The British example demonstrates that even poor and inegalitarian societies can build egalitarian and effective health care systems. The British live about as long as we do, although they spend only half as much on health care—and despite their climate and the ingestion of ice cream made from fish fat. We should be able to do far better with our vast resources, even without adopting British forms of finance and delivery. Canada and most of Western Europe have done so for years. Our public would support equity in health care even if this required paying more money; happily, it does not. We should move in this direction.

For decades, we have been told that national health insurance must await cost control. Today, we are controlling cost in ways that reduce equity of access and effectiveness of care, while increasing waste. In the process, we are undermining care giver morale, their livelihoods, and trust between care giver and patient. A health care system built on insecurity harms all. We can control costs through better knowledge and financing systems and divert the savings to pay for care for all. We should think about how to move in this direction, so that when the obvious harm of competition prompts another spasm of policy, we will be able to point it in the right direction.

Upheaval and Adaptation

Ross M. Mullner, Odin W. Anderson,
and Ronald M. Andersen

The last decade has witnessed a number of changes that are bringing about a transformation of the economics and politics of hospital care in the United States. These changes create dilemmas that must be addressed by health policymakers. The changes can be categorized according to whether they pertain primarily to the financing of hospital care, to the organizational structures of the hospitals themselves, or to the systems for the delivery of hospital services.

There have been major changes in the way hospital care is being financed. By the beginning of the 1980s the cost of hospital care had escalated to such an extent that both the public and private sectors were driven to initiate cost containment measures. In the public sector, a far-reaching new attempt has been adopted to control the costs of Medicare, the nation's largest health insurance program. In the past, Medicare was open-ended, reimbursing hospitals for whatever costs had been incurred in the provision of inpatient care. In 1983, however, as part of the new social security amendments, the United States Congress adopted the Medicare prospective payment system (PPS), this system reimburses hospitals according to a fixed fee established in advance for categories of medical conditions.

Congress adopted the Medicare PPS because Medicare expenditures were rapidly rising and serious deficits were likely to occur in the program's hospital insurance trust fund. The goal of the Medicare PPS is to slow the rate of increase of federal expenditures for the program. It is to accomplish this by rewarding hospitals for keeping costs under set prices while making them subject to loss if their costs are higher. In theory, unlike the former system of cost reimbursement, prospective payment gives hospitals incentives to greater efficiency.

As its basis for setting prices, the Medicare PPS uses the patient classification system of diagnosis related groups (DRGs). The DRG system assumes that hospital patients can be classified into clinically coherent groups and that the patients in each art reasonably similar in their consumption of hospital resources. Medicare patients are classified into one of 468 DRGs based on their principal diagnosis. principal operating-room procedure, other diagnoses, discharge status, gender, and age at admission.

Hospitals are paid a prospectively determined amount for each Medicare patient per DRG. For example, assume that an eighty-one-year-old male Medicare patient belongs to the DRG of those with a circulatory disorder without myocardial infarction, with cardiac catheterization, with complex diagnoses, which is treated medically for two to five days. Assume further that the Medicare price for this DRG is $1,420. If the patient stays just three days and the care costs the hospital $1,200, then the hospital collects the DRG price of $1,420 and keeps the $220 difference. On the other hand, if the patient stays five days and has many diagnostic tests and other ancillary services, with total costs of $ 1,600, the hospital suffers a $180 loss.

From the hospital's perspective, the DRG prospective payment system creates two challenges: the need to increase efficiency and the need to reduce service utilization. Increased efficiency is achieved by controlling the unit costs of individual services. Reduced service utilization requires that hospitals work with their physicians to control patients' length of stay and use of services.

Because the program is so new, and because it is being gradually phased in over several years, it is difficult to predict the ultimate effects of the prospective payment system. During the program's first year, it does appear to have helped in slowing the rate of increase in expenditures, mainly by reducing the average length of time patients stay in the hospital. The U.S. General Accounting Office has recently found in a sample study of hospitals that the average length of stay for Medicare patients declined from 9.5 days before the prospective payment system to 7.5 days in the first year of the program. At the same time, their study found indications that some patients may be being discharged prematurely and in a poorer state of health than before the PPS program.

State governments, as a result of their own fiscal problems and declining federal funds, have also attempted to control their medical costs by cutting back on their Medicaid programs. The federal government shares the cost of Medicaid with the states, paying an average of 55 percent of the program's costs. The federal share varies with a state's per capita income, ranging from a high of 78 percent in Mississippi to a low of 50 percent for the higher income states in the country. As the federal government limits its contribution as part of an overall effort to reduce the national deficit, states have borne a larger share of the costs.

Medicaid is one of the largest items in most state budgets; in efforts to control costs, many states are limiting the number of reimbursable days of hospital care the poor may receive. For example, in Mississippi, Medicaid will not pay for more than fifteen days of hospital care per beneficiary per year, and in South Carolina patients are limited to twelve days per year. The effects of these reductions have not yet been determined. State health officials are quick to point out that since the average length of hospital stay is seven or eight days there will be no effect on the average Medicaid patient. These limits will disproportionately affect chronically or extremely ill patients, who will most likely exceed the limits.

Significant changes in the financing of hospital care have also been taking place in the private sector. In an effort to brake their rising health insurance costs, a growing number of companies have withdrawn from traditional health insurance carriers and programs and have established self-funded medical insurance programs (run by the companies themselves for their employees). In surveys of the health care cost containment practices of the nation's 1,500 largest employers conducted in 1979, 1981, and 1983, the Health Research Institute found that the number of companies with traditional health insurance programs declined from 45 percent in 1979 to 17 percent in 1983.

The advantages of self-funded insurance programs include the elimination of state premium taxes (which average 2 to 3 percent of premiums), improved cash flow, and the earning of higher interest rates on reserves held to pay benefits. Like traditional insurance programs, they too use third-party administrators to manage benefit claims and to monitor and control costs.

Companies that have continued to provide traditional health insurance coverage are also attempting to hold down their hospital and medical costs. They are increasing their deductibles, offering their employees choices of care including lower cost options, and establishing a number of cost containment features in their group coverages. A growing number of employers that previously paid the entire premium for comprehensive major medical insurance are now requiring their employees to pay a deductible—typically $100 to $200 a year per family member—before receiving benefits. Other companies with deductibles are raising them to as much as $500 a person. Many companies are also encouraging their employees to participate in health maintenance organizations (HMOs), which in many cases provide all care without any deductibles but contain medical expenditure costs by limiting hospital inpatient use by their enrollees. Still other employers are starting to use preferred provider organizations (PPOs). Usually organized by insurance companies, PPOs offer employers contracts with hospitals and physicians that agree to provide care to their employees at a reduced price. As an incentive to employees to use these less costly providers, deductibles are eliminated or reduced.

Employers are increasingly using such cost containment features as: reimbursing prescriptions on a generic basis only; requiring a second opinion prior to surgery; paying the full cost of laboratory tests needed for hospitalization only if they are performed before admission; paying the total costs of certain operations (for example, tonsillectomies) only if they are performed in a doctor's office or surgery center, without an overnight hospital stay; and waiving the deductible for hospitalization if and only if it is approved by the company's insurance carrier or other so-called preadmission certification agency. These cost containment measures appear to have also limited the rate of increase in hospital costs by making potential hospital patients more price-and-cost conscious. Some fear that they may make a significant number of people reluctant to seek even needed care because of the personal out-of-pocket expenses and inconvenience involved.

Changing Organizations

Hospitals are changing their organizational structures. In the 1970s the environment of hospitals had become such that a large number of often conflicting pressures were being brought to bear upon them. On the one hand, they were encouraged to contain costs and reduce unnecessary duplication of facilities; on the other hand, they were encouraged to increase the availability and accessibility of care and to improve quality. One of the most significant trends that has emerged from attempts to deal with these pressures has been the development of multihospital arrangements, often accompanied by a shift in hospitals' ownership status from not-for-profit to for-profit.

In the past, the traditional hospital was a community-based, not-for-profit, freestanding facility which for the most part developed in clinical and managerial isolation from other hospitals. Now, hospitals are becoming parts of collaborative multihospital systems. For example, hospitals are establishing affiliations, developing shared services, contract-managing other facilities, and purchasing other hospitals to form multihospital chains.

Multihospital arrangements can be divided into two broad categories according to the degree to which they achieve the status of an integrated system. The less integrated arrangements link subsystems of independently owned hospitals. They include formal affiliations, shared or cooperative services, and consortia for planning or education. Multihospital arrangements that attain a higher degree of integration include the various types of multihospital systems, two or more hospitals contract-managed, leased, or owned by a single corporate office. Approximately 20 percent of the nation's hospitals are now members of a multihospital system.

The most highly integrated and comprehensive types of multihospital systems are those in which the hospitals are completely owned by the corporate office; among these are the multihospital chains. Although the number of multihospital chains in the United States has decreased slightly in recent years, from 267 in 1980 to 249 in 1984, the number of community hospitals in them has increased rapidly, from 1,787 hospitals in 1980 to 2,050 in 1984. Some observers predict that over half of United States community hospitals will be in multihospital chains within the next ten years.

The last decade has witnessed a dramatic growth in for-profit hospital chains. For example, in 1978 there were 31 for-profit hospital management chains which owned 433 hospitals and accounted for 61,311 beds. By 1984, the numbers rose to 41 companies, 755 hospitals, and 100,113 beds. In addition to constructing or purchasing hospitals, for-profit chains have also entered into contracts to provide management services for non-profit community hospitals. In 1978, 22 chains managed 239 hospitals with a total of 27,098 beds. By 1984, the numbers were 29 companies, 302 hospitals, and 37,434 beds. At present. approximately 14 percent of the nation's hospital beds are owned or managed by for-profit chains and it is predicted that this will increase to 20–25 percent in the next decade.

The great expansion of these for-profit management chains has sparked a heated public debate about the ethics of for-profit corporate medicine. The following questions are being raised: Will the cost of medical care rise? Will the quality of care diminish? Will unprofitable but needed services be discontinued? Will the traditional concept that hospitals are obligated to serve local communities vanish? Will the poor be denied access to needed services?

Delivering Health Care

Hospitals have been adopting new roles and devising new methods and systems for delivering health services. Until recently, hospitals concentrated primarily on providing inpatient care, care which is expensive, relatively inconvenient to obtain, and time-consuming to receive. In response to the demand for less expensive and more convenient care, a growing number of alternative medical facilities, services, and delivery systems have developed; the most important of these are free-standing ambulatory care facilities, HMOs, and aftercare facilities.

Free-standing ambulatory care facilities and services have expanded rapidly in recent years. Outpatient alcohol treatment centers, outpatient dialysis centers, urgent or immediate care centers, and ambulatory surgery centers are growing at an enormous rate. In 1984, for example, there were approximately 1,800 immediate care centers in the nation: by 1988 this number is expected to more than double. A similar rate of increase is expected for the nation's free-standing surgery centers.

Much of the growth of HMOs has taken place in the last ten years, partly as a result of the passage of the Health Maintenance Organization and Development Act of 1973. This federal act established a grant and loan program to assist developing HMOs and required employers to offer their employees a dual choice option of either a conventional health insurance benefits plan or membership in a qualified HMO. At present, approximately 15 million individuals are enrolled in one of the more than 385 HMOs in the United States.

HMOs provide a wide range of comprehensive health services to a voluntarily enrolled population. Covered individuals receive care from specified providers for a fixed, prepaid fee, rather than on a fee-for-service basis. There are two basic types of HMOs: the group/staff arrangement and the individual practice association (IPA). The group/staff

HMO delivers health services at one or more facilities through groups of physicians working for a salary or under contract. The IPA contracts with physicians in the community, who maintain their own offices and usually are paid by the HMO on an agreed fee-for-service schedule.

Since physicians are not paid on a traditional fee-for-services rendered basis, they have no incentive to provide more frequent and complex services and hospital care than may be medically necessary. HMOs represent a powerful means of cost containment and one which will greatly expand in the future. By 1990, it is estimated that one out of every nine Americans, or 25 to 30 million individuals, will be enrolled in an HMO.

Aftercare refers to the facilities and services provided to the elderly and chronically ill; it includes nursing facilities and homes, geriatric outpatient care/day care, home health care, and hospice care. Aftercare, chiefly because of the aging of the nation's population, is the most rapidly growing part of the United States health care system. In 1978, nursing facilities and homes accounted for 1.3 million beds; in 1982, for 1.5 million beds—an increase of 11 percent. Home health care, which provides nursing therapy and health aid services in a patient's home instead of in a hospital, grew from 1,981 nonhospital-based programs in 1976 to 3,131 programs in 1982.

Hospitals have found themselves increasingly in competition with these alternatives. In order to compete, they are expanding and diversifying their range of facilities and services. Many of them are now providing birthing centers, health promotion and wellness programs, same day ambulatory surgery, immediate care minor emergency centers, hospice care, and HMOs. For example, in 1974 there were no organized hospital-based hospice programs, but by 1983 there were 548. There were few hospital-run home health care programs in 1975, but by 1982 there were 507. One survey conducted in 1980 found that 70 percent of the nation's community hospitals performed surgery on an outpatient basis and that 90 percent of all outpatient surgeries were done in hospitals. Another survey indicates that the number of outpatient surgeries performed by hospitals rose 77 percent between 1979 and 1983. Hospitals have also entered the HMO market. A recent survey indicates that in 1983 HMO services were provided through 20 percent of the nation's hospitals.

In order to gain a further competitive edge, and at the same time to lower their costs, hospitals are applying industrial concepts and methods to their operations. The hospital field is in the process of what Theodore Levitt has called "the industrialization of service." In a 1976 article in the *Harvard Business Review*, Levitt argued that society must break away from its preindustrial notions about what service is, and does, and adopt the concepts of industry. Adherence to the traditional ideal of service, one person directly and personally attending another, limits efficiency and productivity. The service sector should be more innovative and increase its use of various types of technologies, seek a greater standardization of methods, and in some cases apply a greater division of labor.

Examples of the industrialization taking place in hospitals include: the increasing automation of medical testing and laboratories; the greater use of computers in medical abstracting and billing systems (which in many cases link the patient's bill and medical record information), in inventory control, and in pharmacy services; and the increasing use of standardized cost accounting, which enables hospitals to better determine their true costs of providing services.

Questions and Answers

As a result of all of these changes, a greater profusion of health care facilities and services are now being offered to the American public than ever before—in ways that seek to make their delivery more efficient, and slow the rate of increase of the costs for care. At the same time, the individual citizen is being asked to shoulder a larger portion of the responsibility for choosing, and paying for, the care that he or she receives. Hospitals are being made more conscious of costs, was they are paid prospectively, and have more concern for staying within their budgets.

These changes create problems that must be faced by members of our society in general and by health policymakers in particular. First, who is responsible for providing care to those who are unable to pay for it? Second, what will be the ultimate consequences of what some have termed the "commercialization" of health care? Is there, for example, a danger that hospitals will provide only those facilities and services that are most profitable, and only in those areas where market opportunities are greatest?

Although all hospitals provide some uncompensated care (charity care plus care for which bills are unpaid), a small number of them provide a disproportionate amount. For example, less than 10 percent of the nation's hospitals account for 40 percent of the nation's uncompensated care for the poor. This disproportion is being intensified by the growing trend to transfer indigent patients to local government-funded hospitals, a process known as "dumping." For example, Parkland Memorial Hospital, a county teaching hospital in Dallas, found that of the 2,000 recent transfers it received, 75 percent occurred because the patients lacked financial means. In order to encourage the indigent to seek care in government-funded hospitals, some nongovernment hospitals ration care for uninsured citizens. They refuse to admit uninsured nonemergency cases unless they pay all or part of their bill in advance, admit only the indigent expected to have a short stay, or increase waiting times for charity care patients.

Many of the hospitals that provide a large amount of uncompensated care are public and nonprofit teaching hospitals in large inner cities. They serve high concentrations of the indigent and unemployed. These hospitals are now reeling from uncompensated costs and are facing a crisis. Even by the most conservative estimates, uncompensated care now amounts to billions of dollars a year. As one noted health services researcher has recently commented, uncompensated care is fast becoming the Achilles's heel of the competitive health care system.

Health policymakers must ask, and attempt to answer, a number of questions about this problem. Is it indeed a national problem that should be attacked through public tax supported programs? Should states and local communities take up a larger share of the task of helping the indigent? What role should private health insurance have in helping to solve the problem? At present, there is no consensus on how best to resolve the dilemma of uncompensated costs. Given Congress's struggle to trim the national deficit, it is clear that there is little hope that the federal government will expand existing entitlement programs—especially Medicaid.

In the absence of any federal action, several states have taken steps to solve the problem. Florida, for example, has recently established a trust fund that distressed hospitals can draw from to pay their uncompensated costs. This fund was created by levying a 1 percent tax on net hospital revenues, and supplemented by an annual appropriation from the state. The legislatures of Ohio and Texas are also considering similar strategies. Another proposed solution is that part of the cost of providing care for the poor be factored into Medicare's DRGs. Other proposals include a broad-based tax, such as an excise tax on alcohol or tobacco, a general sales tax, or a tax on health insurance premiums.

Related to this critical policy issue, and yet distinct from it, is the issue of the growth of for-profit corporate hospital care. Although there has always been a segment of the nation's hospitals that have been under for-profit ownership, it was not until the 1970s that the for-profit hospital management companies or chains emerged. These for-profit corporations entered into a predominantly not-for-profit sector of medical care. After concentrating on buying and contract-managing local hospitals, the chains have expanded into other markets as well. They are opening shopping mall surgery centers, purchasing immediate care centers, starting HMOs, home care companies, and nursing homes, and are even selling health insurance. One for-profit chain has even entered into advanced clinical research on artificial hearts.

The expansion of these chains has sparked a lively and sometimes heated debate about the ethics of for-profit corporate medicine, or, as its critics call it the "commercialization of medicine." Opponents of the for-profits have identified several areas of concern. First, the critics ask, if the for-profits continue to expand what will happen to care for the poor? Who will take up this burden? As for-profit hospitals enter a community will they shift all indigent patients to neighboring not-for-profit hospitals and drive them into bankruptcy? Second, will the growth of the for-profits increase the cost of medical services and at the same time diminish the quality of care? Will unprofitable services, which may be important to the community, be phased out? On the other hand, will profitable services be inappropriately emphasized or overused? Third, what will be the long-term future of teaching hospitals, which offer training, research, and community services, if they are forced to compete in price with for-profit hospitals which do not engage in these unprofitable activities? Fourth, will the for-profits shape the behavior of the nonprofits to such a degree that the latter will abandon their historic humane service mission? Fifth, when economic adversity strikes, will a for-profit conglomerate sell or close a local hospital that it owns, even though it may be the only source of care in the immediate geographic region, thus abandoning the community? As one critic puts it, what is good for Wall Street may be disastrous for Main Street.

Proponents of the for-profits make the following arguments in their defense. First, they say that the distinction between for-profit and not-for-profit hospitals is primarily a legal one: nonprofit hospitals often make profits too, but unlike for-profits do not distribute gains to shareholders and cannot raise equity from the sale of stock. Second, there is little difference in the economic and social performance of most for-profit and not-for-profit hospitals. Cost on a per-admission basis is similar, and one type of facility is as likely as the other to "dump" poor patients on the nearest county hospital. Third, only a small number of not-for-profit hospitals conduct research and teaching. Thus, changes in the ownership of United States hospitals will have less impact on patient care, teaching, and research than other changes, such as stricter public and private reimbursement policies. Fourth, much of the health care system is already organized on a for-profit basis. For example, most physicians, dentists, half of the private health insurance market, and about three-fourths of all nursing homes operate on a for-profit basis. Also, all makers of pharmaceuticals, medical devices, eyeglasses, and hospital supply companies are for-profit firms. Why, then, should there be so much concern over the growth of the for-profit hospital chains?

The ethical issues raised by the growth of the for-profits are complex and are not easily answered. Part of the problem is the lack of specific data to compare and evaluate the claims of either side so that few conclusions can be made. Some of these issues may be clarified by the current study being conducted by the Institute of Medicine of the National Science Foundation. Its final report is scheduled to be completed and released this year.

The diversity of new forms that hospital care is taking in response to financial and political pressures is testimony to the vitality of the health care system in this country. But fears that evolutionary gains in efficiency and cost effectiveness may be accompanied by losses in the traditional values of compassion and charity are perhaps well-founded. As an absolute minimum, what is needed to assure that those who need care the most will be assured of receiving it in these times of rapid changes in the health care field is the speedy passage and implementation of a comprehensive national health insurance program. Unfortunately, this is unlikely to come about in the near future.

Discharge Planning:
No Deposit, No Return

Martin Hochbaum and Florence Galkin

In the last half dozen years, the operations of nursing homes have been examined thoroughly by legislative committees, investigative bodies, newspapers, university public policy centers, and others. In spite of all this activity, one aspect of the operations of nursing homes, their implementation of government-mandated discharge-planning policies, has received relatively little attention. This is so even though both the federal and state governments, in theory at least, have committed themselves to a discharge-planning program for nursing-home patients. On the national level, federal law requires that patient-care policies "effect awareness of, and provision for, meeting the total medical and psychological needs of patients including...discharge planning." Under New York law, operators are required to "maintain a discharge planning program" and "develop and document in the resident's medical record a multidisciplinary discharge plan for all residents; and review...the plan as indicated by change in the patient's...medical condition." What actually occurs is a compliance which fails to consider adequately the individual patient's potential for discharge. Once admitted to a nursing home, the patient has lost his options; he has arrived at his last residence.

Discharge planning is based on the assumption that each patient has needs and potentials which will be most effectively met by evaluating "the total person and not just his immediate medical needs," in the words of a report published by the Commission on Professional and Hospital Activities. Ideally, the process should begin at admission with an assessment of medical, nursing, social, and emotional needs. This should be followed by evaluation of the patient's rehabilitative potential and review of alternative care plans to meet his needs. Once this is completed, the patient's potential for discharge can be ascertained. Discharge planning is not, however, a one-time process. A patient's potential for discharge must be reevaluated periodically to reflect his current state, needs, and resources. For example, a newly admitted patient may have multiple medical and nursing needs which could be compounded by disorientation. This patient may only be eligible for discharge after months of rehabilitation. Recognizing this, the New York law mandates that the patient's discharge plan be reviewed and revised every 90 days "as indicated by change in" medical conditions or needs. This is obviously a time-consuming process. The discharge planner must gather information from a variety of sources to compile "a total picture of the patient's needs and his discharge potential," again in the words of the Commission on Professional and Hospital Activities report. For example, the discharge planner must be familiar with the availability and effectiveness of such community-based programs as visiting nurses, homemakers, home delivery of meals, public welfare, housing, and home visitation. He must also be able to overcome the pervasive fragmentation of services in these areas.

We concentrate here on discharges from health-related facilities (HRF) because patients in these institutions are better off physically and mentally than those in skilled nursing facilities (SNF) and, therefore, stand a better chance of being discharged to their homes. HRF patients, for Medicaid reimbursement purposes, must have scored between 60 and 180 on a New York State patient assessment scale; SNF patients must have scored at least 180. In 1977, out of 17,126 patients discharged from HRFs in New York State, only 1,483 were discharged to their homes. When one discounts the 732 patients "discharged" by death, out of the 16,394 people discharged, only 1,483 (nine percent) were discharged to their homes. The others were discharged to hospitals and facilities offering other levels of care. The figures for 1978 are not very different. Out of 15,908 patients discharged from HRFs in New York, 1,296 were discharged to their homes. Again, discounting deaths, in this case 822, out of the 14,612 patients discharged, only 1,296 or nine percent were discharged home. Most of the others were discharged to hospitals and locations affording other levels of care.

In many cases, the problem begins with the admissions process itself. Most patients are admitted to nursing homes following discharge from a hospital. With hospitals under pressure to empty their beds to satisfy utilization review requirements, there is little opportunity to consider community-based, long-term care options. Moreover, even if there is interest in such alternatives, the chronic nature of the patient's condition often requires multidimensional treatment which the home-care system cannot adequately deliver. The patient is usually confronted with a host of fragmented services with diverse eligibility requirements, rather than a one-stop supermarket mechanism, to meet his varied needs. It frequently becomes simpler to arrange long-term care in a nursing home than in the community. Nursing homes therefore admit patients who lack the ability to live independently or to piece together, from an unorganized and fragmented home health-care system, a solution to their needs. Thus, even for patients who do not require institutionalization, the nursing home may represent the best solution for the individual with chronic conditions. Moreover, it frequently is, or appears to be, the only solution. Once the patient is institutionalized, there is a failure to implement an effective discharge-planning program. This results from a number of interrelated factors:

- Government financial benefits are greater for nursing-home care than for home health care.
- Nursing-home services are not rehabilitative, but aimed at maintaining the patient in the institution.
- Institutionalization is not viewed as part of a continuum of care, but as the end of care.
- Care, including pre-admission assessment, is based on a medical model which ignores alternative long-term care possibilities.

Obstacles to Discharge Planning

Under the present system of Medicaid supplemented by Medicare, the government covers most medical expenses incurred by an elderly indigent person. If the patient lives at home, government payments meet the greatest part of the cost of doctors, nurses, drugs, and certain other medical services. If the patient is placed in a nursing home, Medicaid covers not only all of these expenses but also the cost of lodging, meals, and custodial care normally borne by the patient or his family. This creates a powerful incentive to keep an aged or infirm person in an institution even though better care might be available elsewhere. This situation is compounded by the overwhelming percentage of patients who give up their homes or apartments upon admission to a nursing home. Those on Medicaid no longer possess the financial ability to move from a nursing home to a new apartment because this requires a substantial financial outlay. As Amitai Etzioni has noted, patients become "de facto prisoners of these institutions and of the state since they no longer have…the option of returning to the community, even if their health permits it."

Moreover, the Medicare program, which provides little nursing-home coverage, does not provide comprehensive home health-care benefits. Medicare concentrates on skilled services for the acutely ill, rather than on health-related or basic services for the chronically disabled. Personal care services are not covered. Thus, the limited home health care available under Medicare and the payment of all nursing-home costs for eligible patients through Medicaid create a powerful incentive for institutionalization. Once a person is institutionalized, the system of limited home health-care benefits plus the patient's poverty work to prevent his return to the community.

Many nursing-home patients require specialized rehabilitative services to restore them to their highest physical, psychological, and social functioning and thus bring them to a level of maximum independence. These services should enable them to function effectively within their limitations, prevent deformities, and retard deterioration. A wide variety of services can be provided to meet these goals. They include testing, motivating, and keeping patients physically, mentally, and socially active, as well as improving such functions as toileting, walking, and the use of prosthetic devices.

Three of the principal rehabilitative services for which some data are available are physical, occupational, and speech therapy. According to a national HEW study—based on a review of patients' diagnoses, observed functional status, medical records, and discussion with staff, patients, and others—relatively few patients in skilled nursing facilities receive such services (many respondents in a survey of California's facilities suggested that they "did not have the professional staff to carry out active rehabilitation efforts"). The HEW study demonstrates that, in relation to need, only 11 percent of those requiring occupational and speech therapy and 31 percent of those requiring physical therapy actually receive it. Viewed from another perspective, 89 percent of those requiring occupational and speech therapy and close to 69 percent of those requiring physical therapy were in skilled nursing facilities where they did not receive these services. The HEW study also shows that few of those receiving physical therapy had written plans which were coordinated with rehabilitation programs and that accurate baseline data with which to judge progress is nonexistent.

Where rehabilitative services are available, they are frequently little more than efforts to comply with government regulations aimed at enabling the patient to function in the institution, not in the community. One witness before a congressional committee observed that while the New York State Hospital Code requires nursing homes to provide such services as occupational therapy, this frequently consists of nothing more than "a weekly visit by the occupational therapist, with little or no follow-up between visits." Further indications of this lack of interest are the New York State Moreland Act Commission's making only passing reference to this subject and Ronald Toseland's conclusion, in "Rehabilitation and Discharge: The Nursing Home Dilemma," that the process of rehabilitation in nursing homes is not focused. Even if a patient is potentially capable of discharge, the unavailability of effective rehabilitative services, which could facilitate return to the community, will lead to continued institutionalization. Without such programs aimed at restoring patients to their maximum potential, it is easy to understand why so few are discharged.

The placement of a patient in a nursing home is not viewed as part of a continuum of care which allows for, and encourages, movement back into less restrictive environments. Rather, it is viewed as an individual's final residence or movement into a more restrictive setting. His freedom of choice and right to service in the least restrictive setting are virtually ignored. This is not surprising, given the fact that perhaps as many as fifty percent of nursing-home patients are admitted from hospitals following acute episodes of a chronic condition. Nevertheless, this view makes it virtually impossible for any effective discharge planning to take place. Almost by definition, a patient can only be discharged by death or transfer to a hospital. The fact that so few patients return to the community reinforces this view and makes it a self-fulfilling prophecy.

Further reinforcement of the view of the facility as the last residence arises from the patient's inability to maintain a domicile in the community. This, plus the Medicaid poverty requirement, makes it difficult to find an acceptable community residence. Moreover, Title III of the Older Americans Act and Title XX of the Social Security Act have not yet achieved what the Federal Council on the Aging termed a "focus on long-term care which might make such services a major element in" its delivery.

According to the General Accounting Office (GAO), it is important to prepare an assessment which "identifies the chronically impaired elderly's long-term care needs, and to match those needs to the most appropriate level of services." Such assessment must include an evaluation of the individual's potential to perform activities of daily living, his family preferences and lifestyles, his financial status and psychosocial factors. The study goes on to note that what usually occurs is a medical examination which "often cannot distinguish the impaired elderly who require nursing home placement from those who have the potential to remain in the community."

Nursing-home care is based on a medical model which is delivered in a scaled-down hospital. This is often the case in spite of the fact that nursing homes contain patients whose problems are chronic rather than acute, long-term rather than transient. Moreover, nursing homes lack the hospital manpower and technical machinery; their business is treatment, not diagnosis. Nevertheless, it is the medical model with its emphasis, according to Robert and Rosalie Kane, on "staffing standards, care plans, and audits of results" which prevails.

Quality care is jeopardized when the whole person is not considered. More significant for our purpose is that concentration on medical needs virtually ignores the possibility for effective discharge planning and precludes a return to the community. This is especially poignant since patients are often placed in long-term care facilities not because of medical problems but because alternative arrangements could not be worked out. Once institutionalized, the possibility of alternative arrangements that consider the patient's total needs are ignored and medical needs receive the most attention. Hence, it is precisely those factors which often precipitate institutionalization which receive the least attention.

Potentials for Discharge Planning

Many more nursing-home patients could be discharged to live in the community, in part because many patients are placed in institutions who do not belong there in the first place. One government analysis of studies concerned with appropriate placement of nursing-home patients concluded that two-fifths of residents of Intermediate Care Facilities (ICF) were receiving more care than their conditions warranted. Another analysis stated that up to one-fifth of the institutionalized could remain in the community if they received adequate services. As the GAO observed, "assessment mechanisms have not enabled Medicaid adequately to control avoidable institutionalization."

The failure to consider, and the limited nature of, community-based alternatives results in a nursing-home population which is similar to the population resident in the community. This has been documented in a number of studies. One author notes that individuals with the same characteristics as nursing-home patients continue to reside in the community. Another concludes that both nursing homes and community populations contained people whose impairments ranged from moderate to total. A third suggests that the medical conditions of elderly nursing-home patients are shared by many of the elderly in the community. Another estimates that with adequate community services, one-fifth of nursing-home patients could get by in the community.

The unnecessary institutionalization of people able to function in the community, and their retention in these institutions, ignores the many familiar reasons for their remaining in their own residences. These include their preference for doing so, avoiding the institutionalization syndrome, and, in some cases, financial savings. Older people, when confronted with the need for institutional versus home-based care, usually choose the latter. They do so to preserve their independence, dignity, and identity and because institutionalization is often viewed as a prelude to death.

People who are kept in institutions in spite of the fact that they could function in the community are deprived of an opportunity to obtain care in a setting which offers maximum reliance on individual potential and resources. They lack privacy and are insulated from the general society. Months of unnecessary institutionalization will frequently lead to the loss of the mental and physical will to handle one's own affairs. For some patients, the unnecessary reliance on others to care for them, unless caught in time, will lead to their premature dependence.

The unnecessary retention of some patients in nursing homes also leads to a waste of public funds. We are not discussing patients who will require twenty-four hours a day of paid supervision in the community. For them, home-based programs of care would probably not produce financial savings. However, for patients requiring more moderate attention—i.e., those for whom discharge is most likely—there would be financial savings. The potential savings are of two types. The first are those produced by avoiding the high cost of institutional care. According to the survey by the GAO, "in terms of public dollars, the cost of home-based long-term care is less than or comparable to the cost of the equivalent level of nursing home care." Another savings derives from the fact that hospitalized patients are often required to undergo long waiting periods of expensive hospital care before a nursing-home bed is available. By discharging increased numbers of patients from nursing homes, this waiting period would decrease and produce shorter stays and concomitant savings in public funds.

To those who are uncomfortable with increasing the discharge of patients to the community because of the fear of an increase in mortality, we would point out that the results of numerous studies on this subject appear to be contradictory. Relocated patients have been found to have mortality rates higher than, lower than, and the same as those who are not moved. Moreover, it is important to understand that we are not talking about a move from one institution to another, but from an institution back to the community. Such relocation is not proposed where there is a lack of community programs, including both formal and informal supports, to follow up with and serve the patients.

In numerous cases, because of massive, unalterable physical and psychological infirmities, the nursing home is the final resting place before the hospital and/or grave. In other cases, however, elderly residents who can function independently outside the nursing home are denied exit from the institutional setting. But because nursing homes see placement as permanent, their services are skewed toward continued institutionalization. In addition, government and institutional policies often hinder the discharge of elderly persons from long-term care facilities. This situation is incompatible with the implementation of meaningful state and national discharge-planning requirements.

Part III

Health Policy and Reform

Medical Ghettos

Anselm L. Strauss

In President Johnson's budget message to Congress this year he proposed a quadrupling of federal spending on health care and medical assistance for the poor to $4.2 billion in fiscal 1968:

> The 1968 budget maintains the forward thrust of federal programs designed to improve health care in the nation, to combat poverty, and assist the needy...The rise reflects the federal governments role in bringing quality medical care, particularly to aged and indigent persons.

Three years earlier in a special message to Congress the President had prefaced reintroduction of the medicare bill by saying:

> We can—and we must—strive now to assure the availability of and accessibility to the best health care for all Americans, regardless of age or geography or economic status.... Nowhere are the needs greater than for the 15 million children of families who live in poverty.

Then, after decades of debate and massive professional and political opposition, the medicare program was passed. It promised to lift the poorest of our aged out of the medical ghetto of charity and into private and voluntary hospital care. In addition, legislation for heart disease and cancer centers was quickly enacted. It was said that such facilities would increase life expectancy by five years and bring a 20 percent reduction in heart disease and cancer by 1975.

Is the medical millenium, then, on its way? The President, on the day before sending the 1968 budget to Congress, said: "Medicare is an unqualified success."

"Nevertheless," he added, "there are improvements which can be made and shortcomings which need prompt attention." The message also noted that there might be some obstacles on the highroad to health. The rising cost of medical care, President Johnson stated, "requires an expanded and better organized effort by the federal government in research and studies of the organization and delivery of health care." If the President's proposals are adopted, the states will spend $1.9 billion and the federal government $1 billion in a "Partnership for Health" under the Medicaid program.

Considering the costs to the poor—and to the taxpayers—why don't the disadvantaged get better care? In all the lively debate on that matter, it is striking how little attention is paid to the mismatch between the current organization of American medicine and the life-styles of the lower class. The major emphasis is always on how the *present* systems can be a little better supported or a trifle altered to produce better results.

I contend that the poor will never have anything approaching equal care until our present medical organization undergoes profound reform. Nothing in current legislation or planning will accomplish this. My arguments, in brief, are these:

- The emphasis in all current legislation is on extending and improving a basically sound system of medical organization.
- This assumes that all those without adequate medical services—especially the poor—can be reached with minor reforms, without radical transformation of the systems of care.
- This assumption is false. The reason the medical systems have not reached the poor is because they were never designed to do so. The way the poor think and respond, the way they live and operate, has hardly ever (if ever) been considered in the scheduling, paperwork, organization, and mores of clinics, hospitals, and doctors' offices. The life-styles of the poor are different; they must be specifically taken into account. Professionals have not been trained and are not now being trained in the special skills and procedures necessary to do this.
- These faults result in a vicious cycle which drives the poor away from the medical care they need.
- Major reforms in medical organizations must come, or the current great inequities will continue, and perhaps grow.

I have some recommendations designed specifically to break up that vicious cycle at various points. These recommendations are built directly upon aspects of the life-styles of the poor. They do not necessarily require new money or resources, but they do require rearrangement, reorganization, reallocation—the kind of change and reform which are often much harder to attain than new funds or facilities.

In elaborating these arguments, one point must be nailed down first: *The poor definitely get second-rate medical care.* This is self-evident to anyone who has worked either with them or in public medical facilities; but there is a good deal of folklore to the effect that the very poor share with the very rich the best doctors and services—the poor getting free in the clinics what only the rich can afford to buy.

The documented statistics of the Department of Health, Education, and Welfare tell a very different story. As of 1964, those families with annual incomes under $2,000 average 2.8 visits per person to a physician each year, compared to 3.8 for those above $7,000. (For children during the crucial years under 15, the ratio is 1.6 to 5.7. The poor tend to have larger families; needless to add, their child mortality rate is also higher.) People with higher incomes (and $7,000 per year can hardly be considered wealthy) have a tremendous advantage in the use of medical specialists—27.5 percent see at least one of them annually, compared to about 13 percent of the poor.

Health insurance is supposed to equalize the burden; but here, too, money purchases better care. Hospital or surgical insurance coverage is closely related to family income, ranging from 34 percent among those with family income of less than $2,000 to almost 90 percent for persons in families of $7,000 or more annual income. At the same time, the poor, when hospitalized, are much more apt to have more than one disorder— and more apt to exhaust their coverage before discharge.

Among persons who were hospitalized, insurance paid for some part of the bill for about 40 percent of patients with less than $2,000 family income, for 60 percent of patients with $2,000–$3,999 family income, and for 80 percent of patients with higher incomes. Insurance paid three-fourths or more of the bill for approximately 27 percent, 44 percent, and 61 percent of these respective income groups. Preliminary data from the 1964 survey year showed, for surgery or delivery bills paid by insurance, an even more marked association of insurance with income.

Similar figures can be marshaled for chronic illness, dental care, and days of work lost.

Strangely enough, however, *cash* difference (money actually spent for care) is not nearly so great. The under $2,000 per year group spent $112 per person per year, those families earning about three times as much ($4,000–$7,000) paid $119 per person, and those above $7,000, $153. Clearly, the poor not only get poorer health services but less for their money.

As a result, the poor suffer much more chronic illness and many more working days lost—troubles they are peculiarly ill-equipped to endure. Almost 60 percent of the poor have more than one disabling condition compare l to about 24 percent of other Americans. Poor men lose 10.2 days of work annually compared to 4.9 for the others. Even medical research seems to favor the affluent—its major triumphs have been over acute, not chronic, disorders.

Medical care, as we know it now, is closely linked with the advancing organization, complexity, and maturity of our society and the increasing education, urbanization, and need for care of our people. Among the results: Medicine is increasingly practiced in hospitals in metropolitan areas.

The relatively few dispensaries for the poor of yesteryear have been supplanted by great numbers of outpatient hospital clinics. These clinics and services are still not adequate—which is why the continuing cry for reform is "more and better." But even when medical services *are* readily available to the poor, they are not used as much as they could and should be. The reasons fall into two categories:

- factors in the present organization of medical care that act as a brake on giving quality care to everyone;
- the life-styles of the poor that present obstacles even when the brakes are released.

The very massiveness of modern medical organization is itself a hindrance to health care for the poor. Large buildings and departments, specialization, division of labor, complexity, and bureaucracy lead to an impersonality and an overpowering and often grim atmosphere of hugeness. The poor, with their meager experience in organizational life, their insecurity in the middle-class world, and their dependence on personal contacts, are especially vulnerable to this impersonalization.

Hospitals and clinics are organized for "getting work done" from the staff point of view; only infrequently are they set up to minimize the patient's confusion. He fends for himself and sometimes may even get lost when sent "just down the corridor." Patients are often sent for diagnostic tests from one service to another with no explanations, with inadequate directions, with brusque tones. This may make them exceedingly anxious and affect their symptoms and diagnosis. After sitting for hours in waiting rooms, they become angry to find themselves passed over for latecomers—but nobody explains about emergencies or priorities. They complain they cannot find doctors they really like or trust.

When middle-class patients find themselves in similar situations, they can usually work out some methods of "beating the system" or gaining understanding that may raise staff tempers but will lower their own anxieties. The poor do not know how to beat the system. And only very seldom do they have that special agent, the private doctor, to smooth their paths.

Another organizational barrier is the increasing professionalism of health workers. The more training and experience it takes to make the various kinds of doctors, nurses, technicians, and social workers, the more they become oriented around professional standards and approaches, and the more the patient must take their knowledge and abilities on trust. The gaps of communications, understanding, and status grow. To the poor, professional procedures may seem senseless or even dangerous—especially when not explained—and professional manners impersonal or brutal, even when professionals are genuinely anxious to help.

Many patients complain about not getting enough information; but the poor are especially helpless. They don't know the ropes. Fred Davis quotes from a typical poor parent, the mother of a polio-stricken child:

> Well they don't tell you anything hardly. They don't seem to want to. I mean you start asking questions and they say, "Well, I only have about three minutes to talk to you." And then the things that you ask, they don't seem to want to answer you. So I don't ask them any thing any more....

For contrast, we witnessed an instance of a highly educated woman who found her physician evasive. Suddenly she shot a question: "Come now, Doctor, don't I have the same cancerous condition that killed my sister?" His astonished reaction confirmed her suspicion.

Discrimination also expresses itself in subtle ways. As Frank Riessman and Sylvia Scribner note (for psychiatric care), "Middle class patients are preferred by most treatment agents, and are seen as more treatable.... Diagnoses are more hopeful...." Those who understand, follow, respond to, and are grateful for treatment are good patients; and that describes the middle class.

Professional health workers are themselves middle-class, represent and defend its values, and show its biases. They assume that the poor (like themselves) have regular meals, lead regular lives, try to support families, keep healthy, plan for the future. They prescribe the same treatment for the same diseases to all, not realizing that their words do not mean the same things to all. (What does "take with each meal" mean to a family that eats irregularly, seldom together, and usually less than three times a day?)

The poor especially suffer in that vague area we call "care," which includes nursing, instructions about regimens, and post-hospital treatment generally. What happens to the lower-class patient once released? Middle-class patients report regularly to their doctors who check on progress and exert some control. But the poor are far more likely to go to the great, busy clinics where they seldom see the same doctor twice. Once out they are usually on their own.

Will the poor get better care if "more and better" facilities are made available? I doubt it. The fact is that they underutilize those available now. For instance, some 1963 figures from the Director of the Division of Health Services, Children's Bureau:

> In Atlanta, 23 percent of women delivered at the Grady Hospital had had no prenatal care; in Dallas, approximately one-third of low-income patients receive no prenatal care; at the Los Angeles County Hospital in 1958, it was 20 percent; at the D.C. General Hospital in Washington, it is 45 percent; and in the Bedford Stuyvesant section of Brooklyn, New York, it is 41 percent with no or little prenatal care.

Distances are also important. Hospitals and clinics are usually far away. The poor tend to organize their lives around their immediate neighborhoods, to shut out the rest of the city. Some can hardly afford bus fare (much less cab fare for emergencies). Other obstacles include unrealistic eligibility rules and the requirement by some hospitals that clinic patients arrange a blood donation to the blood bank as a prerequisite for prenatal care.

Medical organization tends to assume a patient who is educated and well-motivated, who is interested in ensuring a reasonable level of bodily functioning and generally in preserving his own health. But health professionals themselves complain that the poor come to the clinic or hospital with advanced symptoms, that parents don't pay attention to children's symptoms early enough, that they don't follow up treatments or regimens, and delay too long in returning. But is it really the fault of whole sections of the American population if they don't follow what professionals expect of them?

What are the poor really like? In our country they are distinctive. They live strictly, and wholeheartedly, in the present; their lives are uncertain, dominated by recurring crises (as S. M. Miller puts it, theirs "is a crisis-life constantly trying to make do with string where rope is needed"). To them a careful concern about health is unreal—they face more pressing troubles daily, just getting by. Bad health is just one more condition they must try to cope—or live—with.

Their households are understaffed. There are no servants, few reliable adults. There is little time or energy to care for the sick. If the mother is ill, who will care for her or take her to the clinic—or care for the children if she goes? It is easier to live with illness than use up your few resources doing something about it.

As Daniel Rosenblatt and Edward Suchman have noted:

> The body can be seen as simply another class of objects to be worked out but not repaired. Thus, teeth are left without dental care.... Corrective eye examinations, even for those who wear glasses, are often neglected.... It is as though...blue-collar groups think of the body as having a limited span of utility; to be enjoyed in youth and then to suffer with and to endure stoically with age and decrepitude.

They are characterized by low self-esteem. Lee Rainwater remarks that low-income people develop "a sense of being unworthy; they do not uphold the sacredness of their persons in the same way that middle-class people do. Their tendency to think of themselves as of little account is...readily generalized to their bodies." And this attitude is transferred to their children.

They seek medical treatment only when practically forced to it. As Rosenblatt and Suchman put it: "Symptoms that do not incapacitate are often ignored." In clinics and hospitals they are shy, frustrated, passively submissive, prey to brooding, depressed anxiety. They reply with guarded hostility, evasiveness, and withdrawal. They believe, of their treatment, that "what is free is not much good." As a result, the professionals tend to turn away. Julius Roth describes how the staff in a rehabilitation ward gets discouraged with its patients who apparently are unable to be rehabilitated and gives up and concentrates on the few who seem hopeful. The staffs who must deal with the poor in such wards either have rapid turnover or retreat into "enclaves of research, administration, and teaching."

The situation must get worse. More of the poor will come to the hospitals and clinics. Also, with the increasing use of health insurance and programs by unions and employers, more will come as paying patients into the private hospitals, mixing with middle-class patients and staff, upsetting routines, perhaps lowering quality—a frightening prospect as many administrators see it. As things are going now, relations between lower-income patients and hospital staff must become more frequent, intense, and exacerbated.

It is evident that the vicious cycle that characterizes medical care for the poor must be broken before anything can be accomplished.

In the first part of this cycle, the poor come into the hospitals later than they should, often delaying until their disorders are difficult to relieve, until they are actual emergency cases. The experiences they have there encourage them to try to stay out even longer the next time—and to cut the visits necessary for treatment to a minimum.

Second, they require, if anything, even more effective communication and understanding with the professionals than the middle-class patient. They don't get it; and the treatment is often undone once they leave.

What to do? The conventional remedies do help some. More money and insurance will tend to bring the poor to medical help sooner; increased staff and facilities can cut down the waits, the rush, the tenseness, and allow for more individual and efficient treatment and diagnosis.

But much more is required. If the cycle is to be *broken*, the following set of recommendations must be adopted:

- Speed up the initial visit. Get them there sooner.
- Improve patient experiences.
- Improve communication, given and received, about regimens and treatment to be followed.
- Work to make it more likely that the patient or his family will follow through at home.
- Make it more likely that the patient will return when necessary.
- Decrease the time between necessary visits.

This general list is not meant to be the whole formula. Any experienced doctor or nurse, once he recognizes the need, can add to or modify it. An experience of mine illustrates this well. A physician in charge of an adolescent clinic for lower-income patients, finding that my ideas fitted into his own daily experience, invited me to address his staff. In discussion afterward good ideas quickly emerged:

- Since teen-age acne and late teen-age menstrual pain were frequent complaints and the diagnoses and medications not very complicated, why not let nurses make them? Menstruating girls would be more willing to talk to a woman than a man.

• Patients spend many hours sitting around waiting. Why not have nursing assistants, trained by the social worker and doctor and drawn from the patients' social class, interview and visit with them during this period, collecting relevant information?

Note two things about these suggestions: Though they do involve some new duties and some shifting around, they do not call for any appreciable increase of money, personnel, or resources; and such recommendations, once the need is pointed out, can arise from the initiative and experience of the staff themselves.

Here in greater detail are my recommendations:

Increased efforts are needed for early detection of disease among the poor. Existing methods should be increased and improved, and others should be added—for instance, mobile detection units of all kinds, public drives with large-scale educational campaigns against common specific disorders, and so on. The poor themselves should help in planning, and their ideas should be welcomed.

The schools could and should become major detection units with large-scale programs of health inspection. The school nurse, left to her own initiative, is not enough. The poor have more children and are less efficient at noting illness; those children do go to school, where they could be examined. Teachers should also be given elementary training and used more effectively in detection.

Train more sub-professionals, drawn from the poor themselves. They can easily learn to recognize the symptoms of the more common disorders and be especially-useful in large concentrations, such as housing projects. They can teach the poor to look for health problems in their own families.

The large central facilities make for greater administrative and medical efficiency. But fewer people will come to them than to smaller neighborhood dispensaries. Imperfect treatment may be better than little or no treatment; and the total effectiveness for the poor may actually be better with many small facilities than the big ones.

Neighborhood centers can not only treat routine cases and act to follow up hospital outpatients, but they can also discover those needing the more difficult procedures and refer them to the large centers—for example, prenatal diagnosis and treatment in the neighborhoods, with high-risk pregnancies sent to the central facilities. (The Children's Bureau has experimented with this type of organization.)

There must be better methods to get the sick to the clinics. As noted, the poor tend to stick to their own neighborhoods and be fearful outside them, to lack bus fare and domestic help. Even when dental or eye defects *are* discovered in schools, often children still do not get treatment. Sub-professionals and volunteers could follow up, provide transportation, bus fare, information, or baby-sitting and house care. Block or church organizations could help. The special drives for particular illnesses could also include transportation. (Recent studies show that different ethnic groups respond differently to different pressures and appeals; sub-professionals from the same groups could, therefore, be especially effective.)

Hours should be made more flexible; there should be more evening and night clinics. Working people work, when they have jobs, and cannot afford to lose jobs in order to sit around waiting to be called at a clinic. In short, clinics should adapt to people, not expect the opposite. (A related benefit: Evening clinics should lift the load on emergency services in municipal hospitals, since the poor often use them just that way)

Neighborhood pharmacists should be explicitly recognized as part of the medical team, and every effort be made to bring them in. The poor are much more apt to consult their neighborhood pharmacist first—and he could play a real role in minor treatment and in referral. He should be rewarded, and given such training as necessary—perhaps by schools of pharmacy. Other "health healers" might also be encouraged to help get the seriously ill to the clinics and hospitals, instead of being considered rivals or quacks.

Lower-income patients who enter treatment early can be *rewarded* for it. This may sound strange, rewarding people for benefiting themselves— but it might bring patients in earlier as well as bring them back, and actually save money for insurance companies and government and public agencies.

Hospital emergency services must be radically reorganized. Such services are now being used by the poor as clinics and as substitutes for general practitioners. Such use upsets routine and arouses mutual frustrations and resentments. There are good reasons why the poor use emergency services this way, and the services should be reorganized to face the realities of the situation.

Clinics and hospitals could assign *agents* to their lower-income patients, who can orient them, allay anxiety, listen to complaints, help them cooperate, and help them negotiate with the staff.

Better accountability and communication should be built into the organization of care. Much important information gets to doctors and nurses only fortuitously, if at all. For instance, nurses' aides often have information about cardiac or terminal patients that doctors and nurses could use; but they do not always volunteer the information nor are they often asked, since they are not considered medically qualified. This is another place where the *agent* might be useful.

It is absolutely necessary that medical personnel lessen their class and professional biases. Anti-bias training is virtually nonexistent in medical schools or associations. It must be started, especially in the professional schools.

Medical facilities must carefully consider how to allow and improve the lodging of complaints by the poor against medical services. They have few means and little chance now to make their complaints known, and this adds to their resentment, depression, and helplessness. Perhaps the agent can act as a kind of medical *ombudsman*: perhaps unions, or the other health insurance groups, can lodge the complaints; perhaps neighborhood groups can do it. But it must be done.

Treatment and regimens are supposed to continue in the home. Poor patients seldom do them adequately. Hospitals and clinics usually concentrate on diagnosis and treatment and tend to neglect what occurs after. Sometimes there is even confusion about who is supposed to tell the patient about such things as his diet at home, and there is little attempt to see that he does it. Here again, follow-up by sub-professionals might be useful.

Special training given to professionals will enable them to give better instructions to the poor on regimens. They are seldom trained in interviewing or listening— and the poor are usually deficient in pressing their opinions.

Clinics and hospitals could organize their services to include checking on ex-patients who have no private physicians. We recommend that hospitals and clinics try to bring physicians in poor neighborhoods into some sort of association. Many of these physicians do not have hospital connections, practice old-fashioned or substandard medicine—yet they are in most immediate contact with the poor, especially before hospitalization.

Medical establishments should make special efforts to discover and understand the prevalent life-styles of their patients. Since this affects efficiency of treatment, it is an important medical concern.

I strongly recommend greater emphasis on research in medical devices or techniques that are simple to operate and depend as little as possible on patients' judgment and motivation. Such developments fit lower-class life-style much better than those requiring repeated actions, timing, and persistence.

As noted, these recommendations are not basically different from many others—except that they all relate to the idea of the vicious cycle. *A major point of this paper is that equal health care will not come unless all portions of that cycle are attacked simultaneously.*

To assure action sufficiently broad and strong to demolish this cycle, *responsibility must also be broad and strong.*

- Medical and professional schools must take vigorous steps to counteract the class bias of their students, to teach them to relate, communicate, and adapt techniques and regimens to the poor, and to learn how to train and instruct sub-professionals.
- Specific medical institutions must, in addition to the recommendations above, consider how best to attack *all* segments of the cycle. Partial attacks will not do—medicine has responsibility for the total patient and the total treatment.
- Lower-class people must themselves be enlisted in the campaign to give them better care. Not to do this would be absolutely foolhardy. The sub-professionals we mention are themselves valuable in large part because they come from the poor, and understand them. Where indigenous organizations exist, they should be used. Where they do not exist, organizations that somehow meet their needs should be aided and encouraged to form.
- Finally, governments, at all levels, have an immense responsibility for persuading, inducing, or pressuring medical institutions and personnel toward reforming our system of medical care. If they understand the vicious cycle, their influence will be much greater. This governmental role need not at all interfere with the patient's freedom. Medical influence is shifting rapidly to the elite medical centers; federal and local governments have a responsibility to see that medical influence and care, so much of it financed by public money, accomplishes what it is supposed to.

What of the frequently heard argument that increasing affluence will soon eliminate the need for special programs for the poor?

- Most sociologists agree that general affluence may never "trickle down" to the hard-core poverty groups; that only sustained and specialized effort over a long period of time may relieve their poverty.

- Increased income does not necessarily change life-styles. Some groups deliberately stand outside our mainstream. And there is usually a lag at least of one generation often more, before life-styles respond to changed incomes.

In the long run, no doubt, prosperity for all will minimize the inferiority of medical care for the poor. But in the long run as the saying goes, we will all be dead. And the disadvantaged sick will probably go first, with much unnecessary suffering.

A Century of Health Reform

Eli Ginzberg

The daily press is a potent reminder that for a number of years the United States has been engaged in fruitless discussions about how to reform its health care system, discussions that are likely to preempt any action for some time to come. One facet of this talk effort is increasingly frequent references to the health care systems of Western Europe, Canada, and even of Japan as potential models for the United States to follow to put in place a system of universal coverage at a cost that does not risk national bankruptcy. I would be the last to argue against learning what we can from foreign countries but a more promising alternative can be extracted from our own experiences in related areas of societal reforms, particularly employment, housing, and education, which can give a deeper understanding of the dilemmas that we face in seeking to improve our health care financing and delivery system.

A search for clues and answers closer to home derives from the growing appreciation among most scholars that every nation's health care system is embedded in its cultural, political, economic, ideological, and social institutions and that these must serve as points of departure for any meaningful exploration of health care reform. To ignore the concreteness of history in favor of scholastic models, no matter how elegant their analytic apparatus, is certain to lead to frustration and bankruptcy.

Two illustrations will make his clear. I was intrigued when a draft copy of Alain Enthoven's memorandum to President Carter's Secretary of Health, Joseph Califano, crossed my desk in 1977. Enthoven proposed a consumer health plan that would require these adjustments and adaptations in the status quo: hereafter, physicians would practice in prepaid health plans and would compete on the basis of annual risk contracts; employers would establish a ceiling on employee health benefits which did not provide greater reimbursement for those workers who continued to select fee-for-service coverage; the federal government would place a ceiling on the tax-free benefits which employers could deduct from their taxable income and the amounts of health benefits that employees could ignore in calculating their income. Finally the states would have to provide health insurance coverage for persons not covered by private employers.

A decade and a half later the record discloses this: most physicians continue to avoid practicing as members of prepaid plans; employers have altered their health care benefit systems' payment structures to reduce and eliminate most earlier discrimination against prepaid plans. In fact they now favor such plans. Despite support from several administrations and even from the tax-writing committees of the Congress, no ceiling has been placed on tax benefits from employer health care coverage. Of our fifty states only Hawaii has a plan that approaches universal coverage although the most recently covered vulnerable population is entitled to no more than five days of hospital care per year.

In 1977, when Enthoven submitted the draft of his plan, the United States spent $170 billions for national health care. The most recent data from the Department of Health and Human Resources show total outlays for calendar 1991 at just under $740 billion. Allowing for the depreciating value of the health care dollar and the increase in population, this is the per capita outlay in constant dollars: 1977 $1,296; 1991 $2,172.

Although the Carter administration was looking desperately for a health reform plan, it ignored Enthoven's proposal. Although Enthoven has refined his original proposal several times in the intervening decade and a half, the plan's greatest "success" to date has been its influence on the current reforms of the National Health Service in Great Britain.

A more contemporaneous illustration of a scholastic exercise in health care reform was outlined by Nobel Laureate Milton Friedman in the *Wall Street Journal* (November 12, 1991) this way: Since the end of the Second World War outputs have been lagging behind inputs into the American health care system by wide margins, particularly since the passage of Medicare and Medicaid legislation in 1965. The real problem, Friedman observes, is output. How does he measure this? By "length of life"—but then he adds, "the quality of life is as important as its length." To this he quickly adds that he does not know how to measure quality. Nevertheless, he offers a two-fold solution; end both Medicare and Medicaid and force every family to buy a major medical insurance policy with a deductible of $20,000 or 30 percent of the unit's income during the previous two years; and end the tax exemption on employer health care benefits that employees receive. Consider the following obiter dictum:

> I conjecture that almost all consumers of medical services, and many providers, would favor a simple reform that would privatize most medical care.... There is only one thing wrong with this dream. It would displease...the large number of people who are now engaged in administering, studying and daily reviewing the present socialized system...they are sufficiently potent politically to kill any such reform before it could get a real following....

There are other problems, not the least of which the tens of millions of employees who will fight to keep the tax benefits of their current health insurance coverage; the thirty million plus members of the AARP who would oppose demolishing Medicare; and most Americans who would balk at a $20,000 deductible health insurance policy. Friedman made some serious errors in estimating consumer support for his plan.

Enthoven is a sophisticated health care analyst and Friedman won the Nobel Prize in economics. What is wrong, very wrong, with their respective health care reforms? Neither Enthoven nor Friedman took the time and trouble to assess the American health care system within the fabric of American society as it is—not as they want it to be. Moreover, Friedman's gloss that our "medical system has become in large part a socialist enterprise," and "our socialized postal system, our socialized schooling system, our socialized system of trying to control drugs, and indeed our socialized defense system provide clear evidence that we are no better at socialism than countries that have gone all the way."

A closer look at the American experience with employment, housing, and education policy may prove illuminating and instructive for health reform if we do more than hide behind the term "socialism" or even "consumer choice." At least the effort is worth a try. The way a society, American or other, deals with critical issues such as employment, housing, and education reflects basic preferences and prejudices that will condition its thinking and action in the provision of health care.

Employment

In our predominantly, though by no means exclusively, market economy, much of the quality of a person's (and a family's) existence is determined by type of job and income, by type of housing and neighborhood a family can afford to live in, and by the quality of education to which the children have access and, not surprising, by the type of health care services available. Admittedly the sequence also runs, at least in part, in the other direction. The level of education an individual achieves is the single most important determinant of later level of income which in turn determines so many other dimensions of a person's life.

Since most Americans make a sharp distinction between individual responsibility and governmental action, it is important to remind the reader how far government has extended its role into the employment arena. In quick review: (1) government has established the minimum age at which young people are permitted to work; (2) it has limited the number of hours of work; (3) it has established rules and regulations governing the health and safety risks to which employees can be exposed; (4) it has established a minimum wage; (5) it has legislated the rights of workers to join unions; (6) it has a Social Security system in place to provide workers and their families with alternative sources of income in the event that they lose their jobs or reach the age of retirement; (7) it has passed anti-discrimination laws and regulations that have gone a fair distance to lower, even to remove, the pre-existent barriers against minorities and women in both initial hiring and later promotion.

Despite these many interventions, government has stopped short of establishing a right for every adult, able and willing to work, to do so. But this does not mean that government has no role in establishing and maintaining a high level of employment. Since the passage of the Employment Act of 1946, the federal government has just such an obligation. And though it has not been able to prevent the recurrence of various short and long recessions, it has been able to avoid bringing on, or contributing to, a major depression such as engulfed the economy in the early 1930s. The federal government has also provided special assistance to major employers in risk of bankruptcy, such as Lockheed and Chrysler; more broadly, it has taken repeated actions to bail out major banks and financial institutions whose possible collapse threatened massive losses of jobs and income.

It is one of the better kept secrets that a leading Republican ideologue, Arthur F. Burns, the former chairman of the Council of Economic Advisors under Dwight Eisenhower and chairman of the Federal Reserve System under Richard Nixon and Gerald Ford, proposed in the mid-1970s that the federal government become the employer of last resort, offering a job at 10 percent below the minimum wage to every person able and willing to work. Hubert Humphrey, the leader of the liberal wing of the Democratic Party and a strong advocate of a full-employment policy, complimented Burns for his forward-looking contribution but, Humphrey aside, the intensifying inflation resulted in the stillbirth of the Burns proposal.

By far the most important interrelationships between the employment and health care sectors grow out of the fact that the United States backed into private health insurance provided primarily by employers as a result of a Labor Board decision made during the Second World War that unions could bargain for such health benefits without violating the existing wage stabilization policy. The federal government encouraged such bargaining by providing tax advantages to both employers and employees. The fact that in the early 1990s about 1500 private companies sell health insurance policies and provide administrative surveillance of employer expenditures for health care is further evidence of the commingling of the private and public sectors in the financing, administration, and delivery of health care.

Another type of linkage goes back to shortly after the end of the Second World War. The federal government then began sustained financing for biomedical research. In 1991, this exceeded $11 billion of federal outlays, an expenditure that is at the heart of the continuing rapid growth in national health care expenditures. The existence of established pharmaceutical companies and medical supply companies and the launching of many new companies to exploit the enlarged pool of knowledge and technique helped to assure American leadership in high-tech medicine and contributed greatly to the growth and profitability of these private sector companies.

In the early 1990s, employment in the health care sector has topped 9 million. This equals about one out of every thirteen workers. Between 1988 and 1990, employment in the health sector grew by 600,000 jobs, in a period of marked slackening of total employment growth. With substantial overcapacity in the nation's 5500 acute care hospitals, a major challenge all levels of government will face for the remainder of this decade will be assessing the effects on local employment of downsizing the nation's overexpanded hospital plant and responding to it.

Housing

A century or more ago, any physically competent adult male could head West and obtain a land grant from the federal government and, with help from his neighbors, could build a home for his family. Since then the

United States has become an overwhelmingly metropolitan society and about four in five persons reside in metropolitan areas. Most Americans rely on the marketplace to buy or rent.

Since the late 1930s the federal government, cognizant of the difficulties many low-income people face in obtaining an apartment or a house on the private market, has pursued a range of subsidy policies. Various state, and even local governments, have also resorted to tax subsidies to expand the housing stock for low-income families. In recent years, a substantial spurt of investment from the voluntary sector, with governmental assistance dedicated not only to improved housing but also to neighborhood improvement, has occurred. If one asks how successful these governmental subsidy efforts have been, the answers will range from quite successful to total failure, such as the forced demolition of the deserted and uninhabited public housing units in the Pruitt-Igoe complex in St. Louis, Missouri.

Responding to the desire and interest of the veterans returning from the Second World War to become home owners, the federal government initiated a substantial Veterans Administration loan program and followed it with an important tax benefit. Homeowners could deduct from their federal income tax liability both the interest costs of their mortgage and local and state real estate taxes. This tax expenditure benefit has been estimated at about $70 billion annually, exceeding the tax expenditure benefits for private health insurance.

Since most purchasers of a new home must obtain a substantial mortgage to finance their acquisition, the ability and behavior of the financial intermediaries become a critical consideration. The recent collapse of so many Savings and Loans Associations left the federal government with few options other than a large-scale rescue operation that is estimated to cost the taxpayers several hundreds of billions of dollars before the S&Ls and the banks return to solvency.

Clearly the access Americans have had to desirable housing was greatly influenced by government actions at all levels—federal, state, and local. Government has used public funds, tax benefits, anti-discrimination laws, land-use standards, and a great many other public sector policies and interventions to expand the supply of available housing. As is so often the case with governmental interventions in the United States, for the most part the major beneficiaries have not been the poor but the middle and upper income classes.

One specific link between housing and health care is the growing number of the urban homeless. Most experts see the root of his problem in thoughtless and indiscriminate release over time of almost 400,000 mentally ill from state mental hospitals without adequate alternative housing for the many who had no families able and willing to care for them and who were unable to care for themselves.

A second important linkage between housing and health is mirrored in the great difficulties state and local governments have in locating special facilities for AIDS patients, drug addicts, and other seriously ill people in middle class neighborhoods—the NIMBY ("Not in My Back Yard") syndrome—which impedes treatment and amelioration of their illness. As a consequence government is forced to locate more and more of these facilities in the most depressed neighborhoods, assuring thereby their further decline.

The concentration of ever larger numbers of the seriously disadvantaged with low-income people in a limited number of inner city neighborhoods makes the challenge of assuring their continuing access to essential health care services much more difficult because most physicians shun establishing or maintaining a practice in such areas. Voluntary hospitals, faced with ever larger numbers of uninsured and underinsured, cannot long survive without restricting the amount of charity care they provide. Public hospitals tend to be few and underfunded. Many of the most vulnerable segments in our society, adults and children, are likely to be seriously underserved when it comes to basic preventive and therapeutic care. This is, in considerable measure, a consequence of where they live or as a result of their being homeless.

The federal government has sought to assist localities to provide shelter for the homeless as many courts have mandated. But the discrepancy between supply and need remains so great that many homeless continue to opt for the streets rather than use overcrowded and frequently dangerous shelters. One conclusion is unequivocal: the United States has not committed itself, much less taken action, to providing adequate shelter for every citizen.

Education

Unlike employment or housing, which the individual is expected to obtain through his own efforts (the welfare population and the institu-

tionalized excepted), public education has been a governmentally mandated long established service available to everybody between the ages
of six to eighteen, and selectively for children as young as three and four
(Head Start). Further, access to continuing education is broadly available for qualified high school graduates in community colleges, state
colleges and universities. A variety of second-choice remedial programs
is available for urban high school drop-outs.

Since the Second World War, state and the federal governments have
taken a number of initiatives directed at improving the quality of public
education from kindergarten through high school. The barriers to higher
education have been substantially lowered for large numbers of qualified
young people who, in earlier times, would have been prevented from
continuing their education because of lack of finances.

Prior to the Second World War, revenues for public education were
raised primarily by local taxing authorities via the property tax, a system of financing that made it very difficult, if not impossible, for low-
income neighborhoods to provide an adequate educational experience
for all their children. Consequently, state aid for public education became the norm and in less than two decades—between 1970 and the
end of the 1980s—the proportion of the state's funding increased from
rough equality with local funding to more than half again as much.
Since 1965, the federal government has made some modest contributions to public education. In the late 1980s, the federal contribution
was approximately 8 percent of the total outlays for education. But the
federal government's primary impact on education was via the Supreme
Court decision in *Brown v. Board of Education* in 1954 and the subsequent implementation of desegregation orders. Desegregation of public
schools in metropolitan areas was vitiated to a marked degree by the
ability of many middle class white families to relocate to suburban
areas. During the post-war decades, large-scale expansion of higher
education was underwritten by both the states and the federal government and resulted in the establishment of new and the expansion of
existing state colleges and universities, and community colleges. The
expansion was furthered by extensive student loan programs in which
the federal government took the lead.

There has been much hand-wringing in the 1980s and early 1990s
over the poor quality of American education, particularly the shortcomings of junior and senior high schools. The schools have been held re-

sponsible for the retardation in the international economic position of the United States. However, the linkage in theory between poor schooling and the loss of American competitiveness has not been established. It is true that schools in low-income, disorganized, urban neighborhoods are often dysfunctional to a point that many young people drop out of school. Lacking skills and competencies, they encounter great difficulties in getting regular jobs and many resort to illicit and illegal activities.

With the advantage of a lengthened perspective since government has been involved in providing access to basic education for over a century and a half, we must conclude that the results have been mixed. At the time of the Second World War, when the minimum standard for induction into the Army was the equivalent of a fourth grade education, over a million young men were rejected for what was labeled "mental deficiency" but which should have been coded "lack of educational achievement." In the state of South Carolina about 250 young black men per 1000 were rejected. The proportion of whites in some of rural Southern states was in the 60 to 70 per 1000 range. John Fischer, former president of Teachers College at Columbia University, once observed that public education has served the American people well, except poor whites and minorities. This judgment has not lost its edge, even in the 1990s.

Lessons for Health Care Reform

Increasing numbers of domestic and foreign observers of our health care system are at a loss to understand why the United States is taking so long to adopt reforms to achieve justice, equity, and efficiency. What are the impediments to our following in the footsteps of most advanced nations and acting expeditiously to provide health insurance coverage for the 35 million persons who currently lack coverage?

The United States continues to expect the individual to find a job and earn an income that will enable him to secure housing and other essentials for himself and his dependents. The only governmental commitment that exists to deliver a basic service to the public is to provide schooling for all children and young people up to age eighteen, a commitment that, up to the present, has carried with it little accountability about how well government meets its responsibility.

True, government has moved a considerable way toward putting in place "safety nets" for those who are unable to work—the unemployed, low earners, and many more unable to support themselves. But existing social welfare supports are not responsive to all, or even to most of the poor. Most Americans balk at expanding the role of government in providing jobs, housing, and quality education for all. Since our society has a number of health care safety nets in place such as public health clinics, public hospitals, Medicaid, and charity care funded by nongovernmental hospitals, the political energy to move toward universal coverage is limited. The partial failure of public education after a century and a half of responsibility adds a healthy dose of skepticism to the presumed benefits that would flow from a system of universal health care coverage.

Neither justice nor equity have commanded top-ranking positions in the nation's value scale. Many politicians continue to rail against "welfare cheats." While we have made considerable progress on the discrimination front since the early 1950s, racism continues to pervade every sector of American life.

Cost Containment

Anybody who has looked even superficially at the expenditure trends in the American health care system is startled by the fact that the share of GNP devoted to health has increased from about 4.5 percent to 14 percent since the Second World War and shows no sign of levelling off. The principal payers (other than households) in descending order of importance are: 1) employers and private health insurance (PHI); 2) the federal government; and 3) state governments. Together they account for about three out of every four dollars of health care expenditures. For the better part of the last two decades, each of these three payers has made valiant efforts to curtail outlays, but with limited success.

Clearly the difficulties are considerable and are likely to remain so as long as each continues to go its own way. But most employers, despite unease with steadily rising health costs, are not about to enter into a partnership with the federal government to control these costs. They prefer to keep their distance. The federal government, facing a deficit of $400 billion, is not looking for new responsibilities.

Talented economists find no difficulty in modeling the structure and interactions of an "efficient" health care system, but their models lack the incentives and the specifications that would lead key decision makers—physicians, voluntary hospitals, private health insurance companies and the other interested parties—to cooperate in putting into practice what these analysts have designed. Government may be willing to intervene in the critical areas of employment and housing to moderate the shortfalls in the operation of the market, but only up to a point. Government was careful not to assume responsibility for the economic efficiency much less for the social justice in the production and distribution of the nation's housing stock.

Administrative Waste

All analysts of our current health care system agree that administrative costs are out of control. They differ only about the outer range of their estimates but few would set the figure below 15 percent. If malpractice and defensive medicine were included, the figure could easily approach 25 percent, or even more. Here is a major opportunity for reform. We have 1500 private-sector companies selling basic health care insurance; the Canadians have none. But eliminating administrative waste is more complicated than it seems. The history of the Department of Housing and Urban Development (HUD) shows weakness in terms of financial probity and a neglect of administrative competence. As chairman of the National Commission for Employment Policy in the 1960s and 1970s, I was in a good position to watch the expenditure of $85 billion of federal funds to underwrite the training and employment of the hard-to-employ. While most of the money went to the poor and unskilled, only a small percentage, possibly as little as 10 to 20 percent, of the trainees achieved the goals of the program by obtaining and keeping a regular job. Most seriously, the educational establishment has been charged with permitting the additional dollars to flow into overhead instead into expanding and improving services to students.

No informed person will argue against taking action to reduce the excessive costs that characterize our current health care system. The difficulty arises when one looks for specific remedies. It is not easy for the federal and state governments, which are committed to the competitive market as the preferred instrument for garnering and distributing scarce resources, to move individually or jointly to outlaw private health insurance companies which are the critical players in providing coverage for most Americans under the age of sixty-five.

Quality Control and Efficiency

Despite unflattering comments made earlier about the efficiency of governmental operations in employment, housing, and educational programs, all is not bleak. The Social Security System mails out about 30 million checks monthly involving over $250 billion annually, with relatively few snags or complaints. This gives us some ground for believing that the federal government can play a constructive role in reducing administrative waste in the health care sector as long as its responsibilities are tied to check-writing, not micro-management of service delivery.

The conviction is growing among leaders of American medicine and health services research that many diagnostic and therapeutic interventions are of questionable, if not negative, value to the patient. Medical and surgical procedures can lead to permanent injury or premature death. Small wonder that "outcomes research" has attracted more and more attention of late, including increased, if still modest, funding from the Congress. The aim of this new effort is to learn more about untested interventions in the hope and expectation of developing "practice guidelines" for physicians to inform and improve patient treatment. Some analysts look to outcomes research, not only as a way to improve quality, but also to lower costs.

Here too, as in the area of administrative waste, many opportunities beckon but expectations should be restrained. A key proponent of outcomes research is Paul Ellwood who has set ten years as the time required before useful results will emerge. Pessimists point out that in a dynamic biomedical environment, practice guidelines will always lag behind new therapeutic breakthroughs and advances.

The example of employment and training programs showed a serious shortfall between congressional expenditures and the ability of the prime sponsors to deliver efficient and effective training services to the hard-to-employ. Some did a good job but they were in the minority. In the case of public housing the demolition of Pruitt-Igoe houses in St. Louis is a potent reminder of how large a gap can develop between proposal and execution. Admittedly the St. Louis failure was extreme. More relevant are the continuing shortfalls in quality control and accountability in public education where even today no agreement exists about how well or how poorly the system is performing.

The scope of the challenge facing medicine is revealed by the fact that during the course of a year patients make about 1.3 billion visits to physicians. Physicians are licensed by state governments. Most large hospitals operate with a closed staff. The medical specialty societies are heavily involved in providing continuing educational opportunities for their members. Better control over quality and efficacy is highly desirable but it will remain an open-ended endeavor. There is no question that our health care system calls for major reforms directed to providing universal coverage, cost containment, the elimination of administrative waste, and quality improvement. But before we go any further it is important to point out that two out of every three Americans are reasonably satisfied with the quality of medical care to which they have access and they are unlikely to support major reforms unless they become worried about the prospective erosion of their present coverage.

That leaves one out of every three Americans at risk in accessing the health care system or in obtaining essential health care services, preventive, therapeutic or rehabilitative. But we must place this shortcoming in perspective. The American people have repeatedly demonstrated their unwillingness to make more than marginal adjustments to broaden opportunities for the unemployed to obtain jobs, for the homeless to obtain shelter, for many poor children to obtain adequate education.

Our recent presidents have opposed expansion of government programs that would serve the unemployed, the homeless, and the illiterate. They have railed against higher taxes although Americans carry a lower tax burden than the citizens of any other advanced country but have been silent about our historic commitment to "equality of opportunity" for every American child and adult. Significant health reforms are not very likely to be implemented until the United States remembers *E Pluribus Unum,* the words on the Great Seal of the United States.

Health Care for the Homeless

Drew Altman, Ellen L. Bassuk, William R. Breakey,
A. Alan Fischer, Charles R. Halpern, Gloria Smith, Louisa
Stark, Nathan Stark, Bruce C. Vladeck, and Phyllis Wolfe

This supplementary statement was prepared by ten members of the Institute of Medicine's Committee on Health Care for Homeless People, not in opposition to the committee's report, *Homelessness, Health and Human Needs,* but from concern that the report is too limited in its discussion of the broader aspects of the issues it addresses. We endorse the report and its recommendations. We especially feel that the fact-finding efforts it embodies were thorough and thoughtful. But the report fails to capture our sense of shame and anger about homelessness, and it incompletely addresses the context in which all discussions regarding the health of homeless persons should be placed.

Any Institute of Medicine (IOM) report necessarily must undergo a process of negotiation among committee members, and then between the committee and external reviewers; such a process assures the objectivity, credibility, and defensibility of the report and its principal findings. This is just as it should be in order for the IOM and the National Academy of Sciences (NAS) to fulfill the critical role of providing objective expert advice. There are invariably frustrations in such a process, but they too are an expected part of a committee's and the institute's work. Another frustration, however, affected the work of this committee; and while the committee's staff did an excellent job of managing this frustration within the academy's ground rules, we feel the need to articulate our feelings in a supplementary statement.

The frustration we all experienced working on the report arises from the nature of the problem we were charged to address. Contemporary American homelessness is an outrage, a national scandal. Its character requires a careful, sophisticated, and dispassionate analysis—which the report provides—but its tragedy demands something more direct and human, less qualified and detached. We have tried to present the facts and figures of homelessness, but we were unable to capture the extent of our anger and dismay. We have summarized available studies on homeless children, but we had no means to paint the pathos and tragedy of these displaced, damaged, innocent lives. We have reviewed the demographic and clinical data and then, walking home, passed men asleep on heating grates or displaced people energetically searching in garbage piles for a few cents' income from aluminum cans. We analyzed mortality data for the homeless but lacked any platform from which to shout that our neighbors are dying needlessly because we are incapable of providing the most basic services.

As the committee's deliberations progressed. we became increasingly aware that homelessness causes some illnesses and exacerbates and perpetuates others by seriously complicating efforts to treat disease and reduce disability. Therefore, only a comprehensive long-term strategy for eliminating homelessness will permanently improve the health status of homeless persons. Because of its charge and its limited resources, however, the committee was unfortunately constrained in its ability to formulate essential long-term recommendations that dealt with the root causes of homelessness.

The most basic health problem of homeless people is the lack of a home; to condemn someone to homelessness is to visit him or her with a host of other evils. Ignoring the causes of homelessness leads to treating only symptoms and turns medical programs into costly but necessary stopgap measures. Attempts to address the health problems of homeless persons separately from their systemic causes is largely palliative.

A broad long-term strategy is needed to solve the health care problems of homeless people. Such a strategy must emphasize the context of homelessness. It must focus on gross inadequacies in four areas: supply of low-income housing, income maintenance, support services, and access to health care for the poor and uninsured.

As the committee observed in its report, the health problems of homeless people that differ from the health problems of other poor people relate directly to their homeless state. We agree with the World Health Organization's 1987 statement on the International Year of Shelter for the Homeless: "Shelter to protect against the elements and to serve as a locus of family life is a basic human need.... At its best, appropriate shelter promotes emotional and social health."

We support the principle that decent, affordable housing is every American's right. This view reaffirms the Federal Housing Act of 1948, which describes the federal government's obligation to assure that every household has access to decent, affordable housing. To this end, we strongly recommend that the federal government work to substantially increase the *supply* and availability of low-income housing. More specifically, we recommend that, as a start, funding for federal housing programs be restored to 1981 levels.

As the committee also observed, people must have income levels that make housing affordable, both to prevent and to end existing homelessness. We were aggrieved to encounter ever-growing numbers of homeless people with full-time jobs, who were unable to afford any kind of housing because they were being paid the minimum wage. It is our judgment that the minimum wage should be set at the level that makes decent housing affordable.

Many people must rely on entitlements for their income and financial support. Not only have these benefits become more difficult to obtain, but today's federal entitlements are not sufficient to support housing for the elderly, the disabled, or those on welfare. If homelessness and its resultant health problems are to be eliminated, those benefits must be significantly augmented.

Many homeless persons are disconnected from supportive relationships and caretaking institutions, as the report notes. Some, such as chronically mentally ill individuals, substance abusers, those with physical disabilities, and the very young and the very old, have special needs. Many homeless people urgently require a wide array of support services, including job training, psychosocial rehabilitation, outreach, and case management.

For the most chronically disabled among the homeless population, psychosocial rehabilitation services must be offered, but for those who cannot be rehabilitated the goal is to provide decent and humane asylum in the community. Disabled people must not be consigned to lives of degradation.

Homeless people encounter many obstacles in obtaining access to health care, but the single greatest problem is one shared by many other Americans; they are unable to pay for health care and therefore often do not receive it. While the Constitution does not promise citizens health care, neither does it guarantee universal free education or old-age pensions. but these rights have long been recognized by policymakers. Additionally, the president's Commission for the Study of Ethical Problems in Medicine and Biomedical and Behavioral Research in their 1983 report *Securing Access to Health Care* concluded that:

> Society has an ethical obligation to ensure equitable access to health care for all. The societal obligation is balanced by individual obligations.
>
> Equitable access to health care requires that all citizens be able to secure an adequate level of care without excessive burdens. When equity occurs through the operation of private forces, there is no need for government involvement, but the ultimate responsibility for ensuring that society's obligation is met, through a combination of public and private sector arrangements, rests with the Federal Government.
>
> The cost of achieving equitable access to health care ought to be shared fairly.
>
> Efforts to contain rising health care costs are important but should not focus on limiting the attainment of equitable access for the least well served portion of the public.

Approximately 37 million Americans, including many of the homeless, are without any form of public or private health insurance. Medicaid has tended to some needs of one large constituency, but we believe the time has come to move toward establishing universal access to health care.

The committee tried to make its report as dispassionate as the IOM/ NAS process requires, but the reality cries out for immediate action. As we witnessed the suffering of America's poorest citizens, we came to understand that the individual health problems of homeless people combine to form a major public health crisis. We can no longer sit as spectators to the elderly homeless dying of hypothermia, to the children with blighted futures poisoned by lead in rat-infested dilapidated welfare hotels, to women raped, to old men beaten and robbed of their few possessions, and to people dying on the streets with catastrophic illnesses such as AIDS. Without eliminating homelessness, the health risks and concomitant health problems, the desperate plight of homeless children, the suffering, and the needless deaths of homeless Americans will continue. We agreed with the recommendations set forth in the committee report, but we felt continuously uneasy because of our inability to state the most basic recommendation: homelessness in the United States is an inexcusable disgrace and must be eliminated.

Health Policy for the Elderly

Steven P. Wallace and Carroll L. Estes

When Ronald Reagan assumed the presidency, both conservative and liberal analysts predicted revolutionary changes in the health and welfare system of the country. When Reagan left office eight years later, major programs affecting the elderly that had been targeted for radical modification or elimination still existed. Medicare continues as a federal program that pays half of the medical bills of the elderly. Medicaid remains a joint federal-state program that pays the medical bills of a large number of elderly poor. Social Security offers federally administered income support, while other programs provide federal funds for social services, food, and other needs.

While the Reagan years did not revolutionize health policy for the elderly, significant structural trends were initiated and/or reinforced. These trends could have long-lasting consequences for the elderly. As the number of elderly grows dramatically over the next fifty years, the federal health policy for the aged will reflect the heritage of New Federalism, fiscal crisis and austerity, and deregulation.

The Demographic "Imperative"

Two factors cause policymakers to worry about the future of health policy for the elderly: the growing number of the elderly and their health status. It is possible to reliably estimate the health-care demands of the elderly at the turn of the century because of two factors. All of those who will be elderly have already been born, and the health of the elderly as a group changes gradually.

The number of elderly in the United States will grow rapidly over the next forty years. In 1980 there were 25.5 million persons age sixty-five and over, accounting for 11.3 percent of the population. That number will double by the early part of the next century; those age sixty-five and over will number 51.4 million by the year 2020. During this time the "oldest old," those age eighty-five and over, will increase threefold, from 2.2 million to 7.1 million.

Because the elderly are more likely to suffer from chronic illnesses than younger people, the growth in the number of elderly raises concerns. Table 1 shows that the elderly are much more likely to suffer from chronic conditions than the general population, even though they are less susceptible to common acute conditions.

Chronic conditions often lead to limitations in the activities of daily living among the elderly, such as dressing, bathing, or walking. Of the younger elderly (those between sixty-five and seventy-four), 37 percent are limited in some way in their activities. For the oldest old, almost 60 percent have limitations. About one-third of the oldest old with limitations are totally unable to carry out one or more activity.

Most of the elderly who have activity limitations remain in their communities. Only about 5 percent of those sixty-five and over reside in nursing homes although this percentage rises sharply to almost 22 percent of those eighty-five and over. Studies have estimated that about 80 percent of all caretaking needs of the elderly are provided by their families.

Chronic activity limitations require long-term care for some, while acute episodes of underlying diseases generate hospital costs. For 1987, U.S. expenditures for health care are projected to total almost $500 billion for the entire population, exceeding 11 percent of the GNP. Over half of the total will be spent on hospital and nursing home care. While the elderly comprise 12 percent of the population, they account for 31 percent of those expenditures. Actually, a small proportion of the elderly are responsible for the lion's share of health care expenses. The last year of life is typically the sickest—only about 6 percent of the elderly die in a given year but they account for 28 percent of all Medicare expenses.

Demographic and health trends are not independent forces on federal health policy for the elderly. Political and economic conditions that frame these trends shape the policy response. The central structural constraints on future health policy for the elderly include the health care system, the changing shape of federalism, the fiscal crisis of the state, and deregulation.

TABLE 1
Acute and Chronic Illness Rates for the Elderly, 1983

	Total Population	65 Years and Over
Acute conditions (rate/1000 population)		
infective and parasitic	20.3	7.3
upper respiratory	40.6	18.1
digestive system	7.6	7.2
Chronic conditions (rate/1000 population)		
heart conditions	82.8	303.0
hypertension	121.3	387.9
arthritis and rheumatism	131.3	471.6

Source: U.S. Bureau of the Census, 1986

The Biomedical Model

While chronic illness has become the nation's primary health problem, the medical care system remains biased towards acute care. The biomedical model is oriented towards treating individuals who have short-term conditions that can be fully reversed. Chronic illnesses, on the other hand, are usually long-term conditions that require supportive and palliative care, and environmental modifications. Federal health policy virtually ignores these needs as it spends the majority of its health funds on institutional and acute care.

Some of the most significant health problems of the elderly are sensitive to social and environmental interventions. The reduction in mortality due to heart disease can be attributed to changes in diet and smoking patterns. The large increase in lung cancer deaths is attributable almost entirely to the increased percentage of smokers in the aging population. Functionally impaired elderly frequently use low-tech equipment to adapt to their illnesses, such as special grab bars or raised toilet seats.

The medical care system individualizes living problems. Illness and functional disability are typically addressed with little attention to the family, community, or social context. Medical research and treatment for the problems of the elderly focuses on the human organism, even though social forces such as poverty, widowhood, or housing conditions may be equally significant.

Changing Shape of Federalism

Federalism denotes the relationships among different levels of government. Since the Great Depression and the New Deal, the federal government has taken an increasingly large responsibility for the health and welfare of the population. The federal government has assumed full responsibility for some programs that address needs of the elderly, such as Social Security for income and Medicare for acute medical care. For other programs, such as Medicaid, which provides health care for the poor, the federal government has developed cooperative relationships with states and localities.

In the 1970s President Nixon initiated policies that increased state and local discretion and responsibilities; President Reagan has vigorously followed this lead by limiting the federal role in health and welfare through block grants, program cuts, and increased state responsibility. Clark C. Havighurst, in *Deregulating the Health Care Industry, Planning for Competition,* reflects New Federalism's ideology that the individual in an open market should be unaffected by government. He states that, "the competitive process, precisely because it is based on choice, validates the outcomes whatever it may turn out to be...[A]n intensely personal matter as what to do about disease should be kept within the realm of private choice." This ideology resulted in proposals to eliminate direct federal involvement in most major health and welfare programs, including Medicare, Social Security, and even the National Institute of Health. In its most basic form, New Federalism challenges the idea that there is any societal responsibility for meeting basic human needs in health, income, housing, or welfare.

New Federalism's goals have been more far-reaching than its achievements. While the Reagan administration has proposed various program changes that would have sharply limited the federal role in the health and welfare of the population, actual changes have followed a historically incremental course. Proposed dramatic changes, such as placing Medicare recipients in the market for private health insurance, have not been successful in Congress. Concurrent policy changes, however, are significantly restructuring the health care system for the elderly.

The *ideology* of the proper federal role has shifted dramatically. The federal government was viewed as the key agent for solving the nation's problem under Johnson's Great Society. Under Reagan's New Federalism, it is seen as a source of the nation's problems. The ideological shift away from a strong federal role provides a powerful constraint on future policy initiatives. This will be significant for the elderly because of their dependence, along with the poor, on federal programs for their health and welfare. While the ideology of New Federalism is to reduce the involvement of the federal government in the lives of citizens, demographic changes in society will increase the pressure on the federal government to take a larger role in the health and welfare of the elderly.

The reliance of the elderly on federal programs is most evident in the importance of Social Security and Medicare to the elderly. If Social Security were eliminated, the poverty rate among the elderly would soar from 12.4 percent to 47.6 percent. Many of those helped out of poverty by Social Security are not far from falling into poverty. Congressional Budget Office analyses of a proposed cost-of-living-adjustment freeze in 1985 estimated that a one-year freeze would have dropped 420,000-470,000 elderly into poverty. The dependence of the elderly poor and near poor on Social Security is shown in Table 2. Low-income couples depend on Social Security for 82 percent of their income, while high-income couples have assets as their primary source of income.

The elderly's dependence on Medicare and Medicaid is similarly large. Medicare paid almost half the medical expenses of the aged in 1984; Medicaid paid an additional 13 percent. Despite these programs, each elderly person had an average of $1,059 in out-of-pocket health expenses, not including insurance premiums. This is a substantial sum, particularly for those living in or near poverty. When the elderly need long-term care for a chronic illness they are particularly vulnerable because Medicare pays for limited nursing home or home health care. The only way for the elderly to get assistance with prolonged long-term-care bills is to spend themselves into poverty and qualify for Medicaid. This threatens the independence of the elderly since few have resources to remain out of poverty after paying for as little as 13 weeks of nursing care.

As a result of their reliance on federal programs for income and health care, the elderly are particularly vulnerable to changes in federal policy that affect the health and welfare of the nation. The needs of the growing number of elderly persons conflict with the antigovernment ideology of New Federalism. While it is unlikely that the federal government will repudiate all responsibility for the health care of the elderly, the legitimation of New Federalism may limit federal government growth to a level below what is necessary to keep up with needs of the growing number of elderly.

TABLE 2
Comparisons of Sources of Income between High- and Low-Income Elderly, 1984

| Source | Percent of Total Income | | | |
| | Couples | | Individuals | |
	Income Less than $10,100	Income Greater than $30,100	Income Less than $4,200	Income Greater than $13,700
Social Security	82	18	75	22
Pension	5	17	1	16
Income from assets	6	38	3	49
Earnings	2	26	1	12
Means-tested cash transfer	3	0	18	0
Other	2	1	2	1
Total	100	100	100	100

Source: U.S. General Accounting Office, 1986

Fiscal Crisis

There are two ways to define a condition of fiscal crisis. One is the objective deficit between revenues and expenditures. This is particularly critical for state governments, since they must normally have balanced budgets. There is also a subjective element to fiscal crises, since "crisis" implies that there are no easy solutions to the fiscal imbalance. The level of taxation that a jurisdiction can support and the level of program reduction that citizens are willing to suffer are political issues. For a condition to be a crisis, therefore, policymakers and the public must perceive a lack of politically legitimate options.

The objective aspects of a fiscal crisis have been observed in local, state, and federal budgets since the late 1970s. The crises have been brought to a head by taxpayer revolts, federal tax cuts, and economic recession. Just as economic crisis provided the context for government expansion during the New Deal, the fiscal crisis of the 1980s is a driving force of New Federalism's attack on government. At the federal level, declining revenues have been caused by massive tax cuts enacted in 1981 and the largest peacetime military buildup ever. This reordering of budget priorities has also led to national debt levels of historic size, both in dollar amounts and as a percent of the GNP.

The subjective component of fiscal crisis is present in the belief that federal spending on the elderly and poor is a major cause of U.S. economic problems. This belief legitimates proposals to decrease the federal deficit by reducing programs for the elderly and poor, even though over half of the current deficit can be traced directly to the 1981 tax cuts. While the tax burden in the United States is lower than in almost all other industrialized nations, austerity is presented as the only possible response to declining revenues. As a result, Social Security and Medicare expenditures, which are funded by a special tax and trust fund, have been used in a political maneuver to reduce the size of the general revenue deficit. In fiscal year 1988, Social Security alone is projected to have a *surplus* of up to $38 billion, with the accumulated surplus growing to an estimated $12 trillion by 2020 when baby boomers will begin to draw it down. Medicare's surplus for 1988 is projected to be approximately $20 billion. On paper this reduces the federal deficit, even though Social Security and Medicare funds can be used only for those programs. The fiscal crisis has entrenched austerity in the public debate, as evidenced by austerity (versus equity) becoming the driving ideology behind health and social policy for the elderly.

Austerity hits the elderly particularly hard because it focuses on governmental finances rather than on total social support for dependents. Attention to the total social support notes that the number of dependents in society (children under eighteen and the aged) has been *decreasing* since the mid-1960s. Children, however, are largely supported by their parents and local programs while the elderly are most dependent on federal programs for their health and welfare. As the aged segment of society grows, and the under-eighteen segment declines, an increasing proportion of society's support for dependent populations will be channeled through the government rather than through the family economy. The dependence on family caused by 65.7 children per 100 adults in 1965 shifted towards dependence on government by 1985, as the *total* dependency ratio (aged and children) fell to 62.1 dependent persons per 100 adults. As the total dependency ratio falls through the end of this century, the proportion of dependents who rely on the federal government will continue to rise.

The elderly are also frequently blamed for the increasing costs of the medical system. Recent data, however, show that factors other than the increasing number of elderly are much more important. A study of 1985 health expenditures and spending projections to the year 2000 indicate that health care costs are rising primarily because of rising prices in the medical care system itself (e.g., rising hospital and physician charges, 55.6 percent of increase), and secondarily to increased intensity of care (higher technology services, 22.9 percent of increase). Increased utilization of services and the much-heralded demographic changes have contributed far less to rising health expenditures. Population growth has contributed less than 8 percent to the rising cost of care, and changes in utilization have no effect. Blaming the elderly for contributing to the fiscal crisis questions the deservedness of those receiving the medical care (the aged) rather than the deservedness of those receiving payments and making profits from providing medical services to the aged.

The politics of fiscal austerity define health and welfare expenditures for the elderly as involved in a zero-sum competition with other sectors of the economy. The argument assumes that if the country is in a fiscal crisis someone *has* to lose out. An alternate way of conceptualizing expenditures on the elderly is to include those expenditures as part of a "citizens' wage." This approach views payment to the elderly as part of delayed wages, rewarding the recipient for previous work. During the post-World War II period, increased health and pension benefits were given to workers as part of wage compensation to promote labor peace and productivity. The broad social benefits of delayed compensation are reconceptualized as burdens on business and society by the politics of austerity. As long as fiscal crisis is the focus of public policy, this dynamic of austerity will continue to define the parameters of the possible.

Deregulation

Deregulation is a hallmark of New Federalism. Minimizing government influence on markets is a key goal of New Federalism since competition and other market forces are seen as maximizing socially valued ends. This approach incorporates the view of people as primarily economic beings. In health care, this approach assumes that health can be treated as a commodity, with the consumer making fully informed rational decisions about the costs and benefits of treatments to prevent pain, illness, and death. A deregulated health market would have little incentive to address the social and environmental bases of many illnesses.

An important example of the impact of deregulation in health care is the eradication of federal restrictions that precluded the entry of for-profit firms in government-financed programs. We are witnessing a federal health policy shift from a concern with benevolence to a concern with economics. With U.S. personal health care expenditures exceeding $400 billion per year (29 percent spent for the elderly), corporate attraction to for-profit markets in medical care for the elderly is obvious. Four proprietary hospital chains already own or manage 12 percent of U.S. hospitals, and some experts predict that in a competitive environment ten giant national firms will capture 50 percent of the medical market to the next ten years.

Deregulation is also giving increased discretion to states in federal-state programs. In 1981, for example, federal funds given to the states for social services (Title 20) were reorganized into a block grant, eliminating most targeting and reporting requirements. Federal regulations have also been relaxed in state-run programs that affect the elderly, such as Medicaid and other health programs.

Deregulation is supposed to foster efficiency in the marketing of services, and give states discretion to shape programs to local needs. The increasing concentration of power in the medical care industry, however, may simply shift the power from the government to corporate board-rooms. While some states have a history of providing adequate benefits to their citizens, states' commitments to and abilities to fund health and welfare programs vary widely and are increasingly disparate.

The structure of the health care system, the ideology of New Federalism, the fiscal crisis of the state, and deregulation are all influences on health policy that have developed or been shaped during the Reagan years. In the years ahead we suggest that these forces will result in future changes in the medical system and health policy, including medicalization, the commodification of health, and the continued growth of the medical-industrial complex.

Medicalization

Medicalization involves the expansion of medical power over social problems. The cost-containment strategies under New Federalism have created conditions that further the medicalization of health services for the elderly. As noted earlier, the major health problem of the elderly is chronic illness that creates needs for supportive care and social services. Families currently provide the majority of the assistance needed by the chronically ill, resorting to institutions only when they are unable to provide the needed care at home. For those without families, services similar to nonmedical family care are necessary to maintain the elderly in the community.

In contrast, cost containment has focused on limiting the use of costly medical services and reducing services for the least disabled. One of the most significant cost-containment actions has been changing Medicare hospital reimbursement to payment of fixed rates based on diagnosis. By fixing reimbursements by diagnosis, hospitals now have an incentive to discharge elderly patients as early as possible, resulting in a decrease in the average length of a hospital stay for the elderly by two days. The release of sicker people into the community has increased the demand for higher technology and skilled services in the community. This increased demand is accompanied by a narrow interpretation of Medicare's home health benefit in an attempt to keep those costs under control. The result is that the skilled nursing paid for by Medicare is being directed towards only the sickest in the community.

The reductions in federal funding for social services (down 42 percent between 1982 and 1988) have forced agencies to reorient their services to be able to obtain reimbursement from other sources, such as Medicare and Medicaid. By shifting their services from social programs to medical support, the agencies reduce their commitment to a "continuum of care" that can offer services at the least restrictive (and least medical) level needed.

Commodification

The biomedical model defines the needs of the aged around a medical-services strategy: as individual medical problems rather than as a result of societal treatment of the elderly, inadequate income, or other social problems. Similarly, the government's response to the needs of the elderly as primarily medical rather than social (e.g., housing, social services, and family care allowances) reinforces the mistaken view that rising health care costs are attributable to the elderly. Contemporary health policies attempt to "solve" the health care cost crisis by addressing only symptoms through medically based management strategies.

There does not appear to be any movement away from the trend of treating the problems of the elderly as primarily medical in nature. Because of the politics of austerity, the expansion of nonmedical community services can only be legitimated if it costs no more than the current medically oriented system. A recent review of demonstration projects that provide community care concludes that programs designed to reduce nursing home use fail to save government money. Noninstitutional care does improve the quality of life of the recipients, but advocating community care based on reducing costs does not appear viable. As long as fiscal crisis defines policy options, it will be difficult to include quality of life as a cost or benefit. Thus, the fiscal crisis, New Federalism, deregulation, and the health care system each support the continuation of health policy that emphasizes an acute medical model in its treatment of the chronic illness and support needs of the elderly.

Rather than treating the health of the aged as a public good that is provided and enjoyed collectively, health is increasingly marketed like other goods and services. Providers of health care to the aged are being forced to abandon charitable goals in the face of the economic "realities" of the market.

Shifting health care into a competitive market is a central aspect of New Federalism. The federal government now allows states to award contracts based on competitive bids to providers of medical care for the poor, with California and Arizona taking the lead in implementing this approach. Other states are using competitive bidding to select providers of community care services for the elderly and social services under Title 20. Entry into the market is typically justified as a cost-containment measure, and is made possible by loosening public program regulations.

As health is treated more as a commodity, health providers come to operate increasingly as do other businesses. We shift from "outreach" programs designed to bring needed services to the community, to "marketing" strategies designed to attract paying customers. This is apparent even in the nonprofit sector, as strategic planning and other business practices become necessary for the economic survival of health care providers. Concern has been raised about what will happen to those unable to pay for their care, an important issue since only one-third of noninstitutionalized poor elderly are covered by Medicaid.

As a commodity, health care relies on the market where access and distribution are based on the ability to pay. As commodification increases, hospitals are shifting their goals from providing services for those in need to offering services to customers. Rather than satisfying a need, medical providers are increasingly in the position of trying to attract profitable patients while avoiding others who may be needy. The structure of medicine as a commodity puts physicians in a particular dilemma since they must balance their role as patient advocates with their role as fiscal agents of hospitals and other health care organizations. As social good (health) becomes a commodity that is valued for its ability to create profit, many of the conditions that maximized the well-being of the elderly are weakened. The growing reliance on the market has intensified a perennial and profound health care question: should health care be provided as a "market good" that is purchased as a commodity by those who can afford to pay, or should it be provided as a "merit good" that is available as a right, regardless of ability to pay? The ideology of New Federalism, politics of austerity. and deregulation are all fostering a situation where health care is increasingly treated as a commodity.

Medical-Industrial Complex

The medical-industrial complex consists of the growing concentration of private for-profit hospitals, nursing homes, and other medical care organizations, along with businesses related to medical goods and services. By 1980 the growth of the medical-industrial complex had become a significant enough force in American medicine to cause Arnold S. Relman, the editor of the *New England Journal of Medicine,* to warn of its impact on the shape of American medicine. In his Pulitzer Prize-winning book, *The Social Transformation of American Medicine,* Paul Starr notes that medicine is losing its basis in voluntarism and local control as a result of the growth of the complex. Not only are an increasing number of hospital beds and other medical services becoming profit-oriented, but even nonprofit hospitals are often establishing for-profit subsidiaries to help generate revenues. Both proprietary and nonprofit hospitals are also integrating both horizontally, into multihospital chains across the country, and vertically, establishing a host of lab, supply, home health, and other services so the patient's medical dollars stay entirely within one company.

The medical-industrial complex has been able to grow because medical care programs for the elderly and poor have bought into the existing medical system rather than establishing a national health service. Since Medicare and Medicaid were designed to provide equal access to "mainstream medicine," government clinics were established only in areas that were unattractive to private providers (via community health centers, Indian Health Service, etc.). While the government philosophy of Johnson's Great Society was expansionist, new programs worked to help the elderly participate in the medical market rather than to change or eliminate the market to meet the needs of the elderly. Publicly funded medical assistance thus greatly enlarged the market for medical providers. The increased number of paying customers for services, and guaranteed profits in some sectors, fueled the expansion and consolidation of medical services.

The medical-industrial complex is best organized to survive and even thrive during a period of austerity. Proprietary facilities are organized around costs, while public and religious facilities are traditionally organized to provide care to needy populations. Profit-oriented providers are therefore more able to respond quickly to cost-cutting policies, as well as to expand into the most lucrative new areas.

New Federalism's emphasis on the market gives the medical-industrial complex an advantage since proprietary hospital chains are the best-positioned to take advantage of a market-oriented system. Hospital chains are moving to "multi-clustering" where a hospital serves as the core of a regional health care network owned by one corporation. These networks can include skilled nursing facilities, home health agencies, durable-medical-equipment centers, and psychiatric, substance-abuse, and rehabilitation units. One large chain, National Medical Enterprises (NME) is already establishing such "multis" in Tampa-St. Petersburg, Miami, St. Louis, New Orleans, Dallas, San Diego. and Long Beach. American Medical International, Inc. (AMI) and Hospital Corporation of America (HCA) have targeted fifteen other cities for their multis. Private nonprofits are also moving in this direction, but they have neither the capital nor the institutional size to create comparable networks nationwide.

With the aging population and a concern with costs, there is an increasing move towards home care services. There are strong incentives for profit-making companies to expand in this area. In 1985, nine profit-making companies, including giants like Upjohn Health Care Services, operated over a thousand full-service home health care offices across the country. Some of these companies, like American Hospital Supply, have integrated their services vertically so that they not only manufacture supplies for hospitals but also deliver those same supplies in individual's homes.

The linkage that will give proprietaries the largest advantage is their merging with or starting insurance divisions. AMI already has its own group health plan, AMICARE, that offers integrated services at its own facilities, and NME is preparing to enter the insurance arena. With insurance companies already among the largest sources of capital in the United States, proprietary chains will be able to further strengthen their market position by accessing the capital made available through their insurance subsidiaries. In contrast, nonprofits face possibly worsening problems in obtaining capital for maintaining their facilities and modernizing care. In addition, Humana and other chains are promoting "brand name medicine" by putting their corporate names on all of the facilities they own. To the extent that health care is deregulated and commodified, providers will do the best by marketing brand name medicine and insurance rather than by emphasizing intangibles like public service.

One of the hazards of a large medical-industrial complex is that the power concentrated within such an industry can shape the direction of health policy to the benefit of the industry, which does not necessarily coincide with the needs of the elderly. A recent example of this is the attempt by the drug industry to defeat the inclusion of drug coverage in the Medicare expansion to cover catastrophic illnesses. Since Medicare has not covered outpatient drug costs, they have been a major burden on the resources of the elderly. Drug companies worried that the inclusion of drugs as a Medicare benefit would lead to a limiting of the costs of drugs, pinching profits.

It should be noted that the growth of the medical-industrial complex is not unique. During the Reagan years, a deregulatory approach to mergers facilitated increased concentration of ownership in a variety of sectors, from transportation to industrials. It is important to keep in mind that many of the structural conditions discussed here extend beyond medicine to affect other sectors of the economy as well.

Hospital Reimbursement for the Elderly

Federal changes in hospital reimbursement for the elderly under Medicare demonstrates how New Federalism, fiscal crisis. and deregulation result in increased medicalization and commodification. and the growth of the medical-industrial complex. When Medicare began in 1966 it paid hospitals retrospectively, i.e., hospitals were paid after providing care for all "reasonable" expenses incurred in treating a patient (including construction costs and profits). In 1983 the federal government began to set limits on the amount Medicare would pay per hospital admission for illness groupings, called diagnosis related groups (DRGs). Establishing payment rates per diagnosis before services are provided creates significant incentives for hospitals to reduce inpatient days by discharging patients "sicker and quicker." Introduced as an austerity measure to reduce federal Medicare costs, DRGs have indirectly raised new discussion about quality of care and access to medical care, both of which were major issues during the 1960s.

The shifting concept of federalism is reflected in the early discharge of ill Medicare patients, shifting care into the community where Medicare pays a smaller proportion of the costs and state and local governments and individuals pay a larger share. Increasing copayments and deductibles for individuals have accompanied DRG-based reimbursement. Out-of-pocket health care costs for the elderly averaged 15 percent of their median income in 1984, while elderly blacks paid 23 percent of their income for health care expenditures in 1981. States and localities also shoulder increased responsibility for expenses not covered by Medicare incurred by the elderly poor.

Although the DRGs regulate payment by diagnosis, decisions about how to cut costs are left entirely to providers, reflecting their deregulatory aspect. Tax laws and deregulation have also encouraged the increased entry of for-profit corporations into medical markets (including both hospital and home health care).

The medical-industrial complex is uniquely positioned to take advantage of DRG-based reimbursements. Proprietary hospital chains, linked to supply companies and post-hospital care services, benefit from economies of scale, mass marketing, and the ability to shift costs. Proprietary chains have pioneered new services to maximize profits such as freestanding emergency rooms, sports-medicine clinics, and drug/alcohol-abuse programs which are well reimbursed or which draw the middle class who can pay the fees. Hospitals have reacted swiftly to the new system, *increasing* their profits after the introduction of DRG-based payment. Investor-owned hospitals made the highest returns on their investments. At the same time, some public hospitals are being closed or bought by investors.

By focusing on the issue of hospital costs, the major component of Medicare expenditures, DRGs perpetuate Medicare's bias towards medically oriented institutional care of the acutely ill. Federal interest in developing an integrated long-term care system that adequately addresses the chronic-illness problems of the elderly remains low since ensuring a continuum of care is not likely to reduce costs or federal responsibilities, nor will it result from deregulation.

The Future of Austerity and Cost Containment

A recent survey of the nation's health system leaders found that those most influential in health care and health policy are divided as to whether cost containment or quality of care will be the most important issue at the turn of the century. These leaders primarily wanted to improve service delivery and financing within the current health system. One in five, however, felt more fundamental changes are needed, including the creation of a national health service or an insurance plan involving federal resource allocation.

Continuing efforts to balance the federal budget indicate that cost containment will remain the central feature of health policy in the near future. Continuing austerity at the federal level was institutionalized by the Gramm-Rudman-Hollings Balanced Budget Act passed in 1985 and revised in 1987. This act required that the federal budget be balanced by decreasing the deficit each year. If Congress does not make budget changes that reduce the deficit by a predetermined amount, automatic expenditure cuts occur. In contrast to tax surcharges that were used in the 1960s to compensate for a growing deficit, this bill embodies an austerity approach to the budget by addressing only spending. The automatic cuts are across-the-board, with the dollar reduction split between military and nonmilitary spending. Program changes are not mandated, only spending levels. This budget-led planning typifies the politics of austerity that is driving health policy.

There are a set of "protected" programs exempt from the cuts, including basic entitlement programs. Inflation and/or increased needs would still create de facto cuts in these programs. Medicare and other health programs were semiprotected by a ceiling on the amount they could be cat automatically. In 1987, Congress avoided the automatic cuts by passing spending and revenue bills that lowered the deficit. The package included increased premiums and deductibles for Medicare recipients, further increasing the out-of-pocket medical expenses of the elderly without modifying the system that generates rising medical costs.

The continued viability of a budget centered around the issue of the deficit ensures that federalism, austerity, and deregulation will remain at the forefront of the policy agenda. Policy concern over medicalization, commodification, and the growth of the medical-industrial complex must wait until the focus of policy concerns returns to the health care system and the health of the elderly and others.

Just as the focus of health policy shifted from access in the 1960s to cost containment in the 1970s, the economics of austerity is leading health and aging policy into retrenchment for the 1980s and 1990s. Retrenchment fits into the ideology of New Federalism, where the federal government is considered primarily responsible only for the national defense. Forcing cutbacks in social programs to help balance the budget would further move the burden of aiding the elderly and disadvantaged citizens to states and localities. The nonprofit health sector will also continue to face increased demand. While about 35 percent of free health care is provided in public institutions, almost all of the balance is provided in nonprofit institutions.

Program changes can only be justified if they save money under the politics of austerity. Unmet needs or inequitable distribution, key arguments for program changes before New Federalism, will continue to be insufficient rationales. Within the last ten years attention has shifted from a proactive discussion of the government's role in ensuring the nation's health via national health insurance to a reactive debate about whether the government should stop regulating health care and let the market control decisions. This debate directs attention away from an adequate assessment of the needs of the elderly and others.

The next significant step likely to be taken in providing health care for the elderly within the framework of New Federalism's limits, the politics of austerity, and deregulation is the further contracting out of services and programs that the government currently provides. Medicare is a likely candidate for contracting out since private companies already play a significant role in administering the program by acting as fiscal intermediaries. Demonstration projects can be implemented under current law to give contracts to insurers like Blue Cross making them responsible for all Medicare recipients in defined geographic areas. These contracts could either be competitively bid (as California did with MediCal—i.e., Medicaid—hospital contracts) or they could be offered at a fixed sum (as current Medicare expenditures are). While the private insurer would have to offer recipients the option of keeping the same Medicare benefits. the private insurer could also offer cost-saving options. Options might include offering recipients reduced copayments if they agreed to go only to specified providers. Contracting out gives private insurers the responsibility of designing options, assuming some underwriting risks, and negotiating with and regulating medical providers. This can be seen as a step towards deregulation since the insurers would be given discretion over program options. The prospect of keeping some or all of any savings (profits) would provide an incentive for the insurers to focus their efforts on costs. A smaller-scale effort in this direction is occurring with the federal interest in increasing the use of health maintenance organizations (HMOs) and other prepaid group practice.

One of the consequences of contracting out is that it removes the program from the political process. This can be seen either as a benefit because it weakens the hands of special interests, or as a disadvantage because it makes the program less sensitive to those affected by it. In the case of a contracted out Medicare, politicians could depoliticize increases in deductibles and copayments by blaming them on insurers' decisions, while the insurers could blame increasing costs on their contracts. The end result would be to defuse the ability of the elderly and other advocates to shape the costs and benefits of Medicare.

Deregulation assumes that the marketplace is the most efficient and effective distributor in society. This implies, a priori, that there is no need to discuss what policies could be enacted to foster the health of the elderly, nor is there a need to carefully evaluate the consequences of deregulation. Thus, to the degree that deregulation is embodied in public policy, it obviates the need for program data or debate about public policy for the elderly.

Another challenge will come from the special health needs of elderly women and minorities in the next century, many of whom will be among those least able to pay for it. The feminization of poverty, coupled with the longer life spans of women, results in older women comprising a higher share of those needing health care while having fewer resources. Similarly, blacks, Hispanics, and other disadvantaged minorities have poorer health, more chronic illnesses, and lower incomes than whites, as well as inferior access to health care. The proportion of minority communities that are elderly, historically small in number, is increasing faster than the proportion of whites who are elderly. Minority elderly will need expanded, culturally relevant, low-cost health care.

If the nation continues to be influenced by New Federalism, austerity, and deregulation, health policies will continue to contribute to the medicalization, commodification, and corporatization of health care. Who will pay for the costs of these "unprofitable" patients is likely to be a growing question. Relegating health care distribution to the market assumes that consumers will be sufficiently informed to make the best choices. Fostering public knowledge of costs, quality, and optimal treatments is problematic.

Unless precautions are instituted, severe fragmentation of health care will occur as companies are drawn to the most profitable sectors of care and unbundled services for the elderly, neglecting unprofitable treatments and populations. This growing fragmentation will decrease the possibility for policies that rationalize the system along criteria of need. Fragmentation of less-powerful interest groups is possible as they are pitted against each other for shrinking government resources. Finally, with federal reimbursements to the elderly made primarily in medical services and with the reduced social service expenditures, broadly conceived "health" care will be a low priority.

Scenarios for Change

The two competing approaches to health policy challenges for the elderly have been based on models of market competition and government regulation. While New Federalism emphasizes market-oriented policies, a return to more regulatory approaches would not necessarily change the trends of the Reagan years. The growth of the medical-industrial complex, for example, may have given it sufficiently concentrated power that it could effectively control local attempts at health planning and regulation. Rather than reforming the present system at the margins through regulation or competition, a substantial restructuring of the health system is needed to best confront the basic problems that affect the health of the elderly.

Because of the power of the medical profession and the medical-industrial complex, restructuring health care for the elderly will require forming coalitions that transcend age and unite groups with common interests (e.g., the elderly and the disabled). These groups could advocate redefining health care away from a strict medical model toward the organization, financing, and delivery of health care along a continuum. This continuum would range from respite care for relieving families who already provide most of the nation's caretaking, to adequate incomes, to acute medical services. In place of austerity and New Federalism, health policy will have to treat health care as part of the Constitution's federal mandate to "promote the general welfare" rather than as a private commodity.

It should be noted that children and the poor do not compete with the elderly in the challenges of health policy, but share these concerns. The medicalization of health care deflects concern with health issues of inner city children such as lead poisoning, nutrition, and mother-and-child health promotion. The commodification of health threatens to widen the gap between the care available to those who can pay and those who cannot, regardless of age. Comparisons between the economic status of the elderly and children are typically made to assert that the elderly have too much, implying that poverty among the elderly should be as shamefully common as it is among children. On the other hand, since the government has been successful in reducing poverty among the elderly, it could be argued that the government should now do the same for children, whether through guaranteed jobs for parents, increased minimum wages, or other income-enhancement policies. If adequate and appropriate health care and an adequate income become federal policy priorities, citizens of all ages would benefit.

In sum, the Reagan years have redirected the course of health policy for the elderly. This change in course has not been the sharp turn hoped for by advocates of the Reagan agenda, but the changes have set up limits to the directions that health policy can take in the coming years. As currently structured, health care for the aged will become increasingly medicalized, commodified, and provided by corporations. Coalition building is needed between the elderly and others concerned with the direction that health policy is taking us if the medical care system is to be reoriented by public policy.

Health policy debate and action for the elderly in the future needs to be indivisible from struggles to:

- Redress restrictions to access to health care that have grown markedly in the 1980s as a result of funding cuts and an increased uninsured and underinsured population. The uninsured population of 30–35 million includes 3 million persons aged fifty-five to sixty-four and almost 400,000 persons over sixty-five. Rising out-of-pocket costs to the elderly will further contribute to access problems as health care increasingly moves out of the hospital, since 60 percent of the elderly's physician charges, for example, are paid out-of-pocket. These statistics challenge the concept that the elderly can bear increased cost shifting and continue to have any reasonable access.

- Develop workable alternatives in providing long-term care services and in preventing the need for institutionalization. The challenge is to strengthen ambulatory care, the continuum of community-based services (e.g., adult day care, congregate meals) and in-home services, and to find mechanisms to bolster the role (acknowledging the limits and personal costs) of family caretaking and other vital sources of personal and social support.
- Refocus attempts at health-care cost containment from the ill to the structure of the medical care system itself. It will be difficult and expensive to target appropriate health services to those most in need as long as health care is increasingly commodified and medicalized. The government needs to reshape the medical care system rather than simply buying into the medical-industrial complex.

Given the scope and costs involved, long-term care and acute care can no longer continue to be financed and developed separately. Piecemeal development of policies based on either market reforms or regulatory cost-containment strategies that leave the basic health care financing system and medical system intact are inadequate. Developing a system that provides universal, quality care at an affordable cost will require concerted federal leadership and a federal role.

The Piper's Tune

Caroline Poplin

Since the defeat of President Bill Clinton's health care reform package last fall, many have breathed a sigh of relief that we dodged a bullet. As Mark Twain once said about his death, however, the demise of health care reform has been greatly exaggerated. Profound reform, maybe even revolutionary change, touching every aspect of health care in this country—who performs it, what is done, how it is financed—continues to sweep the United States unabated. The transformation is called "managed care."

Managed care started a decade or more before Harris Wofford's famous 1991 Senate campaign put health care reform at the top of the national agenda, and it was driven not by consumer demand but by cost. As everyone now knows, health care costs have been rising annually at a double-digit rate since the 1970s, far outstripping the rate of inflation. Health care costs now account for 13 percent of the gross domestic product, the highest percentage in the world. Businesses responsible for health insurance for their employees recognized the problem first. Now the president and Congress realize they must control Medicaid and Medicare spending if they hope to get a handle on the budget. The pressure by payers, both public and private, for relief is becoming irresistible. (It is interesting that the one group *not* demanding radical change are consumers, who, unless they buy their own insurance, have been largely shielded from the cost increase. This in turn may be the reason voters did not respond to frantic appeals from the White House for mass support last year.)

Widespread pressure for cost containment is only increased by the observation that despite our ever increasing investment, Americans do not live longer or healthier lives than do citizens of the other industrialized countries, all of whom spend less. Hence, analysts conclude, there must be waste in the system somewhere, and the solution by far the most

317

appealing to virtually all decision makers, public and private, Republican and Democrat, has been managed care.

A Runaway Medical Market

This solution is not surprising if one considers the genesis of the problem. The United States is a bastion of the free enterprise system, and Americans can be relied upon to respond appropriately to market signals. If the market structure is flawed, however, market incentives may produce a perverse result, as in the case of health care. In a perfectly competitive market, there are many sellers trying to sell high and many buyers trying to buy low. The bargaining between each pair produces the most value for the least cost. For many decades, however, the market for health care services in the United States has worked differently: The patient and the doctor select the service, and a third party, the insurance company or, in the case of Medicare and Medicaid, the government, pays the bill. As long as the patient is covered by so-called indemnity insurance, he or she does not care if the price is high—for the patient, the care is essentially free, and he or she will demand the best. Indeed, patients may feel that they *already* paid for their health care when they bought insurance, and they want to get their money's worth. Health care services become an "all you can eat" buffet. In everyday practice, patient behavior is really quite striking: Individuals who spend hours researching or bargaining for a car, careful shoppers who clip coupons and check for sales, virtually never ask of a proffered medical test or treatment, "How much will that be?" (unless, of course, they have no insurance). Indeed, when an important decision must be made, thoughtful patients will consider risks, benefits, likelihood of success, pain, side effects, impact on others—everything *but* the cost. Patients debilitated after a serious illness or major surgery want to spend a few more days in the hospital (at $700 a day) to rest and regain their strength. Some people request expensive treatments for bothersome conditions they might otherwise tolerate. Families faced with a terminal condition in an aged loved one demand that "everything" be done (and in many situations, the law will back them up). This is, to repeat, perfectly rational economic behavior.

On the supply side, resources—people, capital, expertise—are poured into health care in response to the seemingly endless stream of money, to the point where in many areas, there is now excess: too many doctors, too much equipment, too many beds.

The indemnity insurance system did not simply tend to increase the amount this country spent on health care. It also profoundly affected the character of American medicine. Since cost was rarely an issue, hospitals, manufacturers, and doctors engaged in fierce competition using nonprice inducements: They developed ever more precise imaging techniques; more potent, less invasive tests; more attractive, convenient facilities; and faster service. The indemnity system has surely helped make U.S. medicine the envy of the world—at a price. (It may be significant that one of the few sectors in health care that developed goods whose only benefit was reduced price, *not* quality improvement, was the pharmaceutical industry, which introduced low-cost generic drugs. Medications were among the last benefits to be covered by traditional indemnity insurance, and they still are not covered by Medicare.)

Managed Care Problems

Increasingly, payers in sticker shock are turning to managed care. To harried corporate benefits managers, to insurance companies, to a Democratic president and now increasingly to a Republican Congress, managed care looks like an answer sent directly from heaven.

What is managed care? To understand this concept, some history is helpful. Until the advent of managed care, insurance companies survived and prospered by managing *risk*. In any given year, some 10 percent of the population incurs 80 percent of the medical costs in this country; hence any company thrives to the extent that it can identify and avoid members of this group while insuring the others. This thinking is the origin of insurance physicals, limitations on coverage for preexisting conditions, termination of insurance after illness is diagnosed, and preferential treatment for large employers likely to have many more healthy than sick workers at any particular time.

With continuing expensive improvements in U.S. medical care, however, for many companies risk management is no longer enough to ensure survival; hence some insurance companies are now trying to reduce medical costs directly, that is, "managing care." This is occurring in stages, as insurance companies and health care providers gain experience and sophistication about the market for health care services. First, a company may ask providers—doctors, hospitals, pharmacists—for a steep discount from their usual charges in exchange for a large volume of patients (thus generating a list of "preferred providers"). The company may review the service provided to see if it was necessary ("utilization review") or require a patient to obtain permission for hospitalization or an elective procedure in advance ("preclearance"). These last two techniques have met a storm of resistance from doctors and patients, who believe that they put critical decisions about medical care in the hands of faceless clerks operating under secret protocols. A third approach, even more offensive to doctors, is what is called "economic profiling": Insurance companies review claims generated from services ordered by doctors and may "counsel," or even drop from their provider list, doctors who order "too much." (The extent to which this goes on is hotly disputed by companies and doctors.) In most mature markets, however, companies are avoiding these firefights by going on to the ultimate form of managed care, "capitation."

Under capitation, the managed care company pays a doctor a fixed sum per patient per month, perhaps $11–$14, regardless of the level of service the patient requires. The doctor gets the same payment whether the patient comes every day or not at all, and so the doctor now assumes the risk. If the patient stays well, the doctor does well; if the patient needs or demands a lot of the doctor's attention, the doctor loses and will need the premiums of other, healthy, patients to cover expenses. Doctors may combine with specialists, laboratories, and hospitals to assume the risk for these services as well, so one monthly payment per patient covers them all. In theory, then, the doctor no longer has any incentive to order "extra" tests or treatment, or spend "extra" time with the patient, since the costs will come out of the doctor's own pocket. The insurance company no longer appears to be interfering with medical decisions; rather, the doctor, or the integrated service provider, becomes the insurer, or, to look at it another way, the profit in "retail medicine" comes not from the charge for each service but from the "insurance" part of the business, the excess of premiums paid over costs of services rendered. Since this goes to whoever owns the merged enterprise, the competition for ultimate control between doctors, who provide the expertise, and investors, who provide the capital, is fierce.

Some insurers do allow a patient to see a doctor other than one on the approved list, for an extra out-of-pocket charge. It is widely acknowledged, however, that this so-called point of service option is not profitable and is intended chiefly to help consumers make the transition into fully managed care.

It is no accident that managed care has been enthusiastically embraced, first by employers for their workers, then by economists, and now by policy makers for society as a whole. The system precisely reverses the providers' incentives, which were thought to be driving health care to ruin. (It also changes incentives for research, from better care at higher cost to the same care at lower cost.) Finally, it focuses consumers' attention, to the extent they pay themselves, on the cost of the health care plan and the up-front savings usually available over traditional indemnity insurance. The medical service component, by contrast, is nearly impossible for consumers to evaluate, particularly if they don't know what part of it, if any, they will need. In these circumstances, if he is healthy a consumer is likely to go for the lowest price. (Economic theory predicts this behavior: The more fungible, or interchangeable, a good, the stronger will be the price competition among suppliers.) If the market for health insurance is competitive, this characteristic of managed care should drive down the price and hence the total amount spent on health care. And in fact, in some mature California markets, this is beginning to happen.

Moreover, consumers for the most part seem comfortable with managed care. This may be because the benefits of managed care (the savings) are evident up front, while the possible narrowing of benefits (difficulty in seeing a specialist, for instance) may only become apparent later, if ever. Remember, most consumers will stay healthy.

However, managed care proponents deny they are saving money by reducing quality. On the contrary, they claim they are *improving* people's health as well as cutting costs by emphasizing prevention and the elimination of excessive and harmful practices.

Managed Care Solutions

So managed care has become irresistible; it is sweeping the country. By 1994, 65 percent of workers in medium and large companies were covered by managed care plans. A managed care option is now available—and being strenuously promoted—for Medicare beneficiaries in some cities, and politicians from Bill Clinton to Newt Gingrich are converging on managed care as the only way to save Medicare from bankruptcy in the year 2002.

There is no doubt, furthermore, that for many, managed care is delivering on its promise. Insurance premiums *are* coming down a notch in

California and in some federal government plans. The most successful plans *have* reduced health care costs, as they said they would, by reducing reimbursements to providers, needless duplication of services, and hospital stays. They *have* driven down the prices of many medications for their subscribers, and they have improved health. They *have* increased the use of proven cost-effective preventive measures like immunizations and mammograms. They *have* improved follow-up in some chronic diseases.

That is not, however, the end of the story. We all know, as Milton Friedman says, that there is no free lunch. While the advocates of managed care have been voluble about its very real benefits, they are more discreet about the extent to which this financial reorganization is profoundly changing the face of U.S. medicine. Managed care will affect who is providing medical services and in what setting. More important, managed care will alter what care is ultimately provided, who makes that decision, and how. To look at it another way, there are, at bottom, only so many ways to contain health care costs. One can drive down excess prices to providers; one can redesign services so they are provided more efficiently (lower cost), more effectively (better quality), or both; or one can reduce service. Managed care proudly champions the first two methods. It may also incorporate the third. The industry and academics are aware of these changes. The great Clinton health care debate demonstrated that consumers, by and large, are not. Finally, we need to remember that managed care is not a total solution. There are some problems bedeviling the current system that managed care does not address, like cost shifting, and others, like adverse selection, that it may even exacerbate.

Let us examine these issues in more detail.

Industrialization of American Medicine

In some ways, retail medicine—medicine at the level of a doctor and his patient—is the last cottage industry in America. Until now, most doctors have practiced alone or in groups of two and three, with a nurse or two and a bookkeeper. This has been true not just for primary care providers but for many specialists and surgeons. The system has been almost totally decentralized: Doctors see themselves as the last of the rugged individualists, the prototypical small business owners, something like the craftsmen of the eighteenth century, meticulously tailoring a custom product for each client, doing most of the work themselves. In general, Americans have been pleased with this system, which maximizes provider autonomy, individual attention, and patient control at a time when control is particularly important, that is, when a patient's control over other aspects of his life may be seriously jeopardized.

Nevertheless, a Norman Rockwell doctor can no more survive the economics of managed care than a cabinetmaker could survive the advent of the furniture factory. Although medicine has in some cases arrived at them by a different route, industrial techniques that lowered cost and increased production for manufacturing a century ago are generating the same benefits now for medicine. For example, under managed care it is critically important to a doctor to have a large volume of patients, especially healthy patients. This is not so much because only a small profit is realized on each one but because it reduces the doctor's risk. If one patient "crashes," a doctor with a small practice can be ruined if he or she does not carry (or could not afford) adequate reinsurance, even if the care rendered is impeccable. The only practical way for doctors to avoid this problem is to join together in large groups and sign up the maximum number of patients.

Grouping together provides other benefits for doctors: It gives them greater leverage in bargaining with insurance companies, it allows them to share overhead, and it often improves their overnight call schedules. For patients, however, it may mean more difficulty in getting to see "their own" doctor and a shorter appointment when they get there, typically ten to fifteen minutes (we will return to this). "Continuity of care" may mean being entered in a good computerized tracking system rather than being followed by the same physician over many years.

The spread of managed care has also encouraged vertical integration in medicine, one of the few features of the new system that can be regarded as an unequivocal improvement. We have seen that the provider does best when the patient stays well: It is the provider who pays if a costly hospitalization is necessary to bring the patient back to baseline; hence it now pays for a provider to integrate low-cost techniques, not traditionally within the purview of medicine, into his services. Aides, for example, might be dispatched to a frail customer's home to eliminate safety hazards that could cause a fall and fracture or to help with a complicated medication regimen necessary to keep a patient out of a congestive heart failure or diabetic coma that would require hospitalization. Moreover, if providers control all these so-called ancillary services, they can eliminate duplication, reduce cost, and enhance coordination and thus keep most or all of the insurance premium, the source of the profits under managed care.

Integration may also be proceeding at the level of the physician. Until the 1960s, medicine in this country was largely provided by generalists, who referred unusual or particularly difficult problems to specialists or subspecialists. The complex patient was then worked up completely and often followed independently by two or more separate physicians, an expensive, inefficient, and occasionally dangerous arrangement. The explosion of medical knowledge since then, however, has put increasing pressure on generalists, even those with two or three years of post-internship training. No one can keep up with developments in all the subspecialties of adult medicine (let alone surgery, pediatrics, and so forth), and yet information in these areas often bears on management of common but serious illnesses like heart disease. At the same time, managed care is making a determined effort to reduce the use of expensive specialists. What to do? The best companies are using their specialists not just to see individual patients but to advise the generalists on the newest management techniques in the specialists' area for the generalists' patients and to evaluate current clinic approaches. This, of course, is how lawyers, engineers, and other professionals have been functioning for decades.

Managed care is pushing medicine toward a more conventional industrial organization in other ways that may not be so benign. Until the Japanese revolutionized production management, most manufacturers prospered in this country by breaking down production into standardized tasks requiring little judgment, tasks that could be performed quickly and reliably by workers with relatively low skills. This model could often produce more products, of predictable quality and at lower cost, than could be achieved by the efforts of independent craftsmen. It also reorganized the work place into three classes of people: owners, managers, and laborers. Some managed care companies are moving in this direction and reaping some of the economic benefits. The physicians who have become workers instead of owners are distressed, and the new structure raises questions about responsibility for malpractice. But let us focus for a moment on the drive to standardize medical practice.

Standardization

Standardization is a complex issue in medicine. It was the observation of tremendous variability in the treatment of a given condition, from one U.S. city to another, without any obvious corresponding differences in outcomes, that first suggested to analysts that there was "waste" in U.S. medicine. For example, not too long ago a prominent researcher found that the hysterectomy rate in one city in Rhode Island was three times the rate in a comparable city in Vermont. Total knee replacement was almost twice as likely in Boston as in New Haven, without any obvious differences in underlying patient population. This suggested to many people, economists in particular, that the doctors in Rhode Island were doing "too many" hysterectomies, and doctors in Boston "too many" knee replacements, both profitable procedures.

To eliminate these "excesses" and the associated expense, managed care companies are now encouraging their physicians to standardize their approaches to particular illnesses, limiting tests and treatments to those known to be effective. This "encouragement" takes many forms, from developing practice guidelines for particular illnesses to tracking the prescribing practices of individual physicians, comparing them to others, and discouraging doctors from ordering "too much" or referring or hospitalizing patients "too often." Or the company may simply deduct an "appropriate" amount from the doctors' compensation. The managed care industry argues that it thereby improves the quality of its product, protecting patients from "needless" tests or treatments that might be harmful. And certainly, closer supervision is more likely to catch errors and may be long overdue in a profession not known for vigorous self-regulation.

However, how certain are we of what constitutes the best medical care? How much is "too much"—and how little is "too little"? Just proving that a new drug or treatment is more effective than the old treatment—or than doing nothing—can cost millions and take many years, as any pharmaceutical manufacturer knows. And the results of even the most massive clinical trials are quite limited, often (until recently) restricted to one sex and to patients without other problems that could confound the test results. Because a treatment was shown to work in otherwise healthy young males, does that mean it will necessarily help an elderly lady who also as diabetes and a touch of heart disease? And, of course, under even the best of circumstances, virtually nothing in medicine works all the time: For some conditions, including some very serious ones, a 50 percent success rate is a qualified miracle.

Then there is the question of defining "success." A common illness like coronary artery disease ("heart disease") is the number one killer in this country, and it can also cause debilitating pain, called angina. In the last two decades U.S. medicine has developed and refined a highly effective treatment for heart disease, bypass surgery. Managed care has shown that efficient medical centers can perform this high-quality procedure at lower cost, but this treatment is still not cheap: It runs from approximately $20,000 to $40,000. In certain cardiac patients, it prolongs life. In others, it relieves symptoms but has no effect on mortality. In a third group, it has no advantage over (much less expensive) medication. Whom should we treat? Everyone who can benefit? As it turns out, just to find out into which group a given patient falls costs a pretty penny: The definitive test is an angiogram, and it costs about $10,000. Who should get the test, keeping in mind that heart disease is very common, especially among the elderly? Testing and treating everyone likely to benefit would cost a fortune, probably more than we as a nation are currently spending. Yet we already do roughly two times as many angiograms, and three times as much surgery and angioplasty on heart attack victims (a high-risk group), as do doctors in Canada, with no appreciable improvement in overall mortality.

Hence the variability in the treatment of a given condition from place to place may be due to greedy doctors doing unnecessary procedures, but it may also reflect differences in style—aggressive versus conservative—and considerable uncertainty over what will work and for whom. "Necessity" is in general not immediately obvious: What is "necessary" in any given situation may well depend on who decides and with what goal in mind. Adding "medical"—as in "a medical necessity"—does not change that.

Recall, however, that managed care seeks to reduce costs by reducing "variability," which is thought to reflect "excessive" or "unnecessary" treatment. Moreover, a care manager requires not just effectiveness, difficult as that is to demonstrate, but cost-effectiveness. Clearly, managed care is going to develop, and will be able to justify, test and treatment algorithms with a distinctively conservative bias. The cost will always be clear; the benefit may be less so. If an individual can still work with a touch of angina, does he really need expensive surgery, even though on weekends he has to give up tennis for walking? If he is not going to get surgery, should he have the angiogram?

In the old days, if a patient wanted a full court press when his doctor wanted to wait and see (or vice versa), the solution was easy: Get a new doctor. In fact, that is when choice of physician becomes critical—not when one needs to choose a pediatrician for routine vaccinations but when a loved one is desperately ill and the patient or family is not happy with the doctor's approach, be it too conservative or too aggressive. A good managed care company, of course, will emphasize that it offers a wide choice of physicians. However, recall that its reason for being is to reduce variability—that is, to constrain the doctors' discretion. Hence all the doctors in the plan will be operating by roughly the same set of rules. If a patient wants a different course of action, he or she may need not to change doctors but to change *companies*. Obviously, this will be difficult for a sick patient who has no time to spare and who now has a "pre-existing condition." Finally, recall that a major theme of reform is to encourage price competition between companies by standardizing their offerings. All this should push most patients toward conservative therapy, and the system toward the sought-after cost containment. The patient may not be aware of anything untoward. The insurance company will not say "we don't cover bone marrow transplants for breast cancer"; instead, your doctor will say "I think chemotherapy is the best treatment for you."

Needless to say, this is a radical departure for U.S. medicine, at least from the model publicly propounded by the profession and largely accepted by the public and the courts. Traditionally, our medicine is grounded in the doctor–patient relationship. Together, the doctor and patient decide what the patient shall do, although many doctors emphasize the doctor's knowledge of what is right for the patient while, in modern times, many patients emphasize the patient's right to participate and even to ultimately decide the issues after considering the doctor's advice. Either way, the doctor's only allegiance is supposed to be to the patient. Although managed care may be careful to preserve the appearance of continuing the tradition, however, it adds a third party to the therapeutic partnership: the company itself.

Is the company an 800-pound gorilla? If the patient is dissatisfied with the doctor, the doctor loses one patient. If the managed care company is dissatisfied with the doctor, he or she could lose hundreds of patients or the whole practice overnight. Certainly any conscientious doctor will fight to get the patient something "extra" in a clear case, but, as we see, many cases are likely to be in a gray area where reasonable people might differ. Moreover, the patient is as beholden to the company as the doctor is. If the company tells an employee to see a different, less aggressive, doctor (or if the employer tells him or her to join a less expensive company), the employee must comply or lose insurance coverage.

Adverse Selection and the Consumer

As we noted at the outset, the appeal of managed care is that these cost-cutting mechanisms remain mostly invisible. Traditional structures remain largely in place. The subtlety of the system, however, comes at a price: It is a set-up for litigation. Managed care presents itself to patients as differing from traditional indemnity insurance only in its improved efficiency. So, although the doctor's decision making has been radically altered, the patient's expectations are exactly the same: The patient expects the system to do *everything,* whatever may help, no matter what it costs. Managed care gives no reason to demand less. When there is a bad outcome, and the patient or the family learns that an expensive alternative was rejected without so much as a by-your-leave from them, there may be no twenty-year doctor–patient relationship to hold them back. Indeed, the company's increased involvement in therapeutic decisions will make the company itself, with its deep pockets, that much easier to sue. (Of course, the company's lawyers will contend that medical decisions are made only by the doctor and that the company just does "administration.") Note that the applicable standards of care in these cases are likely to date from the past when cost was an afterthought, if that. This is truly a lawyer's paradise: Tort reform cannot come too quickly to save the hapless doctors.

Despite these quibbles, managed care is reducing some of the excesses of indemnity health insurance. Even its most enthusiastic proponents, however, do not claim that they have the answer for another fundamental problem of health care in this country: the problem of adverse selection. It is adverse selection that is responsible for what *consumers* (as opposed to employers or government) see as the chief problem of health insurance in this country: the inability to get—or keep—health insurance when one really needs it, that is, when one is ill.

Although to a consumer this seems like an anomaly—what use is insurance if it does not cover people when they are sick?—the difficulty follows from an industry that divides people into risk groups or pools and the demographics of illness. As we noted at the outset, some 10 percent of the population is responsible for 80 percent of medical costs. Moreover, many of those who will need care already know who they are—they have already had an illness likely to produce complications or to recur, or they have major risk factors, like a family history of illness. (The insurance companies, of course, know this, too, and try to exclude them.) They will seek a plan with good coverage (because they expect to need it); when they do get sick, they will drive up its costs, and therefore, its premiums. The higher premiums, in turn, will drive away healthy people, who cost the insurance company less and who can therefore obtain insurance for less, and the whole idea behind insurance, of "spreading the cost," will be defeated. Indeed, by facilitating transfer from one plan to another (to encourage competition between plans), most reform scenarios make it easier for healthy people to escape a plan when sick people begin to drive up premiums.

Managed care actually exacerbates this problem in the following way. A characteristic of mature managed care is that it merges the provision of insurance with the provision of health care, that is, in the same decision the consumer chooses health care coverage *and* the doctor, the hospital, and the range and quality of health care services available for the coming year. Hence a consumer who expects serious trouble will buy the plan with the best quality (as well as the most extensive coverage) that he or she can afford. Healthy consumers do not expect to need costly specialists or facilities: They will go, as before (and as intended by employers and policy makers), for the lowest price. Thus, the highest quality plans will attract the sickest people, making them the most expensive, least-desirable for employers and other large payers. If these plans cannot attract and maintain enough premium income to cover their expenses, they will reduce their costs by paying less for services, and when they have exhausted that alternative, they will reduce or ration services.

Unfortunately, that is not the worst of it. While until now, insurance companies survived by screening out the sick, doctors made money by finding and treating them. Managed care, by contrast, "aligns" providers with insurers. Under capitation, the essence of managed care, the doctor, or integrated provider, is paid the same whether the patient is healthy, and never needs care, or is sick. The doctor, however, must now cover the cost of any care in one way or another. Hence, it is now to *the doctor's* advantage to attract as many healthy patients as possible and to discourage or drive away the ill. Therefore, a successful company will structure *care* so as to bring about this result, offering low-cost services of problematic medical value, such as an annual physical, to attract healthy young people (who do not need it) while severely restricting access to specialists important in chronic, expensive diseases. Many managed care companies, such as Kaiser, now limit a doctor's appointment to fifteen minutes or less, which is great for a busy lawyer with the flu or hay fever or a runner with shin splints but frustrating for an older person with high blood pressure, diabetes, a little heart disease, and arthritis, who has some difficulty even getting to the doctor's office. None of the new managed care plans in Boston want to buy the Joslin Clinic, a local center with a national reputation for diabetes management. They all fear the influx of hard-to-control, expensive, diabetics. (High ratings in "satisfaction" surveys, which managed care companies use to impress consumers and employers, may reflect not high quality medicine but large numbers of healthy subscribers who require little except convenience.)

Not only does managed care discourage risk spreading, then, it may be pushing scarce medical resources away from the sick toward the "worried well," where the immediate profit is higher but the ultimate health benefit to society is lower, all the while piously touting "preventive medicine."

Toward A More Impersonal System

So managed care is sweeping through health care like a new information-age Industrial Revolution, gathering political and financial momentum as it goes. However, we see that it is not a panacea. The costs to providers—doctors, hospitals, and pharmaceutical and equipment manufacturers—are obvious to them and in some cases overdue, but there are significant costs even for the putative beneficiaries, society and individual patients. In exchange for more efficiency, patients must accept a more impersonal system, in a field where the personal connection, the "laying on of hands," the doctor–patient relationship, has until now been paramount as a matter of style *and* substance. More important, those who sign a managed care contract make this Faustian bargain: In exchange for choice and savings at the outset, they give up autonomy and control of their destiny at the time when it matters most—when they are gravely ill and the way back is chancy, expensive, and long. The system *intends* that care providers factor cost into diagnostic and treatment decisions, and they may reach a result quite different from the one the patients would have chosen. Indeed, they may never know there was a decision to be made. In any case, this is the private sector, the "market": There is no appeal, except for malpractice after the fact. As for society at large, managed care in its present setting may be diverting scarce resources from the treatable sick to the worried well.

Yet there is no disputing that it *does control costs*, almost by definition; each managed care company can and must tailor the services it provides to the revenue it takes in—by increased efficiency if possible, by internal rationing if necessary.

Do we have any choice? The only obvious alternative to managed care is our old stand-by, fee-for-service medicine. Yet no one so far has designed a fee-for-service system that successfully contains costs. Moreover, in the current competitive private insurance market, fee-for-service may be doomed by the mechanics of adverse selection; ultimately it may be available only to the very healthy and the very rich. Fee-for-service accessible to all may only be possible in a single-payer system. First, a single-payer system eliminates the adverse selection problem. Second, only government may be able to structure fee-for-service so as to get a handle on costs. (The current single-payer systems, Medicare and the Canadian system, have of course conspicuously failed in this regard.)

To be successful, the system would need to incorporate a significant co-pay requirement for all treatment except perhaps basic prevention and comfort measures. The co-pay would have to be enough to force each patient to seriously consider the medical options and compare them to all the other desirable things money can buy. (The co-pay requirement would obviously have to be scaled in some fashion to income, so that the poor could still afford treatment, if they wanted it, and the rich might still stop and think. Clearly the government is in a better position to do this than the private sector.) A requirement like this sounds harsh. However, it is the way we manage all our other affairs in a free-market society. And the benefit is real. Fee-for-service separates decisions about health care from decisions about insurance. A patient can focus directly on individual diagnostic and treatment decisions, rather than being forced to make a one-time all-encompassing decision about both care and coverage. The patient benefits whether the medical option is accepted or declined, so he or she can be discriminating. For example, a person who declines an expensive treatment that has little chance of success or that will leave him unable to function, is rewarded—he or she can send another child to school, take a vacation with the remaining good time, or leave something to charity. If the managed care company makes the same decision for the patient, the money goes to another patient or into its coffers. Conversely, the patient offered little hope who still wants to go for broke can do it. All patients can save money without necessarily sacrificing quality by adding price to their consideration when they comparison shop. Americans are good shoppers. Doctors, hospitals, and other providers will compete for their business as they now compete for Aetna's. Individuals may purchase their services bundled, as in managed care, or they may choose to pay more for care in the traditional setting.

Thus, fee-for-service, supported and contained by single payer, may, as it has in Canada, preserve some degree of decentralization, a place for the neighborhood doctor, small group, or local hospital. More important, it can give individuals real choice all along the line and real authority to make their own decisions, under conditions where they can be relied upon to decide responsibly. In economic terms, it maximizes value to society at minimum cost. Rationing is controlled by patients using the market: They select the tests and treatments that they value most highly rather than authorizing corporations to ration care based on crude cost-effectiveness calculations.

In the final analysis, what the public now considers the most "socialized" system of medicine (although only the financing side is socialized) actually may best preserve the autonomy and choice of the individual. However we do it, though, the recurrent theme of capitalism holds: Who pays the piper ultimately calls the tune.

The All-Frills Yuppie Health Care Boutique

Emily Friedman

The attractive, nicely groomed cowpoke rides resolutely into view on our television screens, traversing beautiful mountain country. He swings off his horse and glares accusingly into the camera. "Some people like to come up here for a couple of weeks to 'get away from it all' and 'get back to nature,'" he says with a sneer. "Well, I live here!" He produces a box of Grape-Nuts from his saddlebag and starts telling us about his with-it, back-to-nature lifestyle and his closeness to the land. While popping bits of cereal into his mouth, he tells us haughtily that Grape-Nuts fits his lifestyle perfectly. He looks down his nose at the presumably quivering television audience and issues a brutal challenge: "You see, it's obvious that Grape-Nuts is right for you. The question is, are you right for Grape-Nuts?"

This is the perfect commercial for an era in which the values associated with young upwardly mobile professionals, or Yuppies, are coming to dominate many consumer markets. Presenting a perversion of core 1960s values that have survived, such as environmental awareness and at least some questioning of the establishment, the commercial is the epitome of the Culture of Inadequacy that has grown up around the Yuppies. It is a culture that says that there is no way a young person today can be attractive enough, accomplished enough, successful enough, rich enough, or possessed of enough resources to really be secure and at the top of the heap. No matter how far you have come, we are told, there is more that you must have and more that you must do, in order to really make it.

This extreme recasting of the American dream is, in many parts of the economy, contributing to the growth (such as it is) of the gross national product. It may actually be doing some good in that if there is money to be made from environmental activism, healthier eating habits, and exercise, little harm will come of it. In health care, however, the Yuppie ethic may have a catastrophic effect on American hospitals and those they serve.

What does the Culture of Inadequacy have to do with health care, which has not traditionally been viewed as a consumer commodity and thus should not be affected by Yuppie consumerism? There is a growing connection. The seemingly unbridled inflation that characterized health care (and especially hospital) costs during the 1970s provoked several governmental attempts to stem the tide, including a stab at health planning in 1976 that today has been abandoned entirely in some states and greatly scaled down in others, and the Joseph Califano-Jimmy Carter cap on hospital expenses that was voted down by Congress. That rejection was based in part on an American Hospital Association campaign, the Voluntary Effort, that promised self-imposed cost restraint by hospitals.

The Voluntary Effort, like most crisis-inspired campaigns, dissipated. Hospitals welcomed the election of Ronald Reagan, who promised an end to regulatory cost containment. He had something else in mind. In 1983, the Reagan administration and Congress implemented, with lightning speed (given the snail's pace at which health care policy is usually made), the diagnosis related group (DRG) method of prospective, payment to hospitals under Medicare. Other federal budget cuts led to a domino effect in the states that in turn reduced the amount of money available for Medicaid and other health programs.

This all began just in time for the recession of 1981–82, during which unemployment contributed to the creation of more medically indigent and Medicaid patients, fewer taxpayers. and growing concern on the part of employers, who found that the negligible amounts of their budgets allocated to employee health benefits were growing faster than their profit margins. Employers' efforts to encourage employees to join health maintenance organizations (HMOs), preferred provider organizations (PPOs), and what Rob Delf of the Multnomah County, Oregon, Medical Society has dubbed OWAs, or Other Weird Arrangements, proliferated. Greater copayments and deductibles for those same employees led to their thinking about health care expenditures more than they had during the glory days of first-dollar coverage of any health care provided by any provider the employee chose.

The effect of all this on patients and hospitals has been significant. First, cost-conscious patients who are paying $100 or $700 or even $500 out of pocket for their care are far more consumer oriented than those who are totally price-insulated. Second, cost-conscious employers, in directing employees to this or that provider, inevitably take away some of the freedom those employees once enjoyed in choosing the location and provider of their care. This is true even if the employer is mandating programs that should be welcomed such as second opinions before elective surgery.

The appearance of a shortage of resources is inevitable under such circumstances; this is the third important effect. Americans equate denial with shortage: this derives from experience with World War II rationing for some and from the old vision of the United States as the land of unlimited plenty for others. The two American beliefs in freedom of choice (in whatever market or setting) and the availability of plenty are not organically connected; but they are connected in the minds of Americans. If we are told we can only use certain hospitals or physicians, or that we must pay a deductible expense, or that another physician must confirm the opinion of the first before a procedure can be performed, we assume that there are not enough resources for us to continue to pursue the unfettered and inexpensive (for us, if not society) freedom of choice we had enjoyed for so long.

Whether this mentality would exist in a population that had never had access to virtually unlimited choice and first-dollar coverage is questionable; the British still view their more limited health care system as a vast improvement over what they used to have. It is too late now for us to find out in America. Whether the resource shortage is real (which is not the case) or perceived (which is the case), when the postwar generation starts seeing what it thinks is a shortage of a resource that it wants, it gets very nervous—far more nervous, probably, than any other generation in the history of the United States.

Easy as it is to take potshots at Yuppies, it is important to understand that there are sound reasons for their nervousness. This generation is the most populous in history; its members have been told over and over again how many of them there are and how much of a population bulge they represent on the demographic scale. Also, they were born to a generation that had endured some of the worst hardships ever visited on Americans. Compared to the horrors that befell most of the population of the Soviet Union before and during World War II, Americans were living a cream-puff life even during the depression: Americans' perception of the period from 1929 to 1946 was that it was about as bad as life could get.

A rural depression was followed by an overall depression that was followed by a war. Resources of all kinds were in short supply for more than a decade. Even when the economy started to recover as a result of wartime activity and New Deal economic policy, the price of that recovery was rationing: bacon, tires, stockings, gasoline—necessities and luxuries alike were parceled out. There was grumbling, but rationing was a simple dividing up of what was available into equal portions, and although people did not like it very much, they accepted it. Unpleasant as it was, rationing was a community burden and a shared experience, and as such it affected most people on pretty much the same level.

Once the war was over and the economy started to improve, that deprived generation started to have babies, and the new parents made a solemn commitment that their children would not go through what they had. "My kid is not going to want for anything!" became the new battle cry, and it looked like an easy promise to keep in the flush 1950s as personal income rose to new highs, the infant interstate highway system began to breed the first suburbs, and the United States established dominance of the world economy.

A disproportionate number of the generation born between 1946 and 1964 were raised in an atmosphere abounding with cars at the age of sixteen, college guaranteed (and paid for without the student having to work), the promise of a professional career for the asking, and a belief that they were entitled to anything they saw or wanted. Rarely has a generation been so betrayed by its parents in terms of unwarranted and unfulfillable expectations. No wonder a futurist recently referred to the children of the late 1940s and 1950s as "the doomed generation." This population went off to college and, coming into contact with various inequities, began to call for the sharing of what seemed an endless cornucopia of resources with the less fortunate. The social movements thus spawned eventually led to enfranchisement in terms of the vote and sponsorship for health care or other benefits for black Americans, the poor, the near-poor, the elderly, and other groups. Later there would be scaled down and less successful efforts to add women and the disabled to that list.

There was even a major movement in the 1970s—the product of an unholy alliance between civil-rights-minded activists and far more cynical government officials—to enfranchise the mentally ill by freeing them from admittedly gruesome institutionalization in mental hospitals to the presumably gentler mercies of community care, which by and large did not then, and does not now, exist. The homeless mentally ill living on our streets, who number in the hundreds of thousands, are among the most visible representations of the naiveté of the 1960s. Advocates and policymakers alike are learning that it is difficult to keep your promises when times, social values, and governmental priorities change—especially when you have made those promises to some of the most politically powerless and socially unpopular groups in the United States.

The mixed fruits of their labor did not affect the Yuppies much one way or another, because they had been enfranchised from birth, and the increasing fiduciary headache their activism produced was, for the most part, unknown to them. What brought them into a head-on collision with the reality of resource constraint was the Organization of Petroleum Exporting Countries and the gas rationing bred by the Arab oil boycott. The generation that was never supposed to even hear the word *rationing* found itself subjected to it.

It is unproductive to point out that the changes in the United States and world economies in the 1970s had to do with a lot more than oil, and that there were many villains, domestic and international, that fueled the crippling inflation of that era. Oil is what got the press attention, and gasoline was what the Yuppies found themselves waiting in line to get. They began to get nervous about the future availability of gasoline, especially with widespread predictions that there would be no more oil at all by 2020 or so—when the majority of the Yuppies would still be alive. In areas such as southern California, where the car passed from being a luxury to a convenience and finally to a necessity decades ago, this was a real threat.

The security of a high-paying professional job proved more elusive than the postwar babies had supposed. In any society, the pay scale is pyramidal in nature: with many low-paying jobs at the bottom, far fewer high-paying jobs at the top. In the United States and most other countries, distribution of the positions at the top is disproportionately (although not totally) determined by education and socioeconomic class. In the United States, race plays a major negative role as well. The pyramid structure must be maintained in order to maintain the society, so although a college degree had been the determinant of higher pay in the past, if millions more young people have college degrees than the market can absorb. the rules change. Now people need a master's degree for a position that once required a baccalaureate: a Ph.D. instead of a master's. As too many postwar academics found out, if there are too many Ph.D.

holders available, even that is no guarantee of a high position in academia or industry. To make matters worse, per capita income began to decline in the 1970s after spectacular increases in the 1950s and 1960s. Today, only 7 percent of those born between 1946 and 1964 earn more than $30,000 a year.

As a result of all this, the 1960s generation, which had once marched in the streets to win a better deal for the vulnerable, began to see itself in direct competition for resources with the people whose cause it had once championed. As has occurred before in the United States, the Yuppies started to reconsider just how deserving the poor and other vulnerable groups, such as the elderly, were. Thus was born the infant science of Yuppie ethics, a much-maligned discipline. Yuppie ethics is, simply put, the study of what happens to a limited resource when a powerful sub-group of the population seeking that resource wants a disproportionate share of it. When the resource is in short supply, be it cars or food or, in this case, health care, that powerful subgroup faces a problem: if it wants more than its share, some other group must receive less than its share. Because that goes against the American grain, the easiest way to justify this reallocation is to convince ourselves that the group from whom we are trying to wrest the resource is undeserving of it.

The First Corollary of Yuppie Ethics is that the level of deservingness of the poor varies in direct proportion to the amount of resources available. The Second Corollary is that if disenfranchising the poor will not free up enough resources to dissipate the fear of shortages, then some other group must also become less deserving.

In trying to define what constitutes "enough" resources in this Yuppie age, we must return to the Grape-Nuts cowpoke and his challenge that the audience prove they are worthy of the breakfast cereal he is hawking. In some cultures, when resources become scarce, quantity supersedes quality as a measure of value. In the Yuppie Culture of Inadequacy, the adequate becomes nothing less than everything. Because the Yuppies were convinced by their parents that they had a right to anything they saw, they are able to glide through the ethical gymnastics required to defend the proposition that the best way to allocate a constrained resource is to give all of it to some people while giving none to others.

The ultimate Yuppie commercial is not the one with the cowpoke. It is the beer commercial during which young professionals prove themselves able to buy and sell stocks, run farms, play softball, raise families, spend lots of time in fashionable saloons, and look perfect, all in the scope of a few hours. It is the commercial that asks the burning question of the 1980s: "Who says you can't have it all?"

In the mature American economy, no sector is immune from the Yuppie resource grab. For health care, and especially hospitals, that fact has far more serious consequences than Yuppies popularizing wine over gin. The new equation of who deserves what resource has pushed hospitals into the hostile arms of individuals and organizations who would like nothing better than to turn health care into a no-holds-barred consumer market dominated by the uncertain mercies of the Yuppie ethic.

Princeton economist Uwe Reinhardt has observed that venture capitalists probably turned to health care because they really did not have anywhere else to go. With an aging population, a predicted (and in some places actual) oversupply of physicians, and generous public and private insurance, health care appeared the perfect plum for venture capitalism. As a result, freestanding urgent care centers, birthing centers, diagnostic centers, surgery centers, and other fragmented, specialized sites of care have blossomed in the 1980s. For-profit hospitals and private not-for-profit hospitals alike have aggregated into multihospital and multiservice organizations that increasingly are offering not only health care, but also health insurance. The boutique mentality has produced a new wealth of frilly, consumer-oriented institutions for the paying patient. These are so commercial in nature that Arthur Caplan of the Hastings Center has dubbed them "designer hospitals."

This is not necessarily all bad: we can hardly complain about patients being able to receive care closer to home, more quickly, in a more humane and intimate environment, at a lower price. We are hard pressed to oppose the offering on an outpatient basis of services that once would have required an inpatient stay that was more costly and often unnecessary. We must applaud the new incentives that have pushed hospitals to consider how they have spent their money; whatever else we can say about competition in health care, it is breeding greater efficiency on the part of institutional providers. It has also bred a profit mentality that may in the end lead not to greater efficiency but to an even weirder allocation of hospital services and revenues—but that is not inevitable. Whatever their motives, as they face a decline in occupancy and stringent demands from insurers and self-insured employers alike, American hospitals are learning to court the Yuppies.

If everyone were a Yuppie, we could all rest content in the knowledge that the revolution in health care has been of great benefit to all. There is evidence that it has not hurt the hospitals very much; according to American Hospital Association data in mid-1985, 82 percent of United States hospitals were operating in the black. Their margins were up to 6.8 percent, a more than 100 percent increase since 1980. Yet inflation in hospital costs had been held to slightly more than 5 percent. Outpatient care is zooming, the length of time a patient spends in the hospital is declining, and everyone is benefiting.

Everyone, that is, except the 18 percent of hospitals that are not operating in the black; the 30 to 35 million uninsured Americans who are at risk of not having access to health care; the more than 20 million Medicaid clients who, because of skimpy payments for their care, are becoming less and less attractive to providers who can afford to eschew them: the 30 million Medicare beneficiaries who are at risk of undercare under the new incentives; and those Yuppies who are now starting to turn forty and are entering the period of their lives when they are at much greater risk of severe illness and injury, including mental, cardiac and other organ ailments, and cancer. Although as much as half of all ill health can be ascribed to unhealthy lifestyles and habits, the rest is probably due to genetics and bad luck. Even the most health-minded Yuppies are going to start needing health care.

How will the Yuppie hospital deal with its healthy young clientele when it becomes an unhealthy older clientele? The payment systems that up until now have benefited hospitals do not recognize that such a change has taken place. The danger in the way many hospitals have positioned themselves in the new consumeristic health care market is that they have surrendered their traditional community service ethic for the more seductive Yuppie ethic. They are not alone in this: physicians in large measure have done the same, as have nursing homes. The newer freestanding organizations were never involved in a community ethic to begin with. Even Blue Cross and Blue Shield, which still hold tax-exempt status (although several congressmen have proposed removing it), are acting more and more like their commercial brethren. They are using selective contracts, forcing discounts, dropping community rating in favor of experience rating, offering HMO contracts at a much lower price, and generally squeezing both subscribers and providers.

The major future focus of American hospitals will not be the young, healthy, employed population; it will be the very population that is now at risk of underfunding or no funding at all. The elderly, the disabled, the poor, and the chronically ill are the market of the future. Robert Butler, chief of geriatrics at Mount Sinai Medical School, told the American Public Health Association annual meeting several years ago that Medicare, which covers the disabled and the over-sixty-five population, was designed as though everyone in the program were forty-years-old. Medicare has chosen to ignore the long-term care needs of the chronically ill elderly to such a degree that those patients are regularly forced to pauperize themselves in order to qualify for Medicaid; more than 70 percent of Medicaid expenditures now go to care of the blind, elderly, and disabled, as opposed to the low-income women and children for whom the program is the only source of care. Although older Americans as a whole are richer than younger Americans, there is a skewing of the level of insurance within the over-fifty population. According to the Senate Committee on Aging, one out of five early retirees aged fifty to fifty-four is uninsured. One age-group most likely to lack adequate health insurance is the population between the ages of fifty-five and sixty-four, who are often not in the bloom of good health.

What we have done, in our zest to make health care conform to the consumerism that has burgeoned in other sectors of the economy, is to embrace three absurdities. First, we have fragmented and recast health care and health insurance so that the most care is available to those who need it least—the healthy, insured, working population—while insurance and, increasingly, health care are denied to those who need them most. Second, in exacting discounts and copayments and directing the least sick away from the hospital, we have stripped hospitals of their ability to provide care to that extremely large population—probably 30 to 50 million people—who for reasons of finance, health status, or location do not have access to any other health care provider. Third, we have bought the Big Lie: that because it would make it easier for some entrepreneurs, venture capitalists, and big purchasers of care to garner huge profits and savings in the face of massive unfunded need, health care can be remolded into a consumer commodity.

The health care system, because of its conservative ideological bent, has brought much of this on itself. Most health care providers are attracted to the idea of being in business and playing in the market, which is ideologically more appealing than regulation. It is difficult to convince them that prospective payment and government budget cuts are simply a different kind of regulation—a more destructive, Social-Darwinian kind.

The public hospitals in the cities, many religious-sponsored hospitals and hospital organizations, and groups representing the patients who are at risk have not joined the general institutional rush to embrace a competitive health care marketplace. So far, their rewards have been penalties in that marketplace and exploitation by others not so bothered by conscience.

The public, 80 percent of whom are privately insured to one degree or another, have so far chosen to ignore the growing threat to the vulnerable because the Yuppie ethic has not yet been satisfied. If policy analysts are correct in theorizing that there is no such thing as a limit to the demand for health care—because so few people are willing to die or sustain permanent damage without a fight—then the Yuppies, and the marketers who have created the values now encircling them, will never again believe that there is enough health care to share with the unfortunate. They are more worried about whether there will be Medicare and social security benefits available to them when the time comes.

Hospitals, which should be serving as advocates for saner long-range planning, are not alone in having blunted their own power by accepting the argument that health care is just another consumer product. Physicians and hospitals alike have done themselves enormous harm by insisting that if costs were contained, the quality of care would suffer. Costs were reduced, and there was little apparent reduction in the quality of care received by most people. As a result, the providers lost their credibility with the public and with policymakers.

Philip Caper of Dartmouth Medical School observed recently:

> Decisions are being made by intermediaries, by employers, and by consultants in terms of what to pay for and what not to pay for. In failing to recognize the legitimacy of concerns about overall health care costs, organized medicine drove society to another solution, which is both less effective and more intrusive than need be...Physician self-restraint has not existed heretofore—nor has it been expected. But I think the alternative to physicians' learning some self-restraint is much worse. Decisions made outside the profession will determine how doctors treat individual patients. That's bad for patients and bad for doctors.

It is also bad for hospitals. Because providers could not see beyond their own noses, brutal cuts in Medicaid, questionable incentives in Medicare that have not been accompanied by reliable quality assurance monitoring, the disenfranchisement of the uninsured, and even the creeping compromise of access to care for the insured as patients' freedom of choice is replaced by restrictive systems and mandated providers—these have largely gone unchallenged.

What happens in the next ten years will determine the fate of the American hospital. There are several factors that could produce a happier result than the dismal scenario now quite likely: half the hospitals and physicians going broke for lack of business while half the population has no access to health care. First, the self-interest inherent in the Yuppie ethic will in the end breed social consciousness. Already, the Yuppies' parents have aged well into the high-risk post-fifty-five-year-old group. With the Medicare deductible having gone up 23 percent to $492 this year, more and more Yuppies are being drawn into their parents' health care financing problems. It is not a long step from there to looking in the mirror and realizing that you are not young anymore. We can hope that the postwar babies will be a healthier senior citizen population because of the positive health habits encouraged by Yuppie culture: but there are no guarantees. Good health habits may only postpone disability. Even though better health produces longevity, the underbelly of that is that the older you are, the more you are likely to need health care.

In seeing their parents struggle with an increasingly skimpy Medicare program, the Yuppies are likely to use their considerable political power to force a strengthening and, it is to be hoped, reconfiguration of the program. It may be too romantic to hope that their brush with vulnerability will also increase their sympathy for the poor; but Medicaid is becoming a program of long-term care for the elderly so fast that support for Medicaid may well become inextricably merged with support for Medicare. There is even some possibility that the Yuppie obsession with good health will breed what it should have bred years ago: an understanding that a commitment to early-intervention preventive health care, especially among low-income mothers and children, saves resources. Given that the Yuppies are interested in having access to resources, they may yet make some bargain with the poor.

As the considerable savings being reaped by insurers, employers, and provider-insurers begin to shrink (as is inevitable with an aging population and a hospital system that is rapidly cutting the fat out of its budgets) the problems of a thoroughly fragmented health care system are likely to become more apparent. At one time, HMOs' reported hospitalization rate of 40 percent less than fee-for-service medicine appeared to promise enormous savings to employers; what happened instead was that the HMOs, in many instances, simply priced themselves slightly below the fee-for-service market and kept most of the savings themselves. There is evidence that the bloom is starting to wear off some of the new organizations.

What is likely to be a more lasting provider of care is a reconfigured hospital—be it public or private, for-profit or not—if it is willing and able to become the coordinator of care for its community or neighborhood. This would require massive changes on the part of the hospital: in mission, in financing, in behavior, and above all in philosophy and sense of community. Focusing care under the coordination of the hospital is the most palatable and communitarian choice. In a game with this many players, someone has to be the referee, and there are really no qualified candidates other than physicians and hospitals, which, after the current skirmishes, are going to be closer partners than in the past.

Their image has suffered much in recent years, but American hospitals are still as trusted as any institution is likely to be in an anti-institutional age. With proper incentives and safeguards, they are still the best candidates to organize, monitor, and provide coordinated health care. Certainly the days of the inpatient-only hospital are over: inpatient care in the future will be only for the very sick. If the payment system is recast to recognize all this, the lost dream of continuity of care might yet become a reality. Those who no longer trust hospitals may find this a naive and dangerous proposal; but it need not be so. It is certainly less dangerous than proposing that third-party payers, with their huge fiduciary interest in the outcome, should direct the future of health care. Undercare is enough of a risk in the current system without a massive financial conflict of interest being injected into the proceedings.

As for government, it is a risky arbiter on two counts. First, politics is a creature of changing times, values, and attitudes; as a result its promises, no matter how sincere, may be short-lived. That has been amply demonstrated in the sad history of the Medicaid program. Second, American government on all levels has demonstrated in the past few years that it will disenfranchise anyone and anything if it believes that is what the people want. As long as government policy is reactive and neither prescriptive nor visionary, allowing government to determine the future nature and financing of health care bodes ill for the millions who are vulnerable.

We are left with the providers, governed and directed by patients and the community, as probably the best chance for the future of health care.

As Robert Sigmond, adviser on hospital affairs to Blue Cross and Blue Shield, observed in paraphrasing Winston Churchill. "Hospitals are the worst possible candidates for community change agents—until you examine the alternatives."

If there is anything to be learned from the erratic course of American health policymaking—what there is of it—it is that the pendulum swings broadly, but it always comes back. There is much to criticize in the Great Society health programs—chiefly the separation of the poor from the elderly in separate programs and the concentration of resources on acute, late-intervention institutional care—but they do represent a set of values. The basis of those values is that health care is not a market commodity but a special service that should be extended as broadly as possible. Today, only the United States and South Africa among developed nations do not recognize access to health care as a right of citizenship; it is unlikely that this will always be the case. Although there will be many casualties in the meantime, health policy will return again to an understanding that frailty, pain, and suffering transcend class and income distinctions, and that ignoring the plight of those who suffer is to ignore our own humanity.

When that time comes, the Yuppie hospital—the hospital that abandoned its community—will be called to account. The fat profit margin and the free champagne with childbirth will no longer serve as a competitive edge. Hospitals will be judged on how well they honored the expectations of those they served, how well they understood the special status that society has traditionally conferred on them, and how much they fought to keep their doors open—not to the healthy but to the fragile. Those hospitals that can pass these tests will still be with us when the Yuppies become, in columnist Arthur Hoppe's lovely phrase, the Grumpies, or Grown Up Mature People. Those hospitals that chose to become slaves to a transient consumer market will be doomed along with that market. They will have proved themselves unworthy of a lot more than Grape-Nuts, and they will not be missed.

The Pitfalls of "Fetal Protection"

David L. Kirp

Just moments before the oral argument in United Autoworkers (UAW) versus Johnson Controls in federal appeals, Judge John Coffey turned to University of Wisconsin law professor Carin Clauss, who was arguing the UAW's case: "This is about the women who want to hurt their fetuses." Judge Coffey's observation puts on display the passions generated by the increasingly widespread corporate practice of "fetal protection" keeping all fertile women out of jobs where exposure to toxic chemicals may mean fetal vulnerability.

Coffey's perspective that, more judiciously put, only a self-centered woman would opt to work in an environment that could menace her future offspring is not uncommon. In this calculus, there is no place for women's choices because there are no choices to be made. Would we grant mothers the right to take away their child's curiosity, the argument runs? Do they have a right to starve a child's brain? For a woman to insist on her right to make batteries becomes a selfish pleasure, morally indistinguishable from her maintaining a drug habit. Both women, the judge's comment suggests, are murderers.

This way of thinking oversimplifies a treacherous policy terrain marked at every juncture by competing interests and obligations, a terrain not well defined by either the language of discrimination or the rhetoric of benign paternalism. Everyone is anxious to minimize birth defects. But women, who know very well what it means to be treated as marginal workers, don't want to be forced out of lucrative jobs at least not without a thorough exploration of the alternatives. For their part, men exposed to toxins have reason to worry about their own reproductive futures. Employers have moral concerns about safeguarding potential offspring and fiscal concerns about avoiding future liability suits on behalf of deformed or stillborn fetuses.

The Johnson Controls case happens to involve a battery manufacturer whose workers are handling lead, a chemical whose toxic properties have been well understood since Hippocrates' day. The issue of fetal protection is not confined to a handful of women in the declining blue collar sector of the economy, where jobs are more likely to be lost due to overseas competition than to arguments about fetal vulnerability.

From the perspective of fetal risk, lead is not the only nor even the most potent toxic. The Bureau of National Affairs estimates fetal protection policies could deny more than 20 million jobs to women in industry alone. Countless millions more jobs, for X-ray technicians and taxicab drivers, radiologists and housepainters and those who work with videodisplay terminals, are also potentially at stake. These too entail exposure to such metals as mercury, boron and arsenic; chemicals including benzene, vinyl chloride, carbon tetrachloride, carbon monoxide and carbon disulfide; physical factors like x-rays and biological agents such as Hepatitis B. All of these and potentially hundreds more elements carry possible, though at present largely unknown, reproductive hazards.

Small wonder that this case has been characterized by one judge as "likely the most important sex-discrimination case in any court since 1964, when Congress enacted Title VII." Positions in the fetal protection debate do not fall neatly along conventional political lines. While Judge Coffey's conservative credentials are impeccable, so are those of the key dissenters, Frank Easterbrook and Richard Posner, both prolific advocates of the assimilation of legal rules to University of Chicago-style market economics. The interesting differences reside in what the Office of Technology Assessment terms "the management of uncertainty." This means examining how risk is understood, and who—company, worker, or government—is best qualified to make the critical choice about risk.

While UAW versus Johnson Controls is nominally a case at law, as both sides acknowledge, there is little in the law itself, or its "developed theories," to guide the analysis. The ban on sex discrimination in Title VII of the 1964 Civil Rights Act was added as an afterthought—a joke that misfired, some contend—about which there was little debate generally and none at all on the particulars of fetal protection. Lawsuits like this one, says the Equal Employment Opportunity Commission, make up "a class unto themselves." These puzzlements are reflected in several appeals court opinions.

Nondiscrimination is the touchstone but not the absolute rule of Title VII. Sex-based exceptions on the grounds of "business necessity" are warranted, the majority in Johnson Controls asserts, if an otherwise sensible and humanely motivated policy—in this case, one that promotes the health of the offspring of both sexes—happens to affect men and women differently. Dissenters insist that, where one sex is singled out by company policy, any claim of "business necessity" is legally irrelevant. Only if the company can demonstrate that sterility is a "bona fide occupational qualification" (a "BFOQ" in Title VII parlance) that is "reasonably necessary to the normal operation" of a business can it exclude women from potentially toxic jobs. The minority also points out that, under the Pregnancy Discrimination Act, which amended Title VII in 1978, unless pregnant (or potentially pregnant) workers differ from others in their "ability or inability to work, " they must be treated just like everyone else. This difference, says the minority, has not been demonstrated. In a bit of legal legerdemain the majority counters that the "business" of this company to which a BFOQ applies is not just making batteries but manufacturing batteries as safely as possible, and that legitimates fetal protection policies.

These are the unsettled questions of law the Supreme Court will have to settle. Behind the thrusts and parries of the lawyers, as behind the questions of what is "reasonably necessary" and whether, in the law, "normal" means just "profit-making," as Easterbrook would have it, or can it also, as Posner proposes, encompass "civilized" and "humane" treatment, resides the deeper issue of risk and public policy. Both sides accept, at least for purposes of argument, that fetal protection is legally unacceptable discrimination "unless the employer shows (1) that a substantial risk of harm exists; and (2) that the risk is borne only by members of one sex; and (3) the employee fails to show there are acceptable alternative policies that would have a lesser impact on the affected sex."

The appeals court majority concludes that "scientific research" on the risks of lead exposure, coupled with the lack of safer options, sustains the company's position. The arguments as simple as a syllogism: lead in blood is dangerous; lead may be passed from a mother to a fetus, where it is also dangerous; therefore, barring women from jobs where they may be exposed to lead is a necessary way to protect fetuses. As it turns out, each step in this argument conceals massive uncertainties and the standard applied by the judges is actually one of zero risk.

At certain levels, the dangers of lead are beyond dispute. In the smelting-houses of the industrial revolution, workers once suffered seizures and loss of consciousness. Their limbs twisted like tree trunks or went limp with dropsy and their minds corroded. Then, the levels of lead carried in the workers' blood reached many hundreds of micrograms per deciliter. Permissible levels are far lower now, fixed for the past decade at a maximum of 50ug/100g by Occupational Safety and Health Administration (OSHA) regulation after thoroughgoing agency review. (At the time, Johnson Controls' medical consultant, Dr. Charles Fishburn, argued that a standard of 200ug/100g offered sufficient health protection.) Not coincidentally, Judge Easterbrook, who was then the OSHA liaison at the Justice Department, was personally involved in the hearings.

Most scientists would accept the OSHA standard as rigorous enough to prevent the familiar signs of lead poisoning: fatigue, constipation, hypertension, diminished sexual drive, memory loss, mood swings. Since researchers have been able to detect the impact of lead at ever lower blood concentrations, there have been calls for radical lowering of permissible blood levels. A scientist from the Environmental Defense Fund, summoned as an expert witness by the UAW, urged a ceiling of 10ug/100g. Yet such a standard would not only be ruinously expensive, it would also require shutting down most cities, where due to lead in the air, blood lead levels typically range upwards from 12 and 20ug/100g.

It has been known for a long time that the offspring of women who carry high lead levels in their blood are also at risk. At the turn of the century, women working in the china and pottery factories who were palsied by lead would conceive a child in order to pass the heavy metal out of their own bodies. These desperate women needed no scientist to tell them a fetus will absorb through the placenta some of the lead that a mother carries. They knew too that the fetus would be spontaneously aborted or be stillborn. Among doctors fear of the impact of lead on the next generation was so great that lead was called "race poison."

This too is history. Yet while lead no longer kills the young, it still can stunt—perhaps arrest—their physical and mental development if absorbed in sufficient amounts. More than 200,000 children, ages 5 or younger, have lead levels above the 25ug/100g specified as a safe ceiling by the Centers for Disease Control. Typically, lead is brought home by the parents, carried away from work on fingers and hair and clothing; or else it comes from old paint pried off walls by small hands or inhaled in the urban air.

The salient questions, how lead is transmitted from mother to child and what are alternative ways of reducing the risks of transmission, go unasked by the appeals court majority in Johnson Controls. Is lead in the mother's blood, at levels to which employees at the firm are actually exposed, dangerous to the fetus? Suppose, for instance, a woman becomes pregnant with a blood lead level of 40ug/100g. It is not known whether the risk, attributable to that exposure, of her having a learning-disabled child is one in three or one in 3,000,000. Among the estimated 50,000 lead-exposed workers and their families whom Dr. Fishburn has treated during his quarter-century of practice with the company, he recalled seeing just one "damaged child" of a high-lead mother, a hyperactive youngster, and Fishburn could be sure the harm was caused during gestation. This does not mean that only one child actually suffered birth defects because of a parent's exposure to lead in the work place. Since other families, Fishburn noted, might have relied on public clinics. What is relevant is that this company acted to keep women off the job without having critical and readily collectible data. Other companies behaved the same way. During the 1970s, American Cyanamid barred fertile women from jobs where they might be exposed to any of 29 chemicals, despite a dearth of evidence about any fetal consequences. When this policy was challenged by the Occupational Safety and Health Administration, the firm narrowed the scope of work place exclusions.

What else might Johnson Controls have done to minimize the possibility of fetal damage, besides denying women access to more than 90 percent of its jobs? For one thing, it could have limited the reach of its policy. The company's rule bars all women between the ages of 17 and 70 from line jobs where lead levels can run high (indeed from all low-lead positions from which workers can bid for line jobs) unless they can prove sterility. Not all women are equally likely to conceive. For blue-collar women over 30, the birth rate is less than 2 percent, and among all women aged 45 to 49, just one in 5000 has a child in any given year. One of the plaintiffs, Ginny Green, was 50 years old, divorced and raising a teenage daughter—not a likely candidate to become pregnant—yet she had been banished to the glorified position of laundress. Even among women who do become pregnant, risk-limiting measures short of banishment are available. Most experts believe that lead crosses the placenta from mother to fetus in the last months of gestation. Since blood lead levels decline sharply in a matter of months, offering women the option of regular pregnancy tests and transferring women workers from the assembly line as soon as they become pregnant would reduce the danger to the fetus from a mother's exposure.

The plant could also make available clearer information on the risks of exposure and the ways an individual worker can lessen those risks. Informing the women on the line that it is dangerous to become pregnant while working in a lead-tainted environment was Johnson Controls' policy until 1982, when the fetal protection rule went into effect. It is as risky as smoking, ran the message, a weak scare at a time when the dangers of smoking while pregnant were not so widely appreciated. Between 1978 and 1982, just seven women with blood lead levels above 30 had borne children, and no birth defects were reported among them. (Amazingly, the record in the case does not reveal how many women were employed by Johnson Controls during the period.) At Johnson Controls plants, most workers holding jobs where a particular individual has lead levels higher than 30ug/100g, the company's trigger for exclusion, has lower lead levels. At any given workstation, lead levels may range from less than 10 to more than 40. The difference has mostly to do with an employee's personal hygiene and willingness to use a respirator. By taking these variations into account, treating workers as individuals rather than defining them entirely in terms of their sex and fertility, all women on the plant floor would not be held to the standard of the least health-conscious. These are all risk-reducing alternatives. Yet for the company, and evidently for the majority of the appellate panel, the tacit rule is that the only acceptable risk level is zero risk, or more precisely, zero risk of fetal harm on the job.

Supporters of the fetal protection rule situate themselves on the moral high ground of protectors of generations to come. "One child born developmentally disabled is a very, very grave injustice to that child and that is a moral risk...we cannot countenance ourselves," testified Dr. Jean Beaudoin, Health and Safety Manager for Johnson Controls, at an administrative hearing on a parallel challenge to the company's rule. Judge Coffey, venturing into the realm of pop psychology, speculated that being a "force in the work place" may warp a working woman's judgment, leading her to "discount this clear risk" to the physical and mental development of her own child.

The women who hold down these factory jobs appreciate that there is no risk-free world. There is only what Judge Easterbrook describes as an individually constructed calculation of net risk. These women are obliged to make their way in the risk pool. They choose this occupation not out of selfishness or a misguided sense of liberation but because they already have children or do not plan to become mothers. They may also intend to stop assembling batteries before becoming pregnant or they may believe the OSHA standard delivers reasonable assurance that having a child poses no undue medical risk even for a woman working on the line. Compared to the realistic alternatives for such women, filing forms in an office or dishing up hamburgers at McDonald's, jobs in the battery plant bring double and triple the hourly wages, deliver better health care benefits, and cause less stress. Although most of the women from Johnson Controls would bristle to be called feminists, having jobs gives them a sense of independence and self-confidence that is otherwise missing from their lives.

Johnson Controls regards those concerns as irrelevant. "If there is a greater risk, that's not our concern," said corporate counsel, when asked during the oral argument about these workers' prospects elsewhere. Yet for the body in question—the fetus—it is surely the fact of risk, not its source, that matters. When it comes to calculating risk, the corporation and the court view male and female workers differently. Consider the story of Donald Penney who, together with his wife Anna May, used to work for Johnson Controls. While the Penneys wanted to start a family, they read about how fathers as well as mothers could conceivably inflict lead poisoning upon the fetus, and they wanted to avoid that potential risk. Anna had a job in a low-lead section of the company, but Don worked on the assembly line. He asked for a three month unpaid leave of absence to bring his blood lead levels down low enough to be reasonably sure he would father a healthy child. Leaves were common in the factory, and one might think that this firm, so concerned with fetal safety, would have applauded Penney's initiative. Instead his request was bluntly rejected, and according to Penney's subsequent complaint, the personnel director berated him for even raising the issue. "If you feel this way, quit."

While a mother can directly intoxicate the fetus, the link between father and fetus is more remote and speculative. At high lead levels, sperm can become misshapen (as can ova). It is uncertain, however, whether sperm remain fertile and, if so, whether sperm damage translates into the chromosome damage that means brain-damaged offspring. The question is what is to be made of this uncertainty.

The Title VII standard adopted by the Johnson Controls appeals court opinion requires that, before adopting a women-only rule, Johnson Controls must demonstrate that lead exposure above 30ug/100 1 in male workers poses no risk to the fetus. A less Procrustean rule would permit the firm to single out women where the risk is, if not zero—at least of relative insignificance—with all the wiggle room that "relative" implies. The evidence does not sustain either the court's approach or the more flexible alternative.

Johnson Control's doctors, who describe themselves as ultraconservative about female workers, dismiss the evidence on the risk from male-to-fetus transmission as too speculative despite OSHA's determination that, at high levels, lead is potentially hazardous to the newborn whether carried by men or women. The paucity of empirical investigations is a testament, not to the dubiousness of the possibility, but to the predilections of the medical researchers. Researchers too habitually look to the mother, not the father, to explain birth defects and design their studies accordingly. Dr. Herbert Needleman, whose research on the link between umbilical cord blood lead levels and children's later development is cited by Johnson Controls in its legal brief, complains in a published commentary that the company misused his findings. "We did not measure paternal exposure and therefore cannot rule this out as a contributing factor. The position that a given level of paternal but not maternal exposure is acceptable is without logical foundation and insupportable on empirical grounds."

The most convincing evidence that lead in men as well as women is hazardous to newborns comes from animal studies. The appeals court majority in Johnson Controls, so deferential to the experts' readings of the data on danger attributable to maternal exposure, refused to take this research seriously. The judges concluded that animal studies are not "solid scientific data" because too "speculative." That finding will surely shock the scientific community (and the Food and Drug Administration), which often relies on animal studies as the best evidence available. Its implausibility suggests that something else is going on here: that the judges, so insistent on a zero risk standard for women workers, have imposed an impossibly heavy burden on those who are concerned about the risks to men.

This judicial double standard, like the company policy itself, has little to do with the law or the evidence, and has everything to do with the conception of the marginality of women in the work place that echoes turn-of-the-century arguments for protecting women workers. The Johnson Controls rule is paternalism, not in its familiar contemporary guise of protecting individuals against marketplace excess—this is, after all, what OSHA's standards entail—but in its older guise of thinly veiled sexism. A famous legal brief, filed by Louis Brandeis nearly a century ago in support of a New York law forbidding the employment of women for night-shift factory work, details the hazards: the awful consequences of "deprivation of sunlight," the difficulty of getting enough rest during the day, the high mortality rates among night workers, the dangers that might befall women walking home at night, the hardships of combining motherhood and night work. Although night work was hard on men too—it brutalized them, often robbing them of a real home life and delivering them to drink—the work had to be done by someone. "Ignorant women can scarcely be expected to realize the dangers, not only to their own health but to that of the next generation from such inhuman usage." Women needed to stay home during the daytime, Brandeis contended, to save their strength for the next generation. All that truly mattered was the biological imperative.

The same argument lies behind contemporary fetal protection policies, as Judge Easterbrook reminded his colleagues. Then and now, efforts at protection have ultimately been powered by the bottom line. Since there was a ready supply of men to fill night-work factory jobs, women became dispensable, but female nurses were too badly needed to be eased out in the name of protection. Similarly, contemporary arguments for fetal protection come most easily at companies like Johnson Controls, where the presence of women is not really required.

Inside Johnson Controls and similar firms, the audible voices—those of foremen and lawyers and doctors will push for the exclusion of women. Shop foremen generally prefer to banish them out of an "Archie Bunkerish" worldview. (Supervisors at American Cyanamid, which instituted similar rules, were reported as saying that the company would get rid of women on the shop floor, "one way or another.") Doctors argue the possible danger to the fetus from maternal exposure to lead.

Perhaps most serious, although never voiced in the course of litigation, is the corporation lawyers' concern that multimillion dollar lawsuits could be filed on behalf of damaged fetuses. In theory, costly mass tort litigation is possible. While suits brought by workers on their own behalf are barred by the workmen's compensation system, litigation on behalf of fetuses is not similarly foreclosed. Yet this legal risk looks to be more theoretical than real. Very few such cases have actually been brought.

Thus far, the lone case involving a female employee resulted in a verdict for the company, even though the firm had violated OSHA standards. The only successful lawsuits were filed a decade ago by men whose sexual functioning was impaired by exposure to the pesticide DBCP. This paucity of litigation may be explained by the fact that, as the Agent Orange litigation showed, it is difficult to demonstrate that on-the-job exposure, not other risky behaviors, caused a fetal defect. It is also unlikely that would-be litigants could show that a corporation that followed OSHA standards had been negligent, and such proof would ordinarily be essential for establishing liability. In keeping women out, a company like Johnson Controls endures no competitive disadvantage since other firms in the business are doing precisely the same thing. No one within the corporate precincts raises the issue of relative risk and no one argues the women workers' viewpoint. In such a setting, discrimination appears entirely rational. Aside from defending what are regarded as nuisance cases like Johnson Controls, the costs appear to fall entirely on the other side of the ledger.

It is easy to sound morally superior when, as at Johnson Controls, women workers are marginal. Businesses that rely on women have been much less scrupulous about the dangers they impose on the unborn. Laundries and dry cleaners use carbon disulfide and benzene, dental offices are often contaminated with mercury. Working in laboratories frequently means exposure to benzene and other potentially dangerous toxins, yet Johnson Controls-type rules have not been introduced in these "women's work" jobs. This selective expression of concern offers a reminder that the very terminology of fetal protection is the language of industrial spin control, the companies' own description of a practice that actually has more to do with corporate protection than fetal protection.

Cytomegalovirus, commonly called CMV, is perhaps the clearest instance of a substance harmless to men, which cannot be transmitted through sperm to a fetus but poses a severe risk to the fetus if the mother is exposed during pregnancy. The virus is passed from young children to pregnant women, a *New England Journal of Medicine* article reports, and then to the fetus, where it wreaks awful neurological damage. There is no way to eliminate CMV, as companies stopped using DBCP once it became apparent that the pesticide caused sterility. Although the risk of contracting CMV is greatest among women who work in day care centers, no one proposes that fertile women not be hired since, obviously and tellingly, no one else would fill these jobs.

The preeminence of market values explains why it is women who staff day care centers and why Donald Penney's request for a leave of absence was treated as a hostile act. "Johnson Controls' standards of ethics provide that it will not engage in any activity...that threatens the physical well being of any person," declares the company, even while insisting that there is no alternative to lead-acid batteries and consequently no way to reduce the risk significantly. Industry experts tell a different story: A less toxic battery could be made, but at much greater cost.

It is surely cheaper to exclude women from manufacturing batteries than to change the process of production itself—even as the risk to indispensable male workers is calculated differently. Yet cost is not the only consideration. Were it otherwise, there would be no Title VII to protect the individual's rights even against, and maybe especially against, efficient forms of discrimination.

One could wish for a world in which no worker, male or female, who contemplates having a child, is exposed to potential hazards. But that is to invent an impossible environment free from stresses, human as well as chemical. While one could also aspire to a set of substantive rules about toxic exposure that confidently guided behavior, the evidence is and will inevitably be imperfect. There are too many distinct hazards to estimate; and the task of gauging their distinctive effects, mediated as they are by genetics and environment and levels of exposure, poses formidable technical difficulties. In a world filled with risks and shaped by uncertainties, the more useful question for policymakers is who is best situated to make decisions.

Standards of nondiscrimination and respect for personal autonomy, on which the standard rests, suggest that, as a matter of principle, affected individuals are generally better able than corporations to calculate the risk of toxic exposure to themselves and their offspring. Yet workers and corporations are not the only interested parties. What is required for sensible fetal protection is a process that allocates risks and cost on a basis broader than considerations of the market or individual liberty, and narrowing the range of choices to assure a work place that is as safe as possible. Safety standards such as those set for lead exposure by the Occupational Safety and Health Administration are necessary as an assurance that safety calculations are not framed in terms of competitive advantage. They also serve to shield individual workers against choices that are too hard to be fairly borne, with health risks set against unemployment. The way OSHA went about fixing the standard for tolerable lead exposure—the agency's meticulous review of the available evidence, resisting both corporate urging for lassitude and unfounded claims of risk stemming from any exposure level—can stand as a model for how government should proceed in the face of unavoidable unknowns.

It makes structural sense for OSHA and not the affected company to fix the ground rules. OSHA has a less direct financial stake in the issue than any particular firm, and can balance cost and safety concerns on an industry-wide, not company-specific, basis. It can assign a value to safety, using techniques more reliable than the after-the-fact and inefficient system of liability law. In setting its standards, the OSHA is not as insulated from politics as is the corporation, but is subject to the push and pull of lobbying by women's groups, unions, and trade associations.

Involving the constituents in the setting of standards does not mean that all rules about reproductive health hazards will be sex-neutral, since science does not mirror principle or ideology so neatly. There are instances in which one sex is so evidently more vulnerable to fetal risk that sex-differentiated rules do make sense—the biological agent CMV is one such instance, the pesticide DBCP another. These determinations are best made by an agency able to appreciate the full implications of such distinctions.

Several reforms are needed to strengthen the present OSHA regime. For one thing, workers are entitled to fuller information on the health risks that toxic exposure still invites, even with feasible safety standards in place. For another, job retraining and medical insurance should be offered to workers who, out of medical concern for the fetus, are removed or voluntarily remove themselves from unavoidably hazardous jobs. Research on reproductive risk, especially studies of paternally-mediated effects of toxins, should be encouraged; the available evidence offers diminishing scientific support for singling out women as vessels of risk. Corporations that follow OSHA's safety standards are entitled to be insulated by federal law against the possibility of mega-judgments in fetal tort suits. Money saved in court costs and lawyers' fees, well over a third of court awards in mass-tort litigation, could be used to help pay for the retraining and health insurance. Modern work places swarm with thousands of substances potentially dangerous to the fetus, everything from manganese to Gamma rays. Sources of danger go far beyond the assembly line, crossing the sex line to affect men as well as women, and leap-frogging the line that separates work from pleasure. Already there are jurisdictions where women who use illegal drugs during pregnancy are jailed as felons; and scientists regularly deliver warnings about what pregnant women eat and drink and smoke. In this sense, lead and crack-cocaine and junk food inhabit the same biological universe.

The more that is learned about these insidious dangers, the more remarkable it becomes that any fetus navigates the perilous voyage from conception to birth healthy and intact. All this knowledge does not really answer the deeper questions. It only sharpens the value choices: between the claims of the generations; between maintaining personal sovereignty and surrendering that sovereignty to those who, whether for profit or out of paternalism, would protect us from ourselves . The Johnson Controls story offers a way of sifting the implications of those choices.

Chemicals and Cancerphobia

Elizabeth M. Whelan

Americans today are nervous. They are worried about funny sound-ing chemicals in our food, water, and air. It is no wonder people are concerned; the popular press has tolled a litany of potential cancer haz-ards in our environment. We have heard that hamburgers may cause mutations, that drinking hair dye is no good for us, that saccharin causes cancer in Canadian rats, and that the mild sedative one needs to digest all this good news has just been banned. There are some times when the only solution seems to be a good stiff drink, as long as it is not Scotch—or beer. These may cause cancer, too!

We have become suspicious, and some of us are so jumpy that we are ready to shout "carcinogen" at the merest hint of trouble, or we are sim-ply fed up with warnings on labels. But American industry has responded to our concerns. We are now told that if it is not "natural," it is best avoided. There are natural clothes, natural foods, natural deodorants, and even natural pesticides. And who could forget natural cigarettes with the Surgeon General's warning naturally displayed? The real issue be-hind this "natural is better than artificial" puffery is not the fact that there *is* concern, but why these concerns exist and what we can or should do about them.

Cancer is an unquestionably serious public health problem in the United States today. In 1980 an estimated 395,000 Americans died from some form of cancer, making it the second leading cause of death behind heart disease. So there is an obvious need for a rational and integrated system to identify and assess cancer risks. This is particularly obvious to those in the chemical or chemical-related industries. But there is substantial disagreement today about the best policy to adopt.

To a large extent, this controversy arises from widespread public mis-conceptions of cancer and its causes. These misconceptions influence research and regulatory priorities and in some cases divert limited economic and technical resources. A solution to these problems, then, depends in part on correcting these misconceptions through education and research. The problem is a complex one, but in an attempt to simplify this discussion, I have identified seven specific areas of cancer misinformation and confusion among the general public. If we are to have any impact on changing our country's current approach to environmental issues, I think it is critical that we first understand—and then proceed to correct—these areas of misunderstanding.

Prevalent Misconceptions

First, there is apparently a very poor understanding about the relative prevalence of cancer in the United States. Surveys indicate that many Americans assume we have an unusually high rate of cancer here—the implication being, of course, that we are paying for the benefits of technology with poor health. The premise is so widespread that it has become part of the popular wisdom. A network television special opened with the statement, "If you live in the United States, your chances of developing cancer are higher than anywhere else in the world." During the debate with Gerald Ford in 1976, Jimmy Carter informed us we had the highest cancer death rate in the world. And when one hears a statement enough, one tends to believe it and to want to take action on the basis of it. The fact, of course, is that the United States has a cancer death rate which is about average for a developed country. In 1980, Scotland held the dubious honor of being Number 1.

Second, the national surveys tell us that people also believe there is a marked increase in the past few decades in the incidence of cancer—enough to warrant the word "epidemic." In 1975 newspapers around the country carried headlines of a cancer epidemic, referring to the possibility that a time bomb was going off. And again, we are back to the implication that as we have developed as a highly technological nation, we have suffered more and more environmentally induced cancer.

Again, however, the popular wisdom does not correspond to the facts. Data from the National Cancer Institute indicate that the overall incidence of cancer (the number of new cases of cancer per 100,000 population) has declined slightly since 1947. There has been an increase in cancer mortality in the past few decades, but certainly nothing on the order of an "epidemic." Most interestingly, only one form of cancer death has increased significantly for all Americans: lung cancer. At a time when American eaters are particularly nervous about chemicals in their food, it is ironic to note that paralleling the dramatic increase in lung cancer, we have been witnessing a precipitous decline in gastric cancer.

Third, it is common cocktail party chatter these days to acknowledge that 90 percent of cancers are caused by factors in the environment. To most laymen, this conjures up the image of a white-coated evil scientist pouring carcinogens into the air, water, food, and work place. The origin of the 90 percent figure was an estimate made by an epidemiologist affiliated with the World Health Organization, who compared international cancer rates by site and concluded that simply being human did not explain the majority of cancers, that differences between countries had to be accounted for by different factors in the environment. In making this estimate he was not referring to "chemicals" around us, but rather primarily to differences in lifestyle factors.

Estimates among epidemiologists now vary somewhat, but there is a general consensus that 40 percent of the cancers occurring today in American men are caused by one specific environmental factor—tobacco (25 percent in women). Additionally, there is a strong suggestion that some aspect of nutrition and diet plays a major role in the development of certain cancers—colon, breast, prostate, and stomach, perhaps accounting for one-third of all these diseases. At this point we simply do not have the answer here, but feel that it is some component of the general diet. And there are some other contributors to environmental cancer: excessive alcohol use, especially in conjunction with cigarette smoking, accounts for a substantial number of oral cancers. A few drugs—most dramatically, DES—have been shown to increase cancer risk. Differences in sexual and reproductive patterns influence risks of cervical and breast cancers. Excessive exposure to radiation—background or manmade—has accounted for some of the environmental cancer toll. And, of course, in some specific instances, exposure to occupational chemicals or conditions has led to increased risk of cancer of a number of sites.

But getting back to perspective, the vast majority of that 80-90 percent environmental cancer figure is accounted for by tobacco and the still undefined contribution of diet. The other factors explain only a relatively small amount of cancer mortality in this country. Although there has been considerable controversy about the subject in recent months, it still appears that well under 5 percent of cancer mortality can be related to occupational carcinogens.

There is no question that a number of industrial chemicals carry potential cancer risks. There is also no question that among them asbestos contributes the greatest risk in terms of exposed populations and widespread use. But if we were to believe Joseph Califano's estimate, there should be an astronomical increase in the number of mesotheliomas, the rare lung cancer almost exclusively related to asbestos. Yet in those states with tumor registries, like New York and Connecticut, these projected increases have not been detected. Perhaps doctors are still misclassifying these tumors as something else, or there is some unknown factor that is delaying their detection. But one thing we do know is that there is a vast amount of difference between the 20 to 40 percent HEW estimate and the 1 to 5 percent estimates of the International Agency for Research on Cancer and another project that reached the same conclusion in a study of the British work force.

There is, however, one point which the HEW paper discussed that has some merit. And that is that we might be misleading ourselves by trying to affix the blame for "X" percentage of cancers to a single chemical or process. The multifactorial nature of cancer seems to argue against this approach. We know, for example, that asbestos is a cancer risk, and we also know that cigarette smoking increases this risk by at least one order of magnitude. Yet it is ironic to read that a court decision declared that a company policy to hire only nonsmokers for work with asbestos is discriminatory. It appears that the court has decided that it is better for the company to risk going out of business to comply with regulatory procedures than to deny a worker the right to kill himself by smoking. But the idea that we should consider the interaction of risk factors in a broader perspective is a reasonable one.

Fourth on the list of common misconceptions about cancer—and related to the one just discussed—is the idea that it is industry, particularly the chemical and manufacturing industries, that causes cancer. Under this misdirected reasoning, one concludes that asbestos and vinyl chloride not only do cause cancer in workers, but also become part of a general polluted environment and cause cancer in the residents of the community as well. A case in point here is the state of New Jersey. It is called "cancer alley," and the recommendation is not to live there—and if you must drive through, hold your breath. If you ask a passerby why the cancer rate is so high in New Jersey, he will tell you, "The chemical industries. That's the price I have to pay to live here."

Actually, however, I have never seen convincing evidence to suggest that general air pollution increases the risk of human cancer. Certainly there are other health and aesthetic reasons for cleaning up our air. But again, the popular misconception about cancer does not correspond to the facts. A careful analysis of the statistics in a state such as New Jersey reveals that it has no different cancer pattern than any other urban area. Of interest to some might be the fact that the lung cancer death rate in some of the more polluted areas of New Jersey is about the same as it is in Rutland, Vermont, where the major industry is tourism.

Fifth on my list of points of concern and misinformation is the general concept of the word "risk." When it comes to discussions of cancer and the environment, most Americans have a very poor concept of the nature of the risks we are speaking of. The problem here is twofold: first, extrapolating from one tragic circumstance to all uses of the substance. Thus a poor understanding of risk assessment might make one conclude that if large amounts of inhaled asbestos increased workers' risks of mesothelioma—and if they smoked cigarettes, of lung cancer—then we should tolerate no exposure to asbestos in the future, no matter how minute the quantities may be and no matter what the cost, in terms of prices and availability of goods, that this reduction would entail.

The second manifestation of public confusion about risk relates to an apparent inability to distinguish between real and hypothetical risks. A risk is something one can identify and quantify, then either accept or reject. Driving a car and flying in an airplane involve risks. People die. At the end of each year we know exactly what the risks of 12 months of use of these conveniences were. Americans appears to have little trouble accepting these real risks. Similarly, cigarettes pose a known health hazard. Epidemiological studies allow calculations of personal risk assumed here. These are real risks. The use of food additives, pesticides, and low-level exposures to occupational chemicals, on the other hand, pose hypothetical risks. Of course it is possible that they contribute to cancer mortality, but we have no evidence at this point that they do. As a society we seem to be drifting toward a policy which tolerates known, major risks chosen by the individual—and rejects hypothetical risks that might be assumed by industry or society as a whole. This was clear to me last year in New York when nearly a quarter million individuals gathered to protest nuclear power. The news clippings I saw revealed that a significant number of them were smoking cigarettes.

Sixth, cancerphobia in America and the dozens of environmental regulations which have stemmed from it are very much tied into what seems to be a new philosophy about cause of disease. If indeed there is one classical attitude about human disease and its causes, it is one based on the assumption that most diseases are unexplainably caused by "bad spirits," "bad air," or simply God's will. Diseases, until recently, just happened. But not so today. Instead, now, we are either guilty or angry when someone close to us becomes ill.

An associate of mine was recently diagnosed as having kidney cancer. For three weeks he asked me the same questions: "What caused it? What did I do wrong? Whose fault was it?" The conversations we have had have been tragically frustrating, with my answer always the same: "We have no information on what causes kidney cancer. We simply don't know." He has posed the same question repeatedly to his physician. Last week the doctor gave in to his pleadings, telling my friend that his use of saccharin might be the cause. Presumably the physician knows that even the darkest picture ever drawn on the issue of saccharin's safety has never implicated the sweetener as a cause of kidney cancer. But the doctor was attempting to fulfill a need; my friend desperately wanted to identify a cause and the saccharin explanation satisfied him, allowing him to place the blame somewhere: on the saccharin manufacturers and on himself for using it. My associate's experience is, I believe, characteristic of a major change in attitude noted during the 1970s, and one which resulted from our new emphasis on cancer and the environment and which has major implications for our economy and standard of living.

While I was a guest on a Chicago talk show last year, a woman called in to tell me her four-year-old son had leukemia. "I know the cause," she told me sadly, "I breast fed him, and my milk was contaminated with DDT. We really have got to ban those pesticides to stop this cancer epidemic." This woman's reaction reminded me of an incident which occurred in New Jersey four years ago: two women from the Bergen County town of Rutherford whose sons had died from leukemia within five months of each other began a personal search for other such cancer deaths. They found a number more, and notified the press that they had identified the "cause" of their children's disease: pollution from the chemical companies in the state. They demanded that some major industries in their neighborhood be closed down. Media coverage of the "cancer cluster" was extensive. Follow-up coverage on the findings of the State Health Department that the frequency of cancer deaths in Rutherford was no more than that expected in any population that size was minimal. In many people's minds the "cause" of those leukemia cases is still the New Jersey chemical industry, although the sobering reality is that we do not know the cause of the overwhelming majority of childhood leukemia cases.

Last year in Oregon a group of 14 women who had suffered a miscarriage or had a child with a birth defect banded together to announce they knew the "cause" of their problem: their area had been sprayed over the past few years with the herbicide 2, 4, 5, T. As a direct result of their announcement, the herbicide was banned, this despite the fact that follow-up reports noted that the miscarriages and birth defects in question occurred in a random manner, with no obvious clustering, within a few months after the spraying. But again, the "cause" of reproductive problems remains in many minds, and again, we simply do not know the real cause of all miscarriages and birth defects. Similarly, Vietnam veterans who now find they have cancer—or children with birth defects—are claiming that this same herbicide, used to defoliate the jungles during the war, is the cause of their problems. And again, the scientific evidence to back up their claims is nonexistent.

In New York City, policemen and firemen have succeeded in passing the so-called "heart bill," which compensates them for any expenses related to the development of heart disease. The assumption here is, of course, that the "cause" of heart disease among these two groups of employees is job stress, and thus the general population of the state should assume all the costs. Actually, however, there is no evidence that "stress" itself is a factor in etiology of heart disease and if, indeed, policemen and firemen do have a higher rate of heart disease than the rest of the New York male population, it is likely to be due to differences in exposure to one established causative factor, cigarette smoking.

We have come a very long way in understanding some of the causative factors in today's major killers. For example, as I have mentioned, we know that cigarette smoking contributes to the causation of one-third of all this year's cancer deaths; that, while the causation of heart disease is complex, cigarette smoking, high blood pressure, and high serum cholesterol are clearly the top three risk factors; that excessive consumption of alcohol increases one's risk of liver and other diseases; that exposure to some occupational chemicals, like asbestos and vinyl chloride, raises cancer risks.

But the fact remains that we simply do not have all the answers. Diseases, and deaths, still occur for reasons unknown to us. Human beings remain mortal. Death and disease are still natural processes. It is unconstructive to blame ourselves in these instances. And it is economically disastrous for a society when there is no proof of guilt.

Seventh, and finally, the cancerphobia which now grips our nation and is dictating federal policy in a number of government agencies seems to be largely traceable to a fear of chemicals. A chemical anxiety. A chemical reaction. Are we eating too many chemicals? Are there too many chemicals in our environment? I met a woman in the supermarket one day who asked me to help her read the label on a box of a low-cholesterol egg substitute. I complied only to have her exclaim, "My goodness, all that aluminum sulfate, sodium and triethyl citrate and emulsifiers. I'd rather keep my cholesterol high than become a walking test tube." Little did she know that the natural organic egg, even if it is laid by a happy hen, contains among other things ovalbumin, conalbumin, globulins, fatty acetic and butyric acids.

Technology and Health

The suspicion over artificial chemicals and complacency over natural ones is silly but seems to be a basis for cancer-chemical phobia. Thus a housewife gets upset about the use of a synthetic estrogen DES sometimes used to stimulate cattle growth and keep prices down, because traces of it have been found in some 5 percent or less of beef livers, and she hears that DES causes cancer. What she does not know perhaps is that any estrogen, natural or otherwise, in high doses will cause cancer, that her body regularly produces it, and that there is 1,000 times the amount of estrogen in a single egg than in a serving of affected liver.

Enough said here. The anxiety, the fear of cancer and its relationship to the environment may be peaking. But misinformation on cancer still abounds. And as it does, and as it directs the policies at the Food and Drug Administration, the Environmental Protection Agency, the Occupational Safety and Health Administration and elsewhere, we are suffering. For businessmen, the implications are clear: more regulation, higher costs, fewer jobs, and limited production. For me as a scientist and consumer the implications are also clear: high prices, higher taxes, fewer products—a diminished standard of living .

When a pesticide is banned, it may make the environmentalists feel good, make them think they are doing something. But as an epidemiologist, I know it is not preventing cancer. And as a consumer it makes me angry that even though the banning has no medical benefits, it means that I will pay more for strawberries and corn next year. Such bannings also serve as a disincentive to an industry that could eventually come up with an even better pesticide—which would help us produce more food, for ourselves and the world. When a food additive is banned, it makes some of the Naderite groups happy, and the government content. But as a scientist I know that, too, will not prevent cancer, but will only serve to remove useful products from the shelves, such as diet soft drinks. When OSHA passes carcinogen standards requiring strict regulation of any occupational chemicals that might cause cancer in laboratory animals, this does not prevent human cancer. That goal could be accomplished effectively and efficiently by giving individual attention to known carcinogens. But what it will mean is that consumers will be paying double or triple for dry cleaning in the next few years.

All of us are consumers. All of us are in favor of good health. If a chemical or processing technique, or any other aspect of our environment, threatens our health, we would all be in favor of restricting or curtailing its use. But what a growing number of us are not in favor of is the passage of laws and regulations that do not protect our health and only serve to remove useful things from the market and raise the prices of those that do remain.

What we need, of course, is a new breed of consumer advocate, one who can effectively explode the myth that we have to choose between modern technology and good health. We can have both. Of course we need to keep health-threatening chemicals out of our food, air, and water. However, with today's consumer advocates leading the show, we are heading toward not only zero risk, but zero food, zero jobs, zero energy, and zero growth. It may be that the prophets of doom, not the profits of industry, are the real hazards to our health.

Reducing Environmental Risks

Robert H. Harris, Robert B. Nicholas, and Paul Milvy

We share Elizabeth Whelan's concern that the public be properly informed about the risks posed to their health by their exposure to chemicals that cause cancer, and that governmental regulatory policies concern themselves first and foremost with those cancer risks the reduction of which will result in the greatest improvement in public health. Where we clearly differ, however, is on the interpretation of the "facts" that underpin the government's current regulatory approach and the "impact" of this approach on the reduction in future cancer deaths.

In the spirit of exposing our "biases," as Whelan clearly does in her article, let us divulge some of ours. We might best do this by discussing how we responded to a recent letter from a consumer whom we will call Mrs. Jones, who worried about her grandson's eating habits. Confused over the recent reports on the cancer hazards associated with charcoal-broiled meat and peanut butter, she related how her daughter became so "panicky" that she did not allow her 12-year old son to eat hot dogs or charcoal-broiled steak and hamburgers at picnics. "If he goes to a ball game, every kid eats hot dogs.... She gives him a peanut-butter-and-jelly sandwich. What is a ball game without a hot dog? Now a report comes out that peanut butter may be carcinogenic."

What are parents to do? Our response, not unlike Elizabeth Whelan's would likely be, was to begin by placing the problem in some perspective. First, we told her that cancer is not unique to our modern society. The earliest known cancer is presumed to be the tumor discovered in the fossil remains of a dinosaur from the Comanchean Period of the Mesozoic Era of geologic time (ca. 125 million B.C.). Traces of bone cancer were also found in the remains of the Java Man (ca. 1 million B.C.), and bone cancer was identified in mummies in the Great Pyramid of Gizeh (2500–1500 B.C.). Such evidence, together with studies of primitive populations free of industrial pollution, makes clear that a certain amount of cancer is a natural component of all living systems (plants also get tumors). But both the amount and type of cancer is highly variable from one region of the world to the next, largely reflecting the different environments to which the various populations of the world are exposed. For example, populations exposed to excessive amounts of sunlight have a higher incidence of skin cancer. Individuals whose diets are rich in certain natural chemicals run a high risk of cancer, which explains the high liver cancer rates in certain parts of Africa and the high rates of cancer of the mouth in parts of Asia. Thus, nature does tempt us with its "forbidden fruits."

Next we reminded Mrs. Jones that cancer rates are usually higher in the more industrialized countries of the world, such as the United States, and that rates have been increasing fairly steadily since the turn of the century. In addition to sunlight, diet, and smoking, exposure to certain man-made chemicals, such as vinyl chloride, asbestos, and benzene, has been shown to cause cancer in workers. The geographical variation in cancer rates in the United States can in part be explained by the differences in industrial activity such as chemical manufacturing. But much of the growth in the manufacture of synthetic chemicals in the United States has been recent (post-World War II). Since 1940, for example, there has been approximately a 200-fold increase in the production of synthetic organic chemicals in the United States (Figure 1). Because there is typically a twenty- to forty-year latency between first exposure to a cancer-causing chemical and clinical symptoms of a tumor, the impact of this chemical revolution on U.S. cancer rates has probably not yet been fully expressed.

Therefore, we emphasized to Mrs. Jones that our risk of cancer is determined by our exposure to certain of nature's carcinogens as well as to those created by humans. We told her that what was important, however, was that scientists are now beginning to identify just what components of the environment, both natural and man-made, are most responsible for our current risk of cancer. Through such identification, certain types of cancer are now largely preventable. Reduced exposure to sunlight will decrease the risk of skin cancer; avoidance of cigarettes and alcohol will diminish the risks of lung, bladder, kidney, mouth, and certain gastrointestinal cancers; and a reduced consumption of animal fats may lower the risk of bowel and breast cancer.

FIGURE 1
Total Synthetic Organic Chemicals, Annual Production (Excludes Tar,
Tar Crudes, and Primary Products from Petroleum and Natural Gas)
Total Chemicals and Allied Products, Annual Value Added

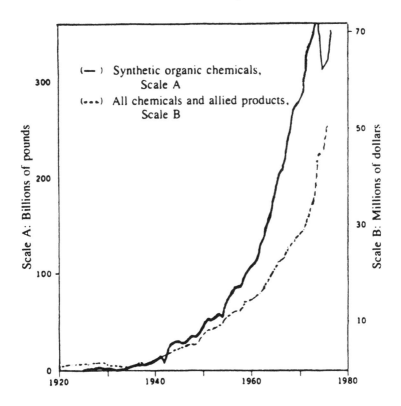

Herein lies the dilemma: avoiding these risks often involves trade-offs which may conflict with our lifestyles. Mrs. Jones's grandson, for example, like most boys, enjoys going to picnics and ball games. Food served at these events, in the true American tradition, often includes charcoal-broiled hamburgers and hot dogs. We now know that certain ways of cooking food, such as charcoal broiling, create certain cancer-causing chemicals in the food. Hot dogs usually also contain nitrate and nitrite preservatives and coloring agents that can lead to the formation of certain potent cancer-causing chemicals. Hamburgers and hot dogs may be contaminated with pesticides that were used to grow the grains that fed the animals. Both are high in animal fat, a high consumption of which may increase the risk of bowel cancer. The alternative food, a peanut-butter sandwich, is likely to be contaminated with low concentrations of aflatoxin, a fungal toxin which ranks as one of the most potent cancer-causing chemicals known to man.

What are the options? First, hamburgers and hot dogs could be cooked in other ways (not charcoal broiled) and at lower temperatures to reduce this hazard. Hot dogs can be purchased that do not contain nitrites and nitrates, and, in both cases, meats can be purchased that were produced with grains for which pesticides were not used. If these options are inconvenient, or judged to be too costly, his parents may decide that his overall diet is not high in animal fats and that an occasional hot dog or hamburger is not inconsistent with that diet. Or a good education on nutrition at home may naturally lead him to feel comfortable in rejecting these foods at social gatherings.

Our answer to Mrs. Jones, in other words, was not a simple yes or no. Life is full of risks and to suggest that we can avoid them all is patently absurd. But this is not to say that if Mrs. Jones, her children, and her grandchildren were better informed they would not be willing to make some trade-offs in their personal lives that could significantly lower their risk of cancer. We are sure that Whelan would agree with our advice to Mrs. Jones that her grandson's overall lifestyle is one important factor in determining his risk of cancer and that some of these risks can be easily lowered. Some cancer risks are easy to avoid and involve little or no expense or inconveniences. For example, when Tris-treated sleepwear was still being sold after Tris [tris (2, 3-dibromopropyl) phosphate] was shown to cause cancer, it could have been avoided since safer alternatives existed at the same or at lower costs. Avoiding certain foods, however, depends on the availability of safer alternatives and the social stigma attached to refusing these foods at social gatherings. Denying a child an occasional hot dog may not be worth the possible conflict he will experience with his peer group. As we told Mrs. Jones, if a battle must be waged over what he can and cannot do with his life, preventing him from smoking cigarettes clearly has greater benefits than preventing him from eating hot dogs.

On the other hand, many cancer risks, such as those associated with air and water pollution, and contamination of our food supply, are difficult, if not impossible, to avoid. Reducing these risks will depend on the collective actions of our society and is clearly dependent on the extent to which society properly perceives the risks. Herein lies Whelan's greatest disservice to her readership. By distorting, misstating fact, and uncritically echoing arguments made by the chemical industry, she seriously misleads the public by downplaying, and occasionally outrightly denying, the generally accepted risks posed by cancer causing chemicals.

As evidence of governmental and public overreaction to chemical exposure, Whelan, while acknowledging the possibility that exposure may contribute to cancer mortality, concludes that "we have no evidence at this point that they do," and downplays the risk by terming it hypothetical. In making this statement Whelan ignores not only the animal evidence she refers to earlier in her remarks but also dismisses the generally accepted epidemiologic evidence on this point. While it is true that the vast majority of chemicals are not known to cause cancer, at least 26 of the 700 chemicals carefully studied by the widely respected International Agency for Research on Cancer have been shown to cause cancer in humans.

Regulation—Costs and Benefits

The recent attacks on government regulation in general, and the regulation of cancer-causing substances in particular, have usually been accompanied by the arguments that the costs of such regulation are excessive (implying that they greatly exceed benefits) and that government regulation has unnecessarily denied the public access to useful products. Whelan embraces this logic when she implies that regulation of carcinogens "only serve[s] to remove useful things from the market and raise the prices of those that do remain." Yet she does not present one single example of a "useful" product that has been banned, leaving higher prices in its wake.

Through a thinly veiled guise of objectivity, Whelan exposes her deeply held prejudices that government regulations are out to get us with statements such as "when a pesticide is banned, I know it is not preventing cancer...the banning has no medical benefits...I will pay more for strawberries and corn next year." Yet we know of no pesticide which has been banned for its cancer-causing properties (and only a handful have been so regulated) whose cancer risk was anything but irrefutable and whose banning resulted in any significant hardship to either farmers or consumers. Take for example the pesticide dieldrin, which was banned by the Environmental Protection Agency (EPA) in 1974. Numerous scientific studies, including several by industry, demonstrated conclusively that dieldrin causes cancer in animals at extremely low concentrations. In fact, laboratory animals were shown to contract cancer at levels typical of those found in human body fat. Furthermore, during the court proceedings that accompanied EPA's banning of dieldrin, industry failed to demonstrate the efficacy of dieldrin for its intended uses, which might even suggest that banning of this persistent pesticide was an economic favor to farmers.

With regard to other "useful" products, such as food additives, Whelan argues that by banning of such products, "...as a scientist, I know that, too, will not prevent cancer, but will only serve to remove useful products from the shelves, such as diet soft drinks." Her target, of course, is saccharin (which has not been banned), and probably other food additives which are only used for cosmetic purposes, such as red dye #2. Cosmetic food additives that are carcinogenic are required to be banned under the Delaney Amendment to the Food, Drug and Cosmetic Act on the logical assumption that the public would rather not bear the cancer risks of continued exposure in the name of enhancing or masking the natural color of foods. Although Whelan's argument assumes that diet drinks and the use of saccharin ward off overweight, the documentation for this simply does not exist. Rather, persuasive studies suggest that no weight reduction results from using saccharin as a sugar substitute. For example, in one careful study obese patients were randomly divided into two diet groups. The diets were identical except that one group consumed artificial sweeteners and the other did not. At the end of the study, those who lost weight, stayed the same weight, or gained weight were unaffected by their use or nonuse of artificial sweeteners. Although it is not clear that saccharin as a sugar replacement reduces dental cavities (another of its suggested virtues), it is easy to demonstrate that for most diabetics whose disease is not extreme the condition can be controlled without the use of diet colas, commercial diet desserts, or the use of saccharin.

That saccharin causes cancer in the male offspring of female rats which had been given very high doses for an extended period is not in dispute. Although it certainly has not been conclusively demonstrated that saccharin is carcinogenic to humans, some recent evidence suggests that high saccharin use is accompanied by a statistically significant increased risk of bladder cancer to women. Other studies have not shown this to be so. Thus, in terms of human epidemiological studies, the situation remains equivocal. This does not mean that it does not cause cancer, only that the evidence is not conclusive one way or the other. In epidemiological studies, scientists tried to show statistically that a few excess cancers are present in a population that consumes saccharin when compared to a similar population that does not. With 22 percent of our population dying of cancer, it is extremely difficult to demonstrate that perhaps 0.01–0.5 percent of them have died because of their exposure to saccharin. Human epidemiology may lack the sensitivity to isolate the effects of this very weak (at least in animal studies) cancer-causing agent from the carcinogens to which we are exposed, many of which are much more potent.

As a complement to the "usefulness" argument, detractors of government regulation of cancer-causing chemicals often cite the alleged high cost to consumers that accompanies such regulation. In an effort to accuse government regulators and "Naderite groups" of overstatement in the name of public safety, Whelan asserts that OSHA's (Occupational Safety and Health Administration) recently developed cancer policy requires regulation of chemicals that "might" cause cancer in animals and "...what it will mean is that consumers will be paying double or triple for dry cleaning in the next few years."

First of all, OSHA's cancer policy has a very strict requirement as to what evidence represents an acceptable basis for concluding that a chemical causes cancer and, as Whelan is well aware, the scientific community is nearly unanimous in its conclusion that chemicals which, in well-conducted studies, unambiguously cause cancer in laboratory animals represent a cancer risk to humans. But her main point is that, apart from whether or not a chemical really represents a cancer hazard to the public, regulation is costly and has been bad economic news to consumers.

While it is undoubtedly true that regulation involves direct cost to industry, the costs are frequently overestimated. Whelan's dry-cleaning example is a reference to the efforts by OSHA and by the Consumer Product Safety Commission (CPSC) to reduce the exposure of workers and the public to the cancer-causing dry-cleaning solvent, perchloroethylene. Contrary to the implications of her statement, modern dry-cleaning establishments have installed very tight machines that allow little "perc" to escape. A new line of dry-to-dry machines has been introduced (replacing with a single unit the two separate "washer" and "dryer" units previously used). Although the newer machines are 30 to 60 percent more expensive than the separate units, their use results not only in a much reduced cancer risk to workers but also reduction in the cost of replacing the lost "perc" as well as reduced operating expenses.

Vinyl chloride, a high-volume chemical used in the manufacture of plastics, is an example of a chemical recently regulated by OSHA, CPSC, and other agencies—regulation that had little or no adverse economic impact on the industry, despite its early claims that regulation would produce devastating economic consequences. As has been the case for several chemicals, vinyl chloride was shown to cause cancer in laboratory animals several years before the tragic human evidence precipitated regulatory action in 1975. In opposing the new OSHA standard, the manufacturers of vinyl chloride (V.C.) had argued that they could meet the new standard only through huge price increases that would make V.C. uncompetitive with other types of plastics. In point of fact, V.C. did not increase disproportionately in price (although inflation has modestly raised the price of all plastics) because industry developed two extremely simple methods for reducing worker exposure that have cost very little and allowed the recapture of most of the V.C. vented to the environment—an economic plus. *Chemical Week* headlined an article on this subject in September 1976: "PVC Rolls Out of Jeopardy, into Jubilation." In this instance we see an example of a new regulation forcing the development of a technological improvement beneficial to all society. This experience is hardly unique.

That decreased human exposure to cancer-causing chemicals results in financial savings to industry is not always true, of course. But for Whelan to talk about higher cost, fewer jobs, reduced productivity, and higher taxes, though factually correct in certain instances, gives the impression that these costs are unjustified. Direct costs imposed by regulation are only part of the story. Pollution control adds to our store of healthy citizens, reducing hospital costs and absenteeism, and creating more useful lives.

Although the aggregate costs of regulating cancer-causing chemicals have not been determined, environmental pollution control in general has added only a modest cost (roughly 0.2 percent per year during 1975–1980) to the production of goods and services, as Figure 2 indicates. Similar calculations reveal that these costs have added only about 0.1 percent to the inflation rate this year, while actually creating about 400,000 jobs. In a study which was prepared for the President's Council on Envi-

FIGURE 2
Percent Annual Increase in Consumer Price Index
with and without Environmental Controls

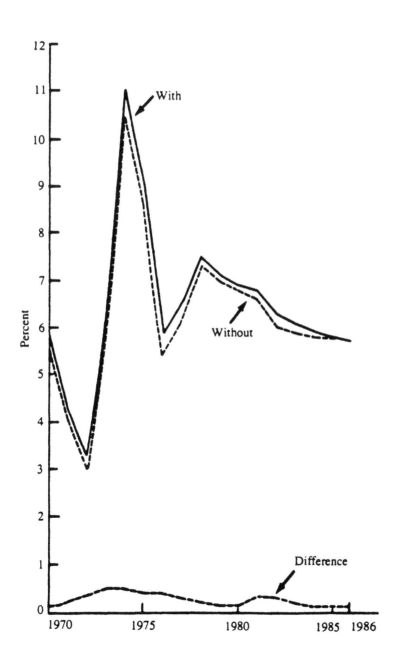

ronmental Quality by Professor Myrick Freeman at Bowdoin College, it was estimated, for example, that the benefits from improvements in air quality amounted to about $21 billion in 1978. (Seventeen billion dollars as a result of reduction of pollution-related deaths and illnesses—asthma, bronchitis, emphysema, and lung cancer—$2 billion in soiling and cleaning costs reductions, as well as smaller savings from corrosion prevention, property value increases, increased agricultural yields, etc.) Despite the large uncertainties in this estimate, including omission of a number of important benefits difficult to assign a dollar value, such as improved visibility, this benefit estimate exceeds the nationwide cost estimate of $19 billion to clean up air pollution in 1978.

Cancer Trends

The cancer debate often revolves around discussion of the proportion of today's cancer rate that is due to various activities such as smoking, diet, occupational exposure, and pollution. But because of the 20- to 40-year latency problem referred to earlier, this debate has only limited usefulness in predicting future cancer patterns. However, recent trends in cancer incidence may reveal important clues to future rates. In discussing these trends Whelan erroneously asserts that the National Cancer Institute (NCI) data show an overall slight decline in cancer incidence during the last several decades. In fact, what the NCI data show, to quote the American Cancer Society's *Cancer Facts and Figures, 1980,* is that "the overall incidence of cancer decreased slightly from 1947 to 1970, but has increased between 5 and 10 percent since 1970" (actually from 1970 to 1976, the latest data analyzed). So cancer trends, which had begun to level off (they have been increasing steadily since the turn of the century, although considerably more slowly after the Second World War), have or may have started again to increase. What is of concern to many cancer specialists, of course, is the possibility that this apparent reversal in trend is due to the public's exposure to man-made chemicals which accompanied the significant increase in the production of synthetic chemicals after the War (see Figure 1), and that this is just the beginning of a significant upward trend in cancer incidence.

In the case of occupational causes of cancer, Whelan attempts to downplay this problem by arguing that worker exposure to carcinogens could not possibly explain more than 5 percent of the cancer mortality rate. Although we would agree that much uncertainty is associated with this estimate, a very strong argument can be made that considerably more cancer in the near future will be related to occupational carcinogens. To come up with a reliable estimate is extremely difficult, but to dismiss this possibility and possibly to err on the side of imprudence, seems to us to be ill advised. Five percent of cancer mortality may, when so expressed, seem relatively minor. Yet it represents 20,000 deaths, more than four-fold more deaths than from job-related accidents. If Whelan would vigorously pursue safety-related measures to decrease accidents on the job, she should also consider reducing long-term cancer risks in the work place.

We would agree with Whelan that smoking is the primary cause of lung cancer. However, her attempt to downplay the potential of chemicals as causative agents in lung cancer is misleading. Whelan seeks to support her position by stating that lung-cancer mortality is identical in the county of Rutland, Vermont, and in the state of New Jersey. The facts are true, but very misleading. Even a state like New Jersey, with its "cancer alley," has large numbers of rural communities which tend to dilute the urban and industrial cancer rates. In Vermont, Rutland's white male cancer rate is more than 20 percent higher than the state average. The explanation for this, according to a representative of the Rutland Hospital's cancer registry, may well be the dust exposure experienced by the large number of men who work in Rutland's important industry, the quarrying of marble, granite, and in earlier years, slate. The wide range of variation among Vermont counties can be illustrated by comparing Chittenden and Essex. Chittenden County, which has considerable industry, has an incidence of lung cancer equally as high as Rutland County's; but rural Essex County has a lung cancer rate 60 percent lower than Rutland's. Similar variations in counties are seen in New Jersey. Nevertheless, it remains true that New Jersey is, in general, more industrialized than Vermont. And, according to NCI, the total cancer mortality during the 20-year period, 1950–1969, was 18.5 percent higher for men and 8.4 percent higher for women in New Jersey than in Vermont. In the case of lung cancer, 24.7 percent more New Jersey men were dying from lung cancer than Vermont men. This is an extremely large differential cancer mortality rate, especially since it reflects exposures to cancer-causing materials that probably occurred during the 1930–1950 interval when "cancer alley" was not yet even a well-beaten path.

"Toxic Chemicals and Public Protection," a recent report to the president by the Toxic Substances Strategy Committee, presents a comprehensive analysis of cancer trends. The report was endorsed by experts from all federal departments and agencies which had major policy, research, or regulatory responsibilities related to control of potentially hazardous chemicals. We hope that Whelan is correct in her belief that cancer trends are not increasing, but it would be unwise and not in the public interest to ignore the more recent data as set forth in this report and in several recent scientific journals.

Lastly, we take strong exception to Whelan's belief, expressed in the final paragraph of a report she prepared for the American Council on Science and Health, *Cancer in the United States: Is There an Epidemic?*, that cancer is due not to "society and the environment, not [to] cells of the body but either [to] an unwillingness to learn or an inability to act." For what she implies, by indicating our lifestyle as the cause of cancer, is that each of us is individually responsible for acts that lead us to get cancer.

It is undoubtedly true that a significant reduction in cancer risk can result from individual changes in lifestyle—reduced smoking and certain dietary changes, for example. But as importantly, strong and abundant evidence implicates exposures deriving from modern industrial processes in the genesis of a significant fraction of all cancer cases. Most, if not all, such exposures are involuntary—frequently we do not even know when or to what we are exposed—and therefore not within an individual's ability to control.

Even in the apparently simple cases involving better recognized risks—smoking, for example—the lines between individual and collective choice often become somewhat fuzzy. Although composition of our diet, and whether we smoke and drink, are clearly within our ability to control as individuals, how we collectively license the public communications network has an important impact as well. Smoking advertisements (a third of a billion dollars are spent on them every year by U.S. companies) bombard us daily with the message that smoking is sexy, stylish, and "with it." There is no doubt that many smokers are, in a very real sense, both psychologically and physically addicted. To call smoking an individual decision that is freely chosen is simply to ignore the effects of advertising on individuals' values and perceptions. In our view the need for collective action is clear. The only question is the manner in which the authority is exercised.

Over the years, society has strongly supported government's authority to act to prevent substantial risks to public health and safety. The more than two dozen federal statutes covering the routes by which certain chemicals or aspects of chemical use can threaten human health and the environment embody a preventative approach, mandating the testing and evaluating of products before they are allowed on the market. These authorities, as well as embodying a precautionary principle, mandate government action when evidence of a hazard is strongly suggestive but not completely certain, and generally provide that the risk of uncertainty—the lack of knowledge about the safety of a product—be borne by the manufacturer and not by the general public. Public experience with DES, Thalidomide, Kepone, and vinyl chloride amply support the rationale of this approach. While government regulation can and must be improved, we do not believe it should be improved at the expense of public health.

Whelan concludes that the regulatory zealots are leading us toward a society that has no food, no energy, and no growth, albeit a society without risk. We do not believe this dire forecast is at all persuasive. Rather we believe that a society with reduced environmental risks is both compatible with economic growth and necessary for the improvement of the quality of our lives.

Cancer and Corporations

Robert Crawford

For Elizabeth Whelan, the public's fear of cancer seems to have spawned a new disease, more malignant than cancer itself. This new illness, *cancerphobia,* menaces the social body just as certainly as its progenitor imperils the physical body. Now evidently of epidemic proportions, cancerphobia can be traced to an antitechnology irrationalism, a backwater chemical anxiety, a cold-sweat fear of modern living. Whelan perceives the carriers of this newest social pathology as "prophets of doom," the source of the misinformation on cancer which "directs" the policies of the regulatory agencies concerned with health. The consequences are said to be far reaching. Industry suffers from "more regulation, higher costs, fewer jobs, and limited production." Consumers experience "high prices, higher taxes, fewer products—a diminished standard of living." Aligned against these hazards is a new breed of public-health educator—the scientist-consumer, lending perspective to the uncontrollable mass of public confusion.

Unreasonable fears about imagined threats should be discouraged; the appeal for caution, commended. Everything does not cause cancer. The economy cannot be paralyzed. Media coverage, which feeds the public discrete reports and single points of view released to support one or another side, only serves to confuse. Carcinogen-of-the-day humor has become a public nuisance. If people are to make sense of all that is being said about cancer, the cool, disinterested testimony of scientific expertise is welcome.

The trouble is that the experts do not agree. The search for the "facts" invariably runs into the selective presentation of facts, along with a profusion of nonscientific judgments and interpretations hidden in a jungle of jargon. How is the nonexpert to form a sensible assessment when scientific and political perspectives have become hopelessly entangled?

Cancer has become one of the most controversial issues of our time. In such a climate, where charges and countercharges over cause and responsibility are as numerous as the credentials of the adversaries, anxiety becomes almost rational. Matters are further complicated when almost daily one reads or hears corporate advertisements proclaiming the safety of one or another industrial technology and the safety consciousness or record of one or another industry. Why is so much effort being expended, the typical cancerphobe might ask?

While the following is not an appeal to avoid the complex, scientific issues involved, it is an argument that the classical political questions of *who gets what and how* are essential to understanding the cancer issue as well. I have seen credible, opposing perspectives to almost every empirical issue contained (often implicitly) in Whelan's article. Other respondents will address some of these. A political analysis, however, will provide a useful framework, unavoidably entailing a point of view, from which scientific claims and other assertions might be more clearly understood. Attitudes are formed, after all, from experiences which extend beyond the technical discussions of proof, test design and validity, reasonable extrapolations from the data, and perennial questions about the status of Canadian rats. Are such experiences and attitudes to be discounted as irrational? Should policy makers, while necessarily requiring the guidance of scientific expertise, bypass mass public sentiment which cannot possibly be familiar with the detailed scientific debates?

Whelan denies what I take to be axiomatic when she asserts optimistically that "we would all be in favor of restricting or curtailing" threats to our health (implying that health is simply a matter of pursuing the most rational route to agreed-upon goals). My departing assumption is the opposite—that corporations are willing to tolerate health threats to the public as an unfortunate but necessary byproduct of a perceived higher good. If this is true, how corporations then protect themselves from a health-conscious public, a consciousness which threatens corporate objectives, is an urgent analytical task. But first, it would be helpful to look at how prevention, and thus cancer, emerged as a public issue.

Politics of Prevention

Just a decade ago, the public's fear of cancer was the occasion for a proclaimed war. Federal money flooded into cancer research, a multimillion dollar a year enterprise. Now, at the beginning of the 1980s, another war unfolds: in place of a war on cancer, there is today a war *over* cancer. Instead of seeing the public's fear of cancer as a legitimate concern about a "growing epidemic" and mandating the massive injection of governmental research dollars, the experts now debate whether we are faced with an epidemic at all. It is important to note the two periods because they so clearly illustrate the political nature of the public discussion. In 1971, the primary cancer lobby was the biomedical research establishment. In 1981, there was a different set of political-economic interests mobilized, attempting to define the nature of the cancer problem and shape the direction of public policy. What happened in those ten years to change the terms of the cancer debate?

The short answer is that we have moved into the age of prevention. Certainly, the biomedical research scientists continue to be the masters of publicity, more than willing to appear in white coat, explaining new therapeutic advances and carefully avoiding mention of persisting survival rates. A steady diet of "breakthroughs" stirs the imagination. Nonetheless, during the last ten years, medicine's jurisdictional claims in the war against cancer have been steadily eroded. Even voices from within the medical world have begun to proclaim its limitations .

By the mid-1970s, several forces, each with its own history, converged to make prevention a pressing political and policy issue. One of these was the earlier success of environmental and labor constituencies in creating new legislation and agencies whose mission would be the reduction of environmental and occupational health hazards. Another was the proliferation of American and world-wide scientific studies, both laboratory and human, identifying risk factors associated with the major chronic diseases. Especially with regard to cancer, the studies gave the regulatory agencies the ammunition they needed to act. The activities of these agencies, in turn, sparked a revival of interest in public-health issues. Small environmental and occupational health movements grew in size and visibility. Anti-nuclear protests developed into a mass movement. Social action had become health conscious.

Largely due to all this new activity, a number of public health warnings and disasters were brought to public attention: PCBs, kepone, saccharin, pesticides, contamination of drinking water, asbestos, vinyl chlorides, DES, Three Mile Island, Love Canal and toxic wastes, and, of course, the accumulation and dissemination of further evidence about three of America's favorite pastimes—the consumption of high fat and high cholesterol foods, tobacco, and alcohol. For still other reasons, to be discussed below, prevention became, by the late 1970s, a widely discussed topic in health policy and medical circles and among the middle class.

The resulting awareness, concern, and polarization over these issues, along with the opening of the new regulatory arenas, politicized health and disease. Prevention became embroiled with other issues and with an array of political tendencies in American life. By 1980, it had become more difficult for the public to think of illness as simply a medical problem. Among growing numbers of people there was suddenly an inkling that vast economic and political forces were at work to shape the course of health and disease. Unlike the relatively stable politics of medical care, prevention emerged as a political unknown—less institutionalized, less amenable to licensed, professional monopolies, and more fractionated by political and economic groups mobilized to protect or extend their interests. Medicine had clearly failed and thus government, industry, and the public, although each manifesting multiple tendencies, began to forge their own health strategies.

Ironically, industry helped create the prevention issue. In the mid-1970s, sectors of the corporate world, along with government officials and the academic policy sciences, turned their attention to the growing problem of medical-care costs. Inflation in the medical sector had become burdensome for everyone; but for government, faced with increasing fiscal pressures, and industry, encountering rapidly rising premiums, medical costs had become critical. A consensus slowly emerged that the medical monolith needed taming, and a broad-based, cost-control coalition began mobilizing to impose reforms. The politics of expansion of medical services, equality of access, and the extension of entitlements, characteristic of the 1960s and early 1970s, was superseded by a politics which would attempt to curb growth, entitlements, and access. The hospital-medical lobby, however, would not be easily dislodged, and thus, direct cost-control reforms were supplemented with intermediate stratagems: public hospitals were closed and other government programs terminated; Medicaid benefits were constricted; and Medicare and private insurance shifted more of the burden of payments to workers and consumers in hope that additional personal responsibility for costs would act as a deterrent to utilization. Comprehensive national health insurance became a dead issue.

Following the lead of the Canadian Minister of Health, Marc Lalonde, health-policy discussions in the United States turned to the idea of prevention as an antidote to spiraling medical costs. Keeping people out of hospitals by keeping them healthy seemed a promising, long-term solution. Healthier employees, moreover, would help lower industry premium rates, cut absenteeism, and improve productivity.

Health promotion, however, contained an even more important symbolic function. The public discussion of prevention—a prevention campaign—might serve to reassure workers and the general public, who had come to see medical care as a right to be guaranteed by work place arrangements or government financing, that less medical care is not equivalent to less health. Thus, even though work place and government entitlements were being eroded, and national health insurance delayed indefinitely, medical benefits would be replaced by a new corporate and governmental commitment to employee and public health. Further, individual responsibility for health, not national health insurance, could be promoted as the optimal solution to both the cost crisis and health maintenance. As of the late 1970s, prevention linked to cost control would become the *cause cèlébre* of national health policy.

Of course, prevention is a broad concept. It allows for the possibility of widely differing definitions and directions. In the political context of the last several years, there has been a tendency to define prevention with almost exclusive emphasis as either a problem of industrial hazards, or as a problem of individual lifestyles and at-risk behaviors, especially smoking. In the lifestyle approach, health education and individual responsibility are the means to better health. It is this definition, with environmental and occupational hazards relegated to the status of "also rans," which has, outside the regulatory agencies, become the prevailing understanding. Promotional activities equating prevention with lifestyle changes have become standard fare. For the corporations, the need for such an emphasis is obvious. Prevention, like pollution before it, needs to be portrayed as an individual problem.

For government officials, only slightly more complex considerations need be mentioned. First, if gains in prevention are to be made, simple political calculation discourages policy makers from bothering too much about reforms which would require a political realignment which presently does not exist. Even though the evidence for large-scale behavior change is not encouraging either, at least there are fewer political obstacles, the tobacco lobby notwithstanding, to health-education efforts aimed at individual health promotion. Moreover, as will be discussed below, a new and significant cultural interest in personal health may reinforce efforts to change lifestyles.

Second, in the more practical context of building and maintaining support for policy priorities, holding together the coalition for cost control, not prevention, is most essential. If the entrenched political power of the hospital-medical lobby is to be broken, corporate support cannot be jeopardized. Pressing for environmental and occupational reforms as a primary prevention strategy would undermine an already tenuous coalition, especially with regard to regulatory, cost-control policies.

Finally, at a very general but not-to-be-overlooked level, the fiscal vitality of government as well as both short-term political viability of ruling parties and long-term stability of governments are dependent on the health of the corporate-controlled economy. Even before Reagan, many political leaders were convinced of the industry perspective that more inducements, not more constraints, were necessary in order to stimulate growth and investment. Even the smoking issue could not be pressed too far for fear of the economic and political repercussions. Nonetheless, much to the consternation of those industries which thrive from the at-risk behaviors, prevention has become practically synonymous with the campaign against "sloth, gluttony, alcoholic intemperance, reckless driving, sexual frenzy and smoking." (The words come from the late John Knowles, past president of the Rockefeller Foundation.) Perceived as *victim blaming* among environmental and occupational-health activists and their supporters, this formulation of the prevention problem has itself turned into one of the major issues in the debate over cancer and other health risks.

New Health Consciousness

The interest in prevention, and, in particular, a focus on lifestyle and health, can also be seen at other levels of American society. Not only has there been a surge in popular concern about environmental and occupational health hazards—what Whelan refers to as cancerphobia—but a new health consciousness and health movements are beginning to transform cultural values about personal health. The new health consciousness has generated a vocal and often aggressive anti-smoking ethic, the proliferation of popular health magazines, massive consumption of vitamins and other health aids, profound changes in dietary habits, and a transformation of tens of thousands of sedentaries into marathon runners. If one were to conclude anything about popular health attitudes in contemporary America, it would be that people, especially the middle class, are beginning to take matters of individual health promotion seriously. Contrary to corporate phobias of an aroused, industry-baiting public, Americans are directing their energies toward lifestyle changes.

There is no simple explanation for the current "wellness" enthusiasm. Certainly, as suggested, it has been promoted. The media are flooded with guides to better health, health-related television series, health features in magazines, and health themes in advertising. But this phenomenon must reflect, in part, a perceived interest and demand for such material. The promotion of lifestyle-oriented prevention efforts by both government and private groups has also stimulated the growth of professional and entrepreneurial interests, quick to perceive opportunities for expansion and new markets. The health-education profession and consulting firms specializing in employee health promotion are examples. Hospitals have also discovered the public-relations values of health promotion.

But why has the professional middle class particularly been so receptive? And how does one explain why large numbers of people attempt difficult lifestyle changes, like quitting smoking, or other changes, like diet, which require an investment of time and money? And why are there so many joggers? Understanding the new health consciousness is important if for no other reason than to combat reductionistic characterizations of popular health attitudes like Whelan's visions of cancerphobia and chain-smoking anti-nuclear demonstrators. Causal understanding is extremely complex, but here are a few observations.

First, personal-health promotion is likely to appear to many people as the only possible alternative to a health-threatening environment which eludes control. Both the number of health hazards communicated in the last decade and the seeming intractability of most of them leave people with a sense of having few options. In the absence of a clear commitment by society to health promotion, individual responsibility comes to be seen as a necessity. The most difficult individual adjustments will be attempted. As individuals, we all face the same dilemma: we cannot afford to wait for a political solution, so we adopt health practices which we believe will reduce our risk. The loss of control over health is "eased by its endless pursuit. "

Second, much of the new interest in lifestyle and health is connected with the cultural diffusion of two important health movements—self-care/self-help and holistic health. The growth of these movements (and, I would argue, the spread of the prevention-lifestyle ethic in general) derives, in part, from popular disenchantment with medicine. Tracing the disaffection is, again, complex, but anger about costs and iatrogenesis, the lack of significant therapeutic success for most of the major chronic diseases, and an unhappiness about the experience of the medical encounter and the dependence on drugs and doctors are all important. The holistic health and the self-care/self-help movements have articulated these discontents and communicated them to wider publics.

Third, the enhancement and control of personal health finds fertile ground in a middle-class population which in the 1970s was forced to adjust to a world of increased insecurity and uncertainty. Not only did people experience an assault of health hazard warnings, but the long wave of post-Second World War economic prosperity began to show the first signs of ebbing. When social life is experienced as eluding control, particularly when people begin to wonder whether a standard of living to which they have become accustomed can be sustained, the need for personal control is often intensified. Personal health has become one area into which people can throw their energies and reassert some sense that they can act on their own behalf. Of course, middle-class people not only have more time and resources for health-promotion activities, they have also acquired fundamental notions about themselves as social actors from work situations and other supporting socializing patterns which predispose them to seeing their achievements as a result of personal effort alone.

Finally, the conception of health which is now applied to prevention retains key medical notions which situate the problem of health and disease at the level of the individual body. In medicine, the individual is the locus of both perception and intervention. Thus, medical perception pushes causal understanding toward the immediate and local, and solution toward the elimination of symptoms and the restoration of normal signs. The new health movements and prevention consciousness modify several important medical concepts, but in one direction only: toward host resistance and adaptation. Social considerations beyond immediate psychological atmospheres are most often neglected. Health promotion remains an individual endeavor.

There are several other explanatory directions one could pursue, connections with social currents both long-standing and recent (e.g., links with the human potential and environmental movements, or cultural traditions about health at least back to the Victorians). What is clear, however, is that the political focus of the environmental and occupational health movements and the public's concern about industrial carcinogens are only part of the total cultural turn toward prevention. Moreover, for complicated reasons, substantial segments of the public, although perhaps holding the more political views as well, have adopted the dominant ideological position that prevention is a problem of lifestyle and requires the assumption of individual responsibility. After all, as we are often reminded, it does make good sense.

Prevention Of Politics

From the foregoing, it can be seen that the age of prevention is evolving and being constructed on several levels. There are powerful forces which converge to define the problem of prevention as a matter of individual behaviors, attitudes, and emotions. Different but overlapping events and forces have given rise to an environmental and occupational understanding of the health problem—a definition which implicates industry. It is difficult to know which way the prevention issue will turn. The ways the public thinks about and acts upon their anxieties and hopes for good health and long life, their understanding of what should be done to promote or maintain health, and their notions of accountability and responsibility are all in flux. The instability of popular perceptions of both problem and solution, especially in a period which will inevitably produce more occupational and environmental health disasters and further discovery of carcinogenic outcomes from industrial products and processes, is the critical ideological and political problem facing the corporations. What is evident is that prevention has become much riskier than corporate executives had ever imagined. The dilemma facing the corporations is that the public discussion and popularity of prevention, even in the form of lifestyle changes and individual responsibility, may reinforce a potentially uncontainable health consciousness. The dilemma cannot be easily resolved since victim-blaming notions of prevention are one of the few ways attention can be diverted from industry. The outlines of an attempted resolution, however, can be seen in Elizabeth Whelan's article. Unlike that of plutonium, the half-life of prevention may have already passed.

Whelan's article contains the classical victim-blaming ingredients: the citation of studies which minimize environmental and occupational health hazards and maximize at-risk behaviors. "As a society," writes Whelan, "we seem to be drifting toward a policy which tolerates known, major risks chosen by the individual—and rejects hypothetical risks that might be assumed by industry or society as a whole." But the real emphasis of her article can be found elsewhere and can be summarized in three points: 1) we are healthier than we think; or certainly, let's not think in terms of epidemics; 2) an irrational cancerphobia—what others sometimes call a Chicken Little syndrome—grips the American public; and 3) we must begin thinking in terms of "acceptable risks"; that is, we must increase our tolerance of an inevitably risky society if we are to continue to enjoy our prosperity. The three are closely linked arguments.

If the primary political concern is to minimize the possibility that the normally quiescent public will become politicized around health issues, the last word one would want thrown about is *epidemic*. It is a mobilizing word, likely to evoke flight or fight. It suggests that all of society's resources and defenses need to be galvanized into action (which is precisely why the biomedical research establishment continues using it). "There has been an increase in cancer mortality in the last few decades," writes Whelan, "but certainly nothing on the order of 'epidemic.'" The fact is that there is no objective way to define *epidemic:* if the "rapidly spreading" part of the definition is emphasized, a usage usually associated with infectious diseases, cancer may not qualify; whereas if the "widespread" or "prevalent" part is stressed, a different determination might be reached. It is not surprising to me that people would assign the term *epidemic* to a disease which, if present trends continue, 25 percent of us will contract and from which 20 percent of us will die. But to Whelan, it is a sure sign of cancerphobia.

Cancerphobia is one of those rhetorical expressions that are clearly designed to stigmatize and belittle political opposition. It is an attribution of both sickness and extremism (combining the best of political slander). Like Spiro Agnew's "nattering nabobs of negativism," cancerphobes are naysayers who neurotically advance the position that "we have to choose between modern technology and good health." Mysteriously, can-cerphobia "is dictating federal policy." For Whelan, the source of can-cerphobia is a combination of anti-technology sentiment, chemical anxiety, and "a new philosophy" which requires the assessment of blame for dis-ease. The latter, in turn, "resulted from our new emphasis on cancer and the environment." Attached to this circular bit of reasoning is the classic lack-of-proof argument. Since Whelan's definitions of the state of the cancer-research art rarely allows us to attribute cause or probable links, the desire to affix responsibility and to restrict exposure to suspected carcinogens amounts to desperation. After all, we are reminded, "death and disease are still natural processes." Finally, the reader is warned that it becomes "economically disastrous for a society when there is no proof of guilt." The prophecy of economic disaster brings us to the *pièce de résistance* of the new ideology: risk acceptability.

Acceptance of Risk

The discussion of risk and health has several dimensions and can only be touched upon here. The application of risk-benefit analysis to regula-tory decisions, for example, would require a thorough discussion of its history and methodology. An excellent critical introduction can be found in an article by David Noble in the July/August, 1980, issue of *Health/ PAC Bulletin*. Despite appearances of scientific rationality, risk-benefit analysis is not likely to result in a less political regulatory decision pro-cess, since methodologies will inevitably reflect subjective judgments with regard to practically every element in the risk-benefit equation. The determination of an appropriate definition and measure of benefit, for instance, is, at core, a political discussion. Noble argues that risk-benefit analysis shifts the locus of decision making into a mode more clearly dominated by business considerations and makes the decision process even more remote from citizen competence and judgment. I will confine myself to the part of the argument aimed at undercutting public support for *any* effort to force the reduction of industrial hazards.

It is legitimate for a society to ask how much risk is acceptable in relation to expected benefit. Choices are made which have consequences for public health at all stages of research, production, use, and disposal of industrial products. The reduction of risks may involve significant added costs—both in terms of time and resources devoted to researching the question and reducing the discovered risk. The presumption on which the need for regulation is premised is that the rational, private firm will reduce only those risks believed likely to cost the firm more if left unreduced. For corporations, which must continually operate in a social and political environment of actual and potential opposition, economic decisions affecting health risks to workers and the public depend unavoidably on the answers to several political questions. Will existing regulations and the successful enforcement of those regulations result in costly recalls, product removals, burdensome fines, or mandated alteration of manufacturing processes? Will liability suits and compensation claims be successful? Are those costs too high? If disasters do occur, can government be counted on to help pay the costs of cleanup or rectification? Will public anger or perceptions of high risk lead to market sanctions?

These calculations involve every facet of potential regulatory, legislative, legal, and public reaction—including, of course, the political and ideological capacity of industry to weaken or neutralize those threats. Thus, the level of "allowed" or acceptable" risk is best understood as a politically determined outcome. It reflects the relative power of corporations, consumers, workers, and the general public. Risk acceptability, in other words, depends on the success of contending ideologies and the political-economic power brought to bear to enforce them. The first objective of corporate-risk ideology is to trivialize the public perception of industrial hazards. Unlike the lack-of-proof tactic, which is aimed at minimizing industrial, causal responsibility, the risk argument stresses the insignificance of industrial hazards by presenting them as comparable to mundane and inevitable risks of everyday life.

Modern living, asserts this new ideology, like living in any age, is characterized by inevitable risks. Taking risks is synonymous with being in the world—getting out of bed in the morning, crossing the street, etc. We take risks because we value the activities we pursue. We ride in airplanes; we drive autos; in other words, we make daily choices which involve risks. These choices follow from explicit or implicit calculations which help us determine whether the risk is acceptable. Essentially, the argument goes, we weigh risk against benefit. Likewise, as a society we are confronted with similar choices and calculations. The contention is made that, in principle, judgments about risk acceptability should be no different for valued social activities, like producing chemicals, than for valued activities pursued by the individual. Since people are willing to assume individual risks, they should also accept equivalent risks from industry. People are irrational or "confused" if they seek a lower level of imposed risks than assumed risks. Elaborate calculations are often made to demonstrate, for example, that driving a number of miles to and from work is equivalent to or much more dangerous than the risk of living next to a nuclear power plant. If industrial risks are really no different in kind or degree from the hundreds of risks assumed daily by everyone, then what is all the fuss about?

Many people will find appealing the argument that the risk of cancer from one or another industrial source is no more probable than being killed driving to work or falling off a ladder. Unless burdened with a family history of cancer, people are likely to believe they will win out in the statistical gamble. The belief in the strength of one's resistance allows many people to smoke without fear of cancer, for example. Familiar risks are more reassuring because it seems, at least in the healthy years of life, we almost always are lucky. Judgments about risks on any one day are far different than for the span of a lifetime. People tend to stop thinking about risks taken daily.

Second, assertions about public confusion regarding risks hide an even more fundamental issue underlying the politicization of environmental and occupational health. Public support for controls on industry may reflect not only a perception of unacceptable levels of risk, but a pervasive lack of trust that corporations will place the health of the public and the work force above considerations of profit. In other words, the issue for many people may not simply be risks to health, but corporate irresponsibility—not a fear of chemicals so much as a fear of chemical *companies*. If an historical mistrust of industry leads to perceptions of negligence, carelessness, or venality, the political issue emerges as very different in kind than if the problem is considered one of acceptable risks and benefits. Is one any less rational than the other? A person need not be an expert in order to reach a conclusion about corporate behavior, whereas risk-benefit assessment is a complex matter more suited to professional policy analysts.

Moreover, most people now seem reluctant to allow any expansion of government power unless some vital aspect of the public's welfare is at stake *and* the institutions responsible for the problem cannot be trusted. Both industry and government compete for lowest ranking in public perceptions of credibility. Issues of credibility have been important in the politicization of almost every major public-health issue. Why did MGM refuse to spend more money on sprinklers in its Las Vegas hotel? Will the utility companies cover up nuclear safety violations or fail to report accidents? Did corporate managers know that asbestos was deadly but continue producing it anyway? Did Ford know about and let stand a Pinto defect that could cost hundreds of lives? What shortcuts were made in the construction or maintenance of DC-10s? Do chemical companies knowingly dump dangerous chemicals, and do they conspire to cover up the evidence? Are the textile companies telling the truth about brown lung disease? Perhaps there would be less of the claimed double standard about assumed and imposed risks if people had more trust. The fact is that they do not. The question of benefit is already on the public's mind, but asked somewhat differently than the corporations would like: Whose benefit is being served when the public is put at risk? The issue is as old as capitalism itself.

The discussion of risk versus benefit bring us to the third, and I think most cynical, objective of risk polemics. In the last decade, so the argument goes, we have been thinking a great deal about risks, but very little about benefits. As a consequence, we are teetering on the edge of economic catastrophe. When everything else fails, the best way to neutralize the public's anxiety about cancer and corporate motives is to introduce into the debate an even greater anxiety. A risk-conscious society and what follows in the form of unreasonable regulation of industry will lead to economic hardship; or as Whelan claims, to "zero food, zero jobs, zero energy, and zero growth." *The prophets of doom, it turns out, are those who see a threat to the profits of industry in a health-conscious public.* America was made great by an entrepreneurial spirit based on risk-taking; and now a public living in morbid fear of cancer and other hazards threatens progress itself. Thus, while the lack-of-proof defense *minimizes* corporate responsibility for cancer, and victim blaming *shifts* the burden of responsibility to the individual, and the first part of the risk argument *trivializes* industrial risks, now this freezing-in-the-dark imagery *maximizes* the public's acceptance of higher risks through crude scare tactics. Americans must begin thinking in terms of trade-offs.

Americans are used to thinking in such terms. Historically, threats of added hardships have been wielded against workers and communities in order to silence voices opposing existing hardships. People have often capitulated to "we-can't-afford-it" polemics, not because they believed the claim, but because of the willingness of corporations to use economic coercion to achieve their objectives. The near-absolute control over production, the national and international mobility of corporations, and the availability of areas where people are more "willing" to accept industry's terms make the threats believable. Factory closures, including the flight of hazardous industries, are already a stark reality for growing numbers of industrial workers and communities. As unemployment increases and real wages fall, the threat of more of the same is a powerful force for inducing acquiescence. Without the threat of economic coercion, and the willingness of industry to act on that threat, the corporate-risk ideology would fall flat.

Under these conditions, people are more likely to "accept" yet higher levels of risk. But Americans will continue to worry about health. Acceptance of higher risks is not the same as believing that those risks are insignificant. I suspect that people will remain mistrustful or angry, even as they become more resigned. Those who have come to believe in prevention might put in an extra mile on the track. If the stress induced by the entire "reindustrialization" effort is not too great, those who are able will drink and smoke less. Public reaction to the inevitable public-health disasters, however, will continue to pose serious problems for the corporate reindustrialization scenario. Barring the discovery of a cure, cancer will remain a political issue. Thus, we will continue to witness the massive investments by industry in health-related defensive advertising and read articles, like Elizabeth Whelan's, which combine the full arsenal of corporate arguments. For, much to the dismay of some, the profits of industry will remain linked with cancer.

Contributors

Drew Altman is president and chief executive officer of the Henry J. Kaiser Family Foundation, one of the nation's largest private foundations devoted exclusively to health. He has also served as vice president of the Robert Wood Johnson Foundation, director of the Health and Human Services program at the Pew Charitable Trusts, and commissioner of the Department of Human Services for the state of New Jersey.

Ronald M. Andersen is Wasserman Professor of Health Services at the School of Public Health, professor of sociology, and chair of the Department of Health Services at UCLA. He is co-editor of *Changing the U.S. Health Care System.*

Odin W. Anderson has served as professor of sociology at the Graduate School of Business of the University of Chicago and the Department of Sociology of the University of Wisconsin, Madison.

Morton Bard is professor emeritus of psychology at the Graduate School of the City University of New York. From 1986 to 1991 he was the American Cancer Society's National Vice President for Service and Rehabilitation. He continues to serve as a consultant to a variety of governmental and nonprofit organizations.

Ellen L. Bassuk is associate professor of psychiatry at Harvard Medical School. She is co-founder and president of The Better Homes Fund, a nonprofit organization started in 1988 by *Better Homes and Gardens* magazine to help homeless families and their children nationwide. She is the author of *Community Care for Homeless Clients with Mental Illness, Substance Abuse or Dual Diagnosis* and the editor of *The Mental Health Needs of Homeless Persons.*

William R. Breakey is professor and deputy director in the Department of Psychiatry and Behavioral Sciences at Johns Hopkins School of Medicine. He has been active at the national level with the American Psychiatric Association and the American Public Health Association, and is a member of several task forces which have addressed health care issues for homeless people. His many articles have appeared in the *British Journal of Psychia-*

try, Urban Health, Psychiatry Research, and *Community Psychiatrist,* among many other publications.

Nancy Wainer Cohen cofounded both C/Sec, Inc. and the Cesarean Prevention Movement. A leading authority on vaginal birth after cesarean (VBAC), she has counseled thousands of women on the subject. Her many articles have dealt with VBAC, cesarean prevention, and positive birthing.

Robert Crawford is associate professor in liberal studies at the University of Washington, Tacoma. He has also served on the faculty of the Department of Political Science at the University of Illinois, Chicago Circle. His articles have appeared in the *International Journal of Health Service* and *Social Science and Medicine.*

Geraldine Dallek is a consultant at Families USA Foundation in Washington, D.C. She is a former health policy analyst at the National Health Law Program, which is a legal services support center specializing in health law issues affecting the poor. She has written extensively on problems of access to health care by the uninsured and Medicaid populations.

Ernest Dernburg is a psychiatrist in private practice in San Francisco. He is assistant chief in the Department of Psychiatry at Mt. Zion Hospital and vice president of the San Francisco Individual Practice Association.

Carroll L. Estes served as chairman of the Department of Social and Behavioral Sciences for 11 years, and is presently director of the Institute for Health and Aging, at the University of California at San Francisco. She is the author of *The Aging Enterprise;* and co-author of *The Nation's Health; Health Policy and Nursing: Crisis and Reform in the U.S. Health Care Delivery System;* and *Long-Term Care Crisis.*

Lois J. Estner has served as an English teacher, a VBAC mother, a La Leche League leader, and a counselor on breastfeeding, childbirth, and cesarean prevention.

Shizuko Fagerhaugh has served as a research associate in the Department of Social and Behavioral Sciences at the University of California, San Francisco. She is the principal author of *Hazards in Hospital Care* and a co-author of *Social Organization of Medical Work* and *Chronic Illness and the Quality of Life.*

Mark G. Field is emeritus professor of sociology at Boston University. He is presently a fellow in the Russian Research Center and an Adjunct Professor in the Department of Health Policy and Management at the School of Public Health, Harvard University. His latest book, with Alphonse d'Houtaud, is *Cultural Images of Health: A Neglected Dimension.*

A. Alan Fischer is founding chairman and professor emeritus of the Department of Family Medicine at the Indiana University School of Medicine. Since 1968 he has held the positions of medical director and staff physician at Lakeview Manor Nursing Home.

Emily Friedman is adjunct assistant professor at the Boston University School of Public Health. She is also a consultant on information dissemination to the Agency for Health Care Policy and Research, U.S. Department of Health and Human Services. She is the author or editor of several books, including *Making Choices: Ethics Issues for Health Care Professionals, The Aloha Way: Health Care Structure and Finance in Hawaii,* and *The Right Thing: Ten Years of Ethics Columns from the Healthcare Forum Journal.*

Florence Galkin is president of MASHOV, an organization dedicated to grassroots organizing in Israel. A member of the executive committee of the American Jewish Congress, she previously served as director of Community Action and Resources for the Elderly.

Eli Ginzberg is director of the Eisenhower Center for the Conservation of Human Resources and the director of the Revson Fellows Program on the Future of the City of New York. He is also A. Barton Hepburn Professor Emeritus of Economics and Special Lecturer in the Graduate School of Business and School of Public Health, Columbia University. He is the editor of *Executive Talent* and the co-author of *Improving the Health Care of New York City's Poor* (forthcoming).

Jeanne Guillemin is professor of sociology at Boston College and the author of *Mixed Blessings: Intensive Care for Newborns,* with Lynda Lytle Holmstrom. She has written extensively on medical technology and women's health, and is currently doing research on public health in Russia.

Charles R. Halpern has served as professor of law at the City University of New York Law School at Queen's College and is currently with the Nathan Cummings Foundation.

Robert Harris has served as a member of the President's Council on Environmental Quality. He is a former associate director of the Toxic Chemicals Program for the Environmental Defense Fund and is the co-author of *Malignant Neglect.*

Martin Hochbaum is director of National Affairs for the American Jewish Congress. His publications have appeared in many journals and newspapers, and he is the co-editor of *Poor Jews: An American Awakening*.

Lynda Lytle Holmstrom is professor of sociology at Boston College and former chairperson of the department. Her books include *The Two-Career Family, The Victim of Rape: Institutional Reactions* (with Ann Wolbert Burgess), and *Mixed Blessings: Intensive Care for Newborns* (with Jeanne Harley Guillemin). Her present research, with David A. Karp and Paul S. Gray, is on family dynamics and the college application process.

Robert G. Hughes is vice president of The Robert Wood Foundation. His articles have appeared in the *Journal of the American Medical Association*, the *New England Journal of Medicine*, and *Health Education Quarterly*.

David L. Kirp is professor in the Graduate School of Public Policy, University of California, Berkeley. His books include *Just Schools: The Idea of Racial Equality in American Education, Managing Education Excellence* (with Thomas B. Timar), and *Our Town: Race, Housing, and the Soul of Suburbia* (with John Dwyer and Larry Rosenthal).

Philip R. Lee has served as professor of social medicine and director of the Institute for Health Policy Studies at the University of California, San Francisco. He has been chancellor of that university and is currently assistant secretary for health, U.S. Department of Health and Human Services. The author or co-author of more than 100 articles and books, his interests include disease prevention, health care for the elderly, and AIDS-related issues.

John Luce has served as associate editor of San Francisco Magazine and public affairs director of the Haight-Ashbury Free Medical Clinic.

Elizabeth W. Markson is professor of socio-medical sciences and community medicine, adjunct professor of sociology, and research professor of medicine at Boston University where she is also associate director of the Gerontology Center. She has authored or edited over 100 articles, reviews, and books, including *Older Women*.

Paul Milvy was a member of the Environmental Sciences Laboratory of New York's Mount Sinai Hospital, working on aspects of environmental and occupational cancer. He is the author of *The Marathon: Physiological, Medical, Epidemiological and Psychological Studies*.

Ross Mullner is associate professor at the School of Public Health, University of Illinois. He has written over eighty articles on various aspects of health care and is currently writing a book on the history of the Radium Dial workers.

Robert Nicholas is former deputy attorney general for the Commonwealth of Pennsylvania, with responsibilities for consumer and environmental law.

Caroline M. Poplin is a physician and attorney. She practiced law for more than a decade at the United States Food and Drug Administration and the Environmental Protection Agency. She is now an internist with the Dewitt Primary Plus Clinic in Virginia.

Alan Sager is professor of health services at Boston University School of Public Health, where he has taught health care finance, administration, and regulation and planning since 1983. He is one of the three principals in the Access and Affordability Monitoring Project, established in 1988 to analyze the causes of health care access and cost problems and to monitor Massachusetts legislation on health insurance.

David Smith is founder and president of the Haight Ashbury Free Clinics and president of the American Society of Addiction Medicine. He is also associate clinical professor of occupational medicine and clinical toxicology at the University of California, San Francisco.

Gloria Smith has served as commissioner of the Michigan Department of Anthropology at Arizona State University.

Louisa Stark has served as adjunct professor in the Department of Anthropology at Arizona State University.

Nathan Stark is Senior Vice Chancellor Emeritus for the Health Sciences of the University of Pittsburgh, and former president and chief executive officer of the National Academy of Social Insurance in Washington, D.C.

Rosemary Stevens is Dean and Thomas S. Gates Professor of the School of Arts and Sciences at the University of Pennsylvania. She has also taught at Yale and Tulane Universities and has held visiting appointments at the London School of Economics and Political Science, Johns Hopkins University, and the Brookings Institution. Her books include *American Medicine and the Public Interest, Welfare Medicine in America,* and *In Sickness and in Wealth: American Hospitals in the Twentieth Century.*

Anselm Strauss is emeritus professor and founder of the Department of Social and Behavioral Sciences, University of California, San Francisco. He is the co-author of several books on problems and issues surrounding health care, including *Boys in White, Time for Dying, Awareness of Dying, Chronic Illness and the Quality of Life,* and *Social Organization of Medical Work.* He has authored and co-authored numerous books and articles on *grounded theory,* the sociological method he developed with Barney Glaser.

Barbara Suczek has served as research associate in the Department of Social and Behavioral Sciences at the University of California, San Francisco. She is a co-author of *Hazards in Hospital Care, Chronic Illness and the Quality of Life,* and *Social Organization of Medical Work.* Currently, she is a mediator for the Family Court in Alameda County, California.

Emanuel D. Thorne is assistant professor of economics at Brooklyn College of the City University of New York and a fellow at Georgetown University's Kennedy Institute of Ethics. His articles have appeared in the *Washington Post,* the *New York Times,* the *Wall Street Journal, Commonweal, Fetal Therapy, The Public Interest,* and the *Journal of Regulatory Economics.*

Bruce C. Vladeck is administrator of the Health Care Financing Administration. He has also served as president of the United Hospital Fund of New York in New York City and chairman of the Institute of Medicine's Committee on Health Care for Homeless People.

Steven P. Wallace is associate professor of public health and is the Borun Scholar of the Anna and Harry Borun Center for Gerontolocial Research at UCLA. His many articles about the impact of race and ethnicity on the use of long-term care have been published in *Gerontologist, Journal of Gerontology, American Journal of Public Health,* and *Journal of Aging Studies.*

Elizabeth Whelan is former executive director of the American Council on Science and Health and former research associate at the Harvard School of Public Health. She is the author of numerous books, including *Panic in the Pantry: Food Facts, Fads, and Fallacies* (with F.J. Stare).

Carolyn Wiener is associate research sociologist at the University of California, San Francisco. She is author of *The Politics of Alcoholism* and co-author of *Social Organization of Medical Work, Chronic Illness and the Quality of Life,* and *Hazards in Hospital Care.* She has published extensively on the topic of sociological and organizational behavior as it relates to health care.

Phyllis Wolfe has served as executive director of the Robert Wood Johnson/Pew Memorial Trust Health Care for the Homeless Project in Washington D.C.

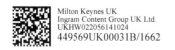